Principles of Family Systems in Family Medicine

Principles of Family Systems in Family Medicine

Edited by

SERGIO HENAO, M.D.

Director, Child and Adolescent Services,
Texas Research Institute of Mental Sciences,
Houston, Texas

and

NELLIE P. GROSE, M.D., M.P.H.

Clinical Associate Professor, Department of Family Medicine,
Baylor College of Medicine,
Houston, Texas

Technical Editor
LORE FELDMAN

BRUNNER/MAZEL, Publishers • New York

Library of Congress Cataloging in Publication Data

Main entry under title:

Principles of family systems in family medicine.

Includes bibliographies and index.
1. Family medicine. 2. Sick—Family relationships.
3. Family psychotherapy. I. Henao, Sergio,
1940- . II. Grose, Nellie P., 1943-
[DNLM: 1. Family. 2. Family Practice. WB 110 P957]
R729.5.G4P7374 1985 616.89'156 85-5909
ISBN 0-87630-388-2

Published by

BRUNNER/MAZEL, Inc.
19 Union Square West
New York, N.Y. 10003

FOREWORD

A tenet of medical education is that it deals with pathophysiological processes within and between many interacting systems at all levels. These include the molecular, biochemical, anatomical, and organ systems. All these, however, are dealt with in the individual patient. A second tenet that unfortunately still exists is the dichotomy between the body and emotions. Despite the intellectual understanding of the relationship and despite the recent advances in psychoneurology, psychoimmunology, and psychoendocrinology, the bulk of medical teaching implies a distinction between the mind and the body. Similarly, despite evidence of the health aspects of bereavement (Osterweis, Solomon, & Green, 1984), and of social support and social isolation (Broadhead et al., 1983), many leaders of medicine have publicly stated that social aspects should be outside the function or teaching of medicine. Engel's statement regarding the need for a biopsychosocial model (1977) is used mainly as a reference in articles, rather than as the basis for medical education. Some of these points were well addressed in the recent General Professional Education of the Physician Report *(Physicians for the 21st Century*, 1984) which, among other things, emphasizes the importance of the study of social sciences and humanities in addition to the natural sciences. Missing in this report, however, is any mention of the family.

The recognition of family practice as a medical specialty in the United States occurred in 1969. In the last decade, the vast majority of U.S. medical schools have created either a department or a division of family medicine. This development was due to a number of social and political factors and did not, and still does not, imply any fundamental change in the philosophy of biomedical, tertiary-care-oriented medical education.

However, the students who were attracted to family medicine and went into practice as community physicians soon realized that many important aspects of primary-care medicine had not been dealt with. One of these is the interaction of the identified or presenting patient and his or her intimate social group, which is usually the family and/or household and occasionally is a wider network of friends, kin, or neighbors. It is obvious to family physicians that everything of importance that impinges on the individual patient affects each individual in his or her intimate environment, as well as the primary system as a whole. Conversely, anything that influences the system as a whole—loss of home, loss or change of employment, move to a new area—affects each member of the system (family). Similarly, many symptoms or behaviors of patients are caused by or are a reflection of family dynamics and functioning. Compliance with treatment and outcome are frequently intertwined and dependent on the interaction of the patient with his or her family.

With this realization comes the process of attempting to understand the individual patient in the context of his or her family and/or the wider environment for diagnostic and management purposes. Family physicians are then beset with many problems. How do we assess a family system that is in a continuous dynamic equilibrium (see Chapter 3) and changes over time through the life cycle? There are very few so-called objective measures but, rather, subjective ones in which the physician's own feelings, attitudes, knowledge, and skills greatly influence and are interwoven into the diagnosis and management. When do we act as catalysts allowing the family to utilize their resources (counseling) and when do we attempt to radically alter part of the system (therapy)? What signs and symptoms are known that will identify high-risk families? What preventive measures have been shown to be beneficial and, dare we say it, cost effective? Will the medical care system compensate family physicians for preventive or therapeutic counseling?

These and many other questions face family physicians who, in order to carry out comprehensive care, must be knowledgeable about the functioning of the family systems of their patients. It is in this context that I welcome this book which attempts to dissect, define, and demonstrate the principles of family systems for application to our discipline. We will be better family physicians if we absorb and digest these principles.

Jack H. Medalie, M.D.,
Dorothy Jones Weatherhead Professor
and Chairman of Medicine,
Department of Family Medicine,
Case Western Reserve University,
Cleveland, Ohio

REFERENCES

Broadhead, W., Kaplan, B., James, S., Wagner, E., Schoenbach, V., Grimson, R., Heyden, S., Tibblin, G., & Gehlbach, S. (1983). The epidemiologic evidence for a relationship between social support and health. *American Journal of Epidemiology, 117*, 521-537.

Engel, G. (1977). The need for a medical model. *Science, 196*, 129-136.

Physicians for the 21st Century: The GPEP Report. (November 1984). Chairman S. Muller, American Association of American Medical Colleges, Washington, DC.

Osterweis, M., Solomon, F., & Green, M. (Eds.) (1984). *Bereavement: Reactions, consequences and care*. Washington, DC: National Academy of Sciences.

CONTENTS

CONTRIBUTORS

Lisa C. Baker, Ph.D.
Assistant Professor, University of Oklahoma Health Sciences Center, Department of Family Medicine, Oklahoma City, Oklahoma

C. Christian Beels, M.D., M.S.
Associate Professor; Director, Fellowship in Public Psychiatry, Department of Psychiatry, College of Physicians and Surgeons, Columbia University and New York State Psychiatric Institute, New York, New York

Donald A. Bloch, M.D.
Director, Ackerman Institute for Family Therapy, New York, New York

James H. Bray, Ph.D.
Assistant Professor, Department of Psychology, Texas Women's University, Houston, Texas

Collier Cole, Ph.D.
Clinical Psychologist, Rosenberg Clinic; Clinical Assistant Professor, School of Allied Health Sciences, University of Texas Medical Branch, Galveston, Texas

Richard Fisch, M.D.
Director, Brief Therapy Center, Mental Research Institute, Palo Alto, California; Clinical Assistant Professor, Department of Psychiatry and Behavioral Sciences, Stanford University School of Medicine, Stanford, California

Ernest Frugé, Ph.D.
Research Specialist, Gerontology Center, Texas Research Institute of Mental Sciences, Houston, Texas

ROY J. GERARD, M.D.
Family Physician; Professor and Chairman, Department of Family Practice, College of Human Medicine, Michigan State University, East Lansing, Michigan

MICHAEL L. GLENN, M.D.
Family Physician in Private Practice, Everett Family Practice, Everett, Massachusetts

THELMA JEAN GOODRICH, Ph.D.
Behavioral Scientist; Assistant Professor, Department of Family Medicine, Baylor College of Medicine, Baylor Family Practice Center, Houston, Texas

NELLIE P. GROSE, M.D., M.P.H.
Family Physician, Private Practice; Clinical Associate Professor, Department of Family Medicine, Baylor College of Medicine, Houston, Texas

J. RAY HAYS, Ph.D., J.D.
Acting Director, Training Division, Texas Research Institute of Mental Sciences; Clinical Associate Professor, Department of Psychiatry, Baylor College of Medicine, Houston, Texas

SERGIO HENAO, M.D.
Director, Child and Adolescent Services, Texas Research Institute of Mental Sciences; Clinical Associate Professor, Baylor College of Medicine and University of Texas Medical School, Houston, Texas

BARBARA J. HOEK, M.A.
Marital and Sex Therapist, Houston, Texas

JUDITH LANDAU, M.D.
Associate Clinical Professor; Director of Family Therapy Training, The Family and Marriage Clinic, Department of Psychiatry, University of Rochester School of Medicine, Rochester, New York

RONALD LIEBMAN, M.D.
Medical Director, Philadelphia Child Guidance Clinic; Psychiatrist-in-Chief, Children's Hospital of Philadelphia; Clinical Associate Professor, Psychiatry and Pediatrics, University of Pennsylvania School of Medicine, Philadelphia, Pennsylvania

William R. McFarlane, M.D.
Assistant Clinical Professor; Associate Director, Department of Psychiatry, College of Physicians and Surgeons, Columbia University and New York State Psychiatric Institute, New York, New York

Jack H. Medalie, M.D.
Dorothy Jones Weatherhead Professor; Chairman of Medicine, Department of Family Medicine, Case Western Reserve University, Cleveland, Ohio

Salvador Minuchin, M.D.
Director, Philadelphia Child Guidance Clinic, Philadelphia, Pennsylvania

Leonora Montgomery, Ph.D.
Parish Assistant, Emerson Unitarian Church, Houston, Texas

George Niederehe, Ph.D.
Chief of Psychological Research, Gerontology Center, Texas Research Institute of Mental Sciences, Houston, Texas

James G. O'Brien, M.D.
Family Physician; Associate Chairman, Department of Family Practice, College of Human Medicine, Michigan State University, East Lansing, Michigan

Frank S. Pittman, III, M.D.
Psychiatrist and Family Therapist in Private Practice, Atlanta, Georgia

Christian N. Ramsey, Jr., M.D.
Professor and Chairman, Department of Family Medicine, University of Oklahoma Health Sciences Center, Oklahoma City, Oklahoma

Donald C. Ransom, Ph.D.
Associate Professor of Family and Community Medicine, School of Medicine, University of California, San Francisco, California

Bernard L. Rosenfeld, M.D., Ph.D.
Assistant Professor, Department of Obstetrics and Gynecology, Baylor College of Medicine, Houston, Texas

John Sargent, M.D.

Associate Director, Pediatric-Psychiatry Liaison Program; Clinical Assistant Professor, Child Psychiatry and Pediatrics, University of Pennsylvania School of Medicine, Philadelphia, Pennsylvania

Gabriel Smilkstein, M.D.

Professor, Family Medicine Department, School of Medicine, University of Washington, Seattle, Washington

M. Duncan Stanton, Ph.D.

Professor and Director, Division of Family Programs, Department of Psychiatry, University of Rochester School of Medicine, Rochester, New York

John H. Weakland

Associate Director, Brief Therapy Center, Mental Research Institute, Palo Alto, California; Clinical Assistant Professor, Department of Psychiatry and Behavioral Sciences, Stanford University School of Medicine, Stanford, California

Donald S. Williamson, Ph.D.

Director, Houston Family Institute; Clinical Associate Professor of Psychology, Department of Psychiatry, Baylor College of Medicine, Houston, Texas

INTRODUCTION

Since we decided to create this volume three years ago, there has been much debate about the treatment of "the family" in family medicine, about the relationship of family therapy to family practice, and particularly about who is the patient in a medical practice run according to systemic principles.

As a psychiatrist (Henao) and a family practitioner (Grose), we have been applying these principles in our practices for years. The integration of this approach into the actual practice of family medicine is a complex task. We believe that it deserves further exploration, and that is our purpose here.

This book is addressed to family practitioners, mental health professionals who interact with family physicians, and teachers and students of family medicine. It is not comprehensive enough to be a text, but we hope that it will contribute to the understanding and refinement of family systems theory in medicine.

Some issues—especially those concerning the usefulness of family systems theory in family medicine—have become clearer to us as we worked with our contributors. They represent many points of view. We, who worked on the book for two years, are now certain that *the individual patient is the unit of care*—not the family, as many writers on family medicine have proposed.

Physicians treat individuals, and family is an arbitrary category difficult to define. Are homosexual or unmarried heterosexual couples, elderly people living together, and single people living in a meditation center examples of families? To quote psychiatrist and family therapist Fred Duhl, "One cannot kiss a system." But we do believe that the individual should be evaluated and treated "systemically" and that the family is one of the strongest and most important systems for all of us.

This is no different, we believe, from looking at heart disease from a systemic point of view. The heart may be the target organ for treatment, but therapeutic orientation and methods clearly are systemic. In essence, then, we advocate the individual as the unit of care, the focus of a systemic view of illness and treatment that includes not only the family but the biological, socioeconomic, and religious-spiritual systems.

The book's first section provides an overview of the theoretical underpinnings of a general systems approach to medicine as well as descriptions of some of the best known systemic models.

Common clinical issues in family medicine as they relate to the systemic and natural evolution of the family are discussed in the second section.

The third section deals with the application of a family systems approach to such clinical problems as substance abuse and psychosis, and also presents family assessment tools and some of the legal issues that may come up in a practice conducted with a family systems orientation.

We acknowledge the help of our technical editor, Lore Feldman, whose skill, tact, and good humor made the work enjoyable, as well as Kathleen Kimball-Baker and Alison Cook. Nellie Grose's thanks go specifically to Harry Goolishian for introducing her to systems theory and for his continued support of her work. We are grateful to Linda Schachter for her expert work in organizing and typing the manuscript and for taking care of the many details involved in bringing this book together.

Sergio Henao, M.D.
Nellie P. Grose, M.D.

Principles of Family Systems in Family Medicine

I.
PHILOSOPHICAL AND THEORETICAL BASIS OF A FAMILY SYSTEMS APPROACH

1

THE EVOLUTION FROM AN INDIVIDUAL TO A FAMILY APPROACH

DONALD C. RANSOM, Ph.D.

No officious slave
Art thou of that false secondary power
By which we multiply distinctions, then
Deem that our puny boundaries are things
That we perceive, and not that we have made.

William Wordsworth, *The Prelude*

The evolution of the horse from *Eohippus* was not a one-sided adjustment to life on grassy plains. Surely the grassy plains themselves were evolved *pari passu* with the evolution of the teeth and hooves of the horses and other ungulates. Turf was the evolving response of the vegetation to the evolution of the horse. It is the *context* which evolves.

Gregory Bateson, *Steps to an Ecology of Mind*

The two epigraphs set the themes for this chapter. The first is borrowed from Ian McWhinney's (1981) excellent text, *An Introduction to Family Medicine*. It captures the arbitrariness of boundaries and sets the tone for a portrayal of family medicine as an approach that can deal with the complexity and meaning of illness without rejecting reductive strategies when they can be useful.

The second captures in an example the hallmark of the interactional perspective that informs the conceptual basis of contemporary systems theory and, by extension, family systems medicine.

This chapter simply traces threads in the evolution from an individual to a family approach in health care. It argues that the family approach (a concrete manifestation of the "contextual" or "systems" view) increases the adequacy of the conceptual basis of understanding health and illness and leads to a new type of practice.

The approach discussed here attempts to reunite patient and disease, and patient, physician, family, and community. This is achieved by providing the conceptual means of approaching the interpenetration of gene, organism, person, family, culture, and so on. Thus, in place of the image of the biomedical organism adapting to an alien environment, the family systems approach provides a language for talking about the way organisms define and shape their environment in the course of living, and vice versa.

Person and family are two aspects of a continuous process of mutually determining change, like horses and the grassy plains in the epigraph. Clinicians working with this model chart a course between the biological, the psychological, and the social characteristics of the patient, looking for points of contact that allow them to be helpful (see Ransom, 1983b). This view provides a persuasive logic for health care professionals to focus on patients and their contexts. In this technical sense, it may be said that the family or the context is the patient.

The Family in Family Medicine

In a 1973 article in the *Journal of the American Medical Association*, H.E. Vandervoort and I asked, "Where is the family in family medicine?", raising what we believed was a crucial issue in the new discipline. We objected to the expropriation of the words *family* and *family medicine* to describe, ipso facto, what family physicians do, if that activity was to represent an unreconstructed general practice. We also addressed the confusion introduced by using the terms *family medicine* and *family practice* interchangeably and suggested that such usage was misleading and was inhibiting the potential development of a new field.

It seemed important to insist that the terms be kept conceptually distinct. *Family practice* designated the recognized medical specialty, a model of primary medical care delivery that was defined according to accepted usage as "a discipline of synthesis, integrating a wide range of medical and personal skills into the practice of a single physician. In theory, family practice means comprehensive, continuing care provided to all age groups by a personal physician" (Ransom & Vandervoort, 1973, p. 1099).

Family medicine, in contrast, referred to a field of inquiry and was defined normatively as:

> an emerging discipline concerned with the *relationship* (emphasis added) of life in small groups to health, illness, and care. Its focus is on the ecology of relations among individuals in families and between families and their surrounding environment. (The term family is used in the broadest sense to describe any group of intimates with a history and a future.) Family medicine aims toward understanding and changing health problems that cannot be managed successfully by dealing exclusively with the individual and his or her illness, abstracted from the pattern of recurrent interpersonal situations that shape and transform a human life.
>
> Proponents of family medicine maintain that any reorganization of medical education into the systems approach should fully include the family as one such system basic to the curriculum, recognizing family patterns as a potential etiologic source in disease as well as recognizing the role of the family in perpetuating "diseased" patterns of behavior. By focusing on those small human systems that affect health so radically, family medicine signals the formal initiation of "microecological medicine." (Ransom & Vandervoort, 1973, p. 1099)

Ten years ago these ideas were ironically foreign to a new specialty that had renamed itself "family" practice. Today they may be controversial but have many advocates. The important point was *not* that the family should *replace* the individual as *the* patient, or that the *exclusive* subject of family medicine should be small social-system behavior. Such responses simply further illustrate the *either/or* reflex the systems approach was proposing to complement with *both/and*. Rather, by placing the term "family" in such high profile we meant to emphasize the dual significance of "family" already established by the revolutions in the mental health disciplines: *family* as a metaphor for the emotional, cognitive, and material reality that makes the patient's condition *socially intelligible;* and *family* as a metaphor for the *thesis of connectedness* and, by extension, for the approach that studies hierarchical ("levels of") organizing relations, the "systems" approach.

Thus, what we tried to say was that the most important development in the new field of family medicine was the viewpoint (the "gaze" of central interest to Foucault, 1975) being constructed to look at health and illness and to design interventions. Such ways of seeing and doing are always self-conscious and clumsy at first, although they eventually make their way to the unnoticed background of beliefs, conventions, and habits embodied in routine skills and practices if they are useful. It was this sort of change we were working toward.

Two Historical Sources

These were by no means original ideas. Both the systems and the family-centered approach had been stressed in medicine at different limited points for more than a hundred years. The gradual emergence from a focus on individuals and parts of individuals abstracted from their contexts, to individual processes and their contexts as interactive and mutually determining (here called the family systems approach), forms a complex and untold story. Two historical sources contribute to the current form of family medicine that embodies this family approach: special interest in family relations and health, illness, and care; and the transformation of general practice to family practice. The remainder of this chapter will trace these separate lines of development to their confluence in present-day medicine.

Family Relations and Health

The history of interest in family and health, or the family as a unit of care, and the history of family practice represent separate developments until the early 1970s. The pioneers who drove to the forefront their interests in these two sets of issues were concerned with different questions and different goals. It was not until the accreditation requirement in 1969 by the American Board of Family Practice to create family practice centers with their own exclusive identity that the two groups found a structure in which to work together on common problems. To clarify this enabling development, it is helpful to trace the interest in the family as a unit of care through a brief description of its main contributing projects.

The Peckham Experiment

The modern history of family-centered care begins with the Peckham Experiment. This remarkable venture left a greater legacy to contemporary students of the family and health than any other project to date. Conceived and guided by the distinguished pathologist George Scott Williamson, the Peckham Experiment was the source of several books (e.g., Pearse & Williamson, 1931; Williamson & Pearse, 1938). A full account of the rationale, methods, experiences, and findings of the project is provided in *The Peckham Experiment: A Study in the Living Structure of Society*, by Innes Pearse (Williamson's wife) and Lucy Crocker (1943). The latter is one of the most rhapsodic pieces on the family ever written. Two modern sequels, reflecting on the whole project and exploring the implication for renewed work, are by Williamson and Pearse (1980) and Pearse (1980).

In 1926 a "family club" was opened in a small house in the southeast

London borough of Camberwell. From modest beginnings, the club attracted an increasing membership and support from philanthropic contributors so that in 1935 a three-story, 58,000 square-foot structure, the Pioneer Health Centre, was built: "It was a great venture; a social structure to be built with a new unit—not the individual but the *family*" (Pearse & Crocker, 1943, p. 13). The Centre contained a large swimming pool, gymnasium, game rooms, a music room, library and quiet room, work rooms, a large dance floor with stage, a theater, a self-service cafeteria and pub, a store, outdoor grounds, and eventually expanded to incorporate a summer camp and a cooperative farm seven miles away. At its peak, enrollment reached 1,400 families, all living within a mile (which they considered to be walking distance), in the principally lower-middle- and middle-class neighborhood.

In the beginning, the aim was research. The plan was to construct a setting "to be furnished with people and their actions" (Pearse & Crocker, 1943, p. 69). It was to be "a biologist's living laboratory." The setting was designed for people to bring their backgrounds with them, since whole families or households were encouraged to enroll. By circumscribing the membership to those who lived within a one-mile radius of the Centre, the research team drew together "a large and representative sample of families capable, by their territorial base, of becoming a community" (Barlow, 1983, p. 2). This community of persons and families could thereby be observed over a long span of time, interacting with one another, using the resources of the environment for good or for ill and developing through the stages of their lives. The goal was to study life *in vivo* and thereby to learn something about *health* rather than illness.

The Pioneer Health Centre was in no way a medical polyclinic of the type familiar in those days. Its most important medical service was to provide annual combined physical examination with laboratory studies and consultation, called "the family health overhaul." A condition of membership was that every member of every family would undergo an annual overhaul, after which the results and their implications would be discussed with the family as a group. The policy was "information without advice," although it is clear in retrospect that much advice was given through both the substance and form of the information provided.

Many health-related activities were sponsored by the Centre, including premarital and prenatal counseling for couples, swimming and exercise classes for pregnant women, and an alternative birth arrangement with a nearby teaching hospital in which mothers could be received for the period of 48 hours covering the delivery, after which they returned home with their babies. This was in contrast with the two-week period of hospitalization customary at the time.

The Centre also sold fresh raw milk and organic vegetables. This sort of activity followed from their concept of the proper role of a health professional as introducing and managing essential resources within the immediate environment so that the availability and use of those resources were enhanced, thereby facilitating growth and development in health.

The commitment to health through human development within the family and community is further exemplified by an experiment begun in the summer of 1939 and cut short by the war. Maria Montessori planned an educational nursery for children one-and-a-half years old and older, including their mothers, "so that in helping with the education of their own children not only might they come through practice to understand the essence of education, but they might also simultaneously renew their own education long since forgotten and foregone" (Pearse & Crocker, 1943, p. 317). Montessori schools are now spread throughout the Western world.

The legacy of the Peckham Experiment is the highly developed model of social organicism which infused everything associated with the project. The family-as-organism idea is appealing in spite of its too literal application of the biological analogy. It is a precursor of the organismic systems theory of von Bertalanffy (1968) that was to evolve into a general systems theory. Like von Bertalanffy and later systems thinkers, the early Peckham project leaders made much of the difference between "physiological operation" and "biological functioning." They were interested not only in the response of organs and tissues under controlled laboratory conditions (Williamson was also a pathologist); they were even more interested in the behavior of whole organisms in an ever-changing natural environment. By organism, they meant "any living entity capable of performing the full cycle of its specific existence." And for them, the family was just such a unit/organism.

Three principles central to the Peckham experience have gained increasing utility. One is the idea of emergent quality. Over and over again Pearse and Crocker give examples of how the couple or the family, acting together, exhibit a new and different quality that cannot be understood or reduced to the individuals acting separately. The principle is illustrated at many levels, including cognitive functioning. For instance:

> When two diverse individuals function as an organism, *all that they encounter* acquires a new significance. It is not merely the addition of the experience of one to that of the other, making the combined view a larger whole seen, but that with new polarity a new *quality* is given to their apprehension. And this quality of perception is given not only to what is experienced at the moment, but that experience itself influences what they in their new functional orientation will in the future experience—hence altering their every action. (Pearse & Crocker, 1943, p. 19)

As the last sentence reveals, the complexity of the model put forward already extends beyond the insight that the whole is greater than the sum of its parts. The whole, under continuous construction, shapes the capacities and actions of the parts, leading to recursive reconstruction of the whole, and so on.

The second principle proposes both a personal and a family life course or life cycle, with a set of stages marked by predictable periods of rapid reorganization. During these times of transition, environmental conditions play an important role in successful and healthy development. In fact, a basic aim of the Peckham Experiment was to provide the kind of environmental conditions that would facilitate the transformation of each of the major stages, as the staff understood them, at the opportune moment. Today, no approach to the study of health would be complete without a full discussion of the interplay of individual and family life cycles.

The third principle proposes an integrated hierarchy of levels of organization composed of parts that maintain themselves through relations with the environment. The Peckham pioneers made two astute complementary observations about this process. The first is that the development of health requires a "fitness" of the environment; the second adds the qualification that the general state of the environment does not determine in a direct way the health of the individuals in it. That state is mediated, for better or worse, by the organized activity of micro-environments—the immediate surround of the person as represented by the family and the local community. The lesson of many years of observation at the Pioneer Health Centre is that "it is, in particular, this inner environmental circle in its influence on the facilitation or inhibition of health that the health professional requires to understand" (Barlow, 1983, p. 10).

The practical implication is that if influencing an individual's state of health is the goal, intervention must be directed not only toward processes within the person and toward the person as a whole, but toward the appropriate social environment as well. Seen in this light, social environments are more than background; they are levels in a hierarchy of developmental activity in which all individuals participate.

Patients Have Families

One year after the Pioneer Health Centre was built, the Josiah Macy, Jr. Foundation funded "The Study of the Family in Sickness and Health Care." Shepherded by Lawrence K. Frank of the Macy Foundation and guided by his ideas (see *Society as the Patient*, 1948, a collection of Frank's essays), the study was a venture among members of the faculties of public health, medicine, and psychiatry at Cornell University Medical College, and included representatives from social work and nursing from New York Hospital. A group of 15 families was studied over a two-year period with the goals of understanding "the interrelationship between illness and the family situation," learning something about the "implications for treatment" following from such an approach, and "exploring the best methods for cooperative treatment" with the family health care team assembled for the study (Richardson, 1945, pp. 312-313). The report of the study, *Patients Have Families,* was prepared by Henry B. Richardson, the project's director.

What the Peckham Experiment provided in commitment to total health and dedication to establishing the family and the unit of living, the Macy Family Study matched with formal elegance in describing the family as a system that functions to influence the state of health of its members and regulates their access to health care and community resources. *Patients Have Families* is an early example of the contribution that social and behavioral scientists can make to the interdisciplinary study of health and illness.

The following passage from Richardson's book has probably come to be the most widely quoted passage in the family medicine literature:

> The idea of disease as an entity which is limited to one person and can be transmitted to another fades into the background and disease becomes an integral part of the continuous process of living. The family is the unit of illness, because it is the unit of living. (p.76)

The word "system" is used in its modern technical sense, as in the following passage:

> The doctor who treats the patient for a chronic disease may be observing one aspect of a reciprocating system of which he may become aware if he inquires into the health of the family. (p. 234)

This formulation was offered more than a decade before Don Jackson gave his now classic lecture on "family homeostasis" (1957). In chapters entitled, "The Family Equilibrium" and "Different Types of Family Equilibrium," and in an appendix called "Concepts Relative to the Family Equilibrium," the general idea of the family as a system was spelled out.

To gain some idea of the sophistication and scope of these early concepts, it is instructive to look at the seven processes Richardson described as "useful partial views" that help "to visualize the essential characteristics of the family equilibrium" (1945, pp. 321-327). The idea of "reciprocating systems," for example, has sustained a position of central relevance to students of the family and health to this day. A reciprocating system in its simplest form is "a behavioral relationship between two persons in a family group, such that the participants tend to react on each other in a predictable manner with specified results" (1945, p. 323). Several good examples are provided in the text. The two-person system is often part of more complicated interlocking systems, which may involve other individuals, and what the research team called "factions" (coalitions, in current terminology). These systems, in turn, are described in ways which sound like contemporary discussions of enmeshment and disengagement (e.g., Minuchin, Rosman, & Baker, 1978) and triangulation (as in Bowen, 1978; Haley, 1977). Reciprocating systems are also interwoven with many of the external relationships of the family and are relevant to health or illness.

Richardson is explicit that "a reciprocating system refers to an interpersonal relationship, and is otherwise meaningless" (p. 324). This emphasis contrasts with what he characterized as the conventional use of terms like "patient" and "diagnosis" in a noninteractional sense:

> Most of these professions tend, for the time being at least, to see the system from their own angle, and through the eyes of one of the members of the family. The result is a view which may be broad or narrow, but tends to be incomplete. The system can be seen best in its entirety by comparing observations from as many angles as are relevant to the situation. (p. 324)

From my first reading of *Patients Have Families* in 1967, I was struck that such an obscure book could contain so pure a model of the family as a system. The conceptual phrasings, in particular, are astonishing considering that they were produced by a classically trained internist who had done animal experimentation, electrocardiography, and bench research on metabolism before directing the Macy Foundation study.

In a brief note in the appendix to *Patients Have Families*, Margaret Mead appears as a member of the study group. Mead was to use the materials by members of each discipline represented, together with records of the research, "and organize them as basic materials upon which Dr. Richardson could write his report" (p. 316).

In an interview arranged to discuss the Richardson project, Mead explained that the final statement of the group's report drew heavily on a major paper she was preparing at the time, "The Concept of Culture and the Psychosomatic Approach" (finally published in *Psychiatry*, 1947), and that the early systems concepts were provided by Gregory Bateson, her husband at the time. Through Mead's contribution to the book's preparation, Bateson was trying out ideas upon which the field of family therapy was eventually to be built.

Richardson and his family study team succeeded in refocusing the "gaze" of medical practice ahead of their time. In the final paragraph of the introduction to *Patients Have Families* they say, "In summary, the profession of medicine progressed from the diseased organ to the total personality of the patient, and is now ready for the concept of the individual as a member of a family in its community setting" (p. xviii). Perhaps they were taken by the excitement of interdisciplinary work or the promise of new ideas from cybernetics, a field whose early development was supported by a series of conferences sponsored by the same people from the Macy Foundation who were supporting their work. Perhaps Richardson's own clinical experiences had persuaded him that family-centered medicine was the next logical step. In any case, World War II intervened. When it was over, the next 20 years were to witness instead the greatest investment in biomedical reductionist research and emphasis on subspecialization in the history of medicine.

The Family Health Maintenance Demonstration

As the Macy-funded "Study of the Family in Sickness and Health Care" was drawing to a close, the Community Service Society and the Milbank Memorial Fund were being persuaded to support what eventually became the "Family Health Maintenance Demonstration" of the Montefiore Medical Group, a comprehensive health care option of the Health Insurance Plan of Greater New York. Located at Montefiore Hospital and affiliated with the Columbia University College of Physicians and Surgeons, the demonstration was planned from 1943 to 1950 and then existed for nine years under the direction of George A. Silver.

On a much wider scale than Richardson's family study, the Family Health Maintenance Demonstration combined research with service. Over a five-year period, a wide range of data was collected from slightly more than 100 families matched against a roughly equal number of controls. Study families were provided with a team consisting of an internist, a pediatrician, a public health nurse, and a social worker, and all available specialty and ancillary services as needed. The centrality of the family and the importance of disease prevention were emphasized. The results for the individuals enrolled were, in general, favorable, but as an experiment in providing health services to families, the demonstration left us with more information about what not to do than how to put the family approach into practice. In *Family Medical Care: A Report on the Family Health Maintenance Demonstration*, Silver (1963) described the project and its results in detail (see also *Family Medical Care: A Design for Health Maintenance* by Silver, 1974, a revision and extension of the earlier work).

Favorable results included improved health status and health habits in the demonstration study group. Family members in the study also reported greater satisfaction with their health care than the matched group of controls and, over time, study families dropped out of the plan at a significantly lower rate than did the control families, who received more conventional care (albeit prepaid, a pioneering venture in the 1950s).

Unfavorable results stemmed from complex circumstances and are subject to interpretation. Silver (1963) cited a number of reasons for the demonstration's struggle, including difficulties in team coordination, the absence of appropriate training, and the reluctance of professionals to try out new roles.

With the kind of hindsight that only the passage of 20 years can provide, it appears now that there were two principal reasons for the Family Health Maintenance Demonstration's failure to produce an enduring model of family-centered health care. First, the planners dismissed out-of-hand the idea of introducing a true family practice built around family doctors and set about instead to invent a kind of "family doctoring" to be provided by multispecialty/multiprofessional health care teams. The synthesis hoped for was never achieved. Some practical consequences of this approach led to provider dissatisfaction, tentative and fuzzy interprofessional relations, and the eventual loss of outside support.

The shortcomings of this multirepresentative team approach in actual practice signaled a need for family practice training and the delivery of services in a defragmented mode that went unheeded by the demonstration's leaders and by policymakers in the New York metropolitan region. Family practice, in the traditional sense, was seen as a symptom of a nostalgic longing for a "Golden Age" physician from an era long gone—a romantic fantasy rather than a practical solution. It is instructive that Silver's footnote in 1963—"In recent years, the American Academy of General Practice has pressed hard for such a family practitioner, both in medical-school training and hospital experience" (p. 347)—was substantially unchanged in the second edition in 1974, failing to notice, or at least to acknowledge, the tremendous strides family practice had taken over the decade, including recognition as a specialty and the establishment of residency training in 1969.

The second reason the demonstration was unable to construct an enduring model was that it could not, intellectually, sustain a family focus. As a result, the family, as an irreducible unit of interdependent intimates, was not a focus of assessment and intervention after all. By Silver's own admission, data on family interaction were sorely missed (e.g., 1963, p. 167). The family was pieced together from extensive contact with the individual members separately, but with the exception of the routine family health conference conducted annually (modeled on the periodic Family Health Overhaul of the Peckham Experiment) there is little evidence that demonstration health teams worked with or directed intervention toward the family group as a whole.

These deficiencies, discernible through the gift of hindsight, are remarkable considering the conceptual models of the family close at hand that the demonstration apparently chose not to draw upon. Even though "the spirit, ideology and goal of the Peckham Experiment informed the Family Health Maintenance Demonstration to a significant degree" (Silver, 1963, p. 5), the "family-as-organism" model of the Peckham Experiment did not influence the work of the demonstration in any significant manner. Neither did the "family-as-system" idea from the Richardson study. A curious fact among the traces of the evolving family systems perspective is that the work of the Macy Family Study team is not mentioned in Silver's reports (1963, 1974). Both groups worked in New York, and Bailey B. Burritt, an original guiding force of the demonstration, was also on the technical committee that oversaw the Macy Family Study. It seems that the use of the kindred models of either the Peckham Experiment or the Richardson study could have advanced the Family Health Maintenance Demonstration's purposes, and could have provided a quantum leap forward for a contextual approach to health care, considering the location and the significance of the demonstration's efforts. The omission is all the more poignant in the light of one of the most revealing statements in Silver's book that the Routine Family Health Conference, in which the members were seen all together, "was perhaps the single most useful device employed by the Demonstration" (1963, p. 199).

Other Contributions

In the 35 years since the writing of *Patients Have Families*, the major conceptual and practical developments for working with families have come from the behavioral sciences, especially from that diverse group of mental health specialists interested in family therapy. Few family therapists wrote about general health matters and few contributors to the primary-care movement wrote directly about the family. One exception, Don Jackson, published two little-known papers on family medicine in 1965 and 1966, calling for the general systems approach and directing attention to the ways medical problems affect and are affected by the family homeostasis. An important extension of this exploration of psychosomatic problems is the work by Minuchin and his colleagues in Philadelphia (e.g., 1975, 1978). Two other important contributions are by Weakland (1977) on family somatics and Sluzki (1974) on training family practice residents to think interactionally. Mauksch

(1974) published an excellent paper, "A Social Science Basis for Conceptualizing Family Health," in the same issue of *Social Science and Medicine* in which Sluzki's paper appeared. Also in that issue, Litman (1974) presented the first major review of "The Family as a Basic Unit in Health and Medical Care."

Over the years, scattered contributions to the development of the family as a focus of health care have also come from pediatrics (e.g., Alpert & Charney, 1973, and their co-workers, Haggerty, Kosa Meyer, Roughman and others, in Boston and Rochester during the 1960s), from traditional general practice, medical social work, medical sociology and anthropology, rehabilitation specialties (especially those involved in home health care programs), and from numerous other groups and individuals who have worked in relative isolation and with little support. Overall, family health research projects and family health programs have had a difficult time in the face of indifference or opposition from biomedically minded subspecialists who generally control funds and space. Few survived, until the establishment of family practice as a medical specialty in 1969.

The contributions of general practice in England (e.g., Clyne, 1961; Kellner, 1963) are consistently instructive, but have had little impact on family medicine in the United States. The British do a great deal of practical work as family physicians, without needing to place much special emphasis on the family as an emergent social system. British medical/social science is skeptical about the proposition that a group of persons can be viewed as a general system and, at that level, be described with such terms as "healthy" and "pathological," which ordinarily apply only to individuals (e.g., Black, 1976; Laing & Esterson, 1964; Marinker, 1976; McEwan, 1974).

The Family Practice Reform Movement

In 1969, the Council on Medical Education of the American Medical Association officially recognized family practice as a specialty. The American Board of Family Practice was established and resident training was systematically begun. More important than the establishment of the specialty for family-centered health care, however, was the insistence by the Board that each residency program create a model family practice unit, separate and distinct from ambulatory care services and "unique to family practice." Accreditation would not be granted without such a structure. The Board also wanted behavioral scientists among the core faculty in family practice training programs. Thus, a special place to work was provided for health care and for research.

It would be natural to assume that the forces behind the creation of this opportunity were specifically interested in the family. The historical evidence is not persuasive. Two other issues led to the establishment of family practice. One involved the "primary-care crisis," a set of problems including the maldistribution of physicians, the excess of subspecialists, and the shortage of providers to practice comprehensive continuing care at a reasonable cost. (By the mid-1960s, a corrective was badly needed for the fragmented episodic care that had grown unchecked since the end of World War II.) The other was the desire to train a new kind of physician, more than a primary-care *specialist*, a physician with a different *style*—one who would view people as the subject of medical practice instead of as necessary bothers who complicate the pursuit of pathology and the requirements of treatment. It was painfully obvious that consumer satisfaction had never been lower and that something had to be done about it.

The issues merged quickly in the 1960s to create a powerful reform movement with roots both inside and outside organized medicine. Cogswell (1981) provides an informative review of this reform movement together with a sociological analysis of the major components of the new role of family physician. In addition, Geyman's *The Modern Family Doctor and Changing Medical Practice* (1971) offers a summary of the three separate blue-ribbon commission reports and other early developments which shaped the rationale and ushered in the official sanction for the new model called family practice.

Early Emphasis: The Family as Background

Several themes are consistently found in the early work of four leading physician contributors to the development of a conceptual basis for contemporary family practice (Lynn Carmichael, Ian McWhinney, Gayle Stephens, and John Geyman): a respect for the usefulness of the behavioral sciences, a preference for the biographical/interpretive approach to patients' lives and to the doctor-patient relationship (thanks to the influential work of psychoanalyst Michael Balint in England), an emphasis on the prevention of health problems and the maintenance of healthy lives, and special importance attached to the personal style of practice developed by the physician.

In contrast, there is little practical or conceptual emphasis on the family or the connection of social relations with health. The family is background, an important factor in certain instances, and, when relevant, discoverable through the patient. Absent is the idea that family relations themselves may be viewed as pathological or therapeutic and that the health or illness of a member might be an embodiment of a property of the group. Absent also is the recognition that such relations, when assessed through the patient, are at best partial, and at worst severely distorted, and that gaining the kind of knowledge one needs about such relations requires direct observation of the relevant participants.

In retrospect, it seems there was resistance to the "family-as-patient" suggestion, in part because this construct was feared as an *alternative* rather than a *complement* to the "person-as-patient" and because it threatened the exclusive and confidential nature of the relationship between physician and patient (see Carmichael, 1983, and Ransom, 1983a, for an exchange on this issue.) In any case, a framework for viewing person, family, and physican as conjointly producing states of mind and body through their interactions initially was missing.

The Merging of Family Systems Approaches and Family Practice

The past five years have seen the beginning of a merging of systems concepts as applied in family therapy with the discipline of family practice. A new synthesis is taking place, resulting in a primary-care family-centered approach that is distinguishable from both general practice and family therapy, its two major predecessors. This *family systems medicine* is closing the gap that existed since the Peckham Experiment and the Richardson study.

Three recent events stand out as evidence of this new synthesis, the publication of two books, *Family Medicine: The Medical Life History of Families* (Huygen, 1982) and *Family Therapy and Family Medicine: Toward the Primary Care of Families* (Doherty & Baird, 1983), and the creation of a new journal, *Family Systems Medicine*, in 1983.

For 30 years, Huygen was the only family physician for virtually everyone in three urban villages in the flower district of the Netherlands. His book, a report of his observations and experiences in that time, persuasively illustrates the features of *social intelligibility* and *connectedness* characterizing illness, referred to earlier in this chapter.

Huygen has complete records for all visits and all problems spanning three generations in many families. The number and types of visits by each member each year can be plotted against a parallel account of significant family events. The result is the discovery of a "familiarity of illness" in which significant association is found between family life events, illness in the parental generation, and illness in the children. For example, differences in the frequency of illness in children between families could not be accounted for by housing, financing, or hygiene, but rather by the psychological stability of the parents and the quality of marital and family relationships.

The uniqueness of Huygen's data is illustrated in that he had 20 families in his practice in which two brothers had married two sisters. Two of these families are described in detail. In both cases, one couple was healthier and got along better with each other and the world than its counterpart. Huygen is able to show that, although they begin with similar genetic material, their roles in the larger family and the organization of family behavior are what account for their differences in health in the long run. It is the *pattern* of illness that Huygen presents compellingly, a level of analysis and insight unavailable to those who do not see families in action.

At the close of his book, Huygen professes that "family medicine promotes a way of thinking about health and illness with revolutionary consequences" (p. 145). His definition of family medicine is allied with that of Ransom and Vandervoort in 1973. What is different this time is that the proposition comes from a family physician of long standing, not from a social scientist and a psychiatrist who witnessed an earlier revolution brought about by family therapy.

Doherty and Baird are a family therapist and family physician, respectively, who combined their skills to write the first book on "how a family systems approach can be applied to a wide range of problems that patients bring to their family doctors" (1983, p. vii). The result is a useful synthesis that can stand on its own as a new contribution to the primary-care field. Several ground-breaking contributions stand out. First, Doherty and Baird can demonstrate that a new kind of practice is actually going on in their own work. They also draw a useful distinction between doing family therapy and providing family-centered primary care. The message is that a family physician need not be a family therapist to practice good family medicine. Their summary and application of systems theory is cogent and practical. The usefulness of their approach is illustrated through case examples of a variety of common clinical problems. New questions raised by the application of this framework will undoubtedly stimulate research along novel lines.

Family Systems Medicine published its first issue in the spring of 1983. The journal's subtitle indicates its focus: "A Journal at the Confluence of Family Therapy, Systems Theory, and Modern Medicine." The aim of this quarterly is to unite insights from family therapy and selective approaches within the social and behavioral sciences with the experiences of family-oriented medicine. It seeks to bridge theory and practice in the development of a new perspective that may eventually extend far beyond primary care.

The potential scope of this expanded view of thinking about health, illness, and intervention is illustrated by an example in an editorial in the third issue by Donald Bloch. Bloch quotes William C. DeVries, the head of the team that implanted an artificial heart in Barney Clark. In the *New York Times* of April 17, 1983, DeVries revealed that an earlier biologically suitable candidate could not be chosen because he "had four daughters and a wife, none of whom were interested in whether he lived or died." Apparently, "he wanted to live but he wasn't given a chance because he had no family support system, and the artificial heart is one of the rare instances where a support system is required for medical treatment." Here, in the farthest reaches of tertiary care subspecialty medicine, Bloch finds the "biopsychosocial model *in statu nascendi*."

Summary

Family systems medicine confronts a true dilemma at this stage of our social and economic history. At a time when it has never been more important to view patients in context and to deal with their lives if we are to influence their states of health, never has it been more expensive, more intrusive, and more unconventional to do so. Two currents move in opposite directions. Dedicated clinicians and researchers disagree about the appropriate focus for future work. Contributors to this book would argue that much can be gained by approaching the social environment, yet the press of modern medicine is still narrowly directed toward technocratic, specialized, interchangeable, and reductionist solutions to health problems. Family therapy and family medicine look toward and engage the wider context. By expanding rather than reducing the context of care, we can expect that more effective and lasting approaches to health problems will be constructed.

One indirect result of an expanded and enlivened approach is a subtle but profound effect on patients' abstract and complex learning—deutero-learning (Bateson, 1942)—the construction of mind sets which finds the participants walking away from an encounter with a changed idea of what health and illness are about, what health care is, and what is expected of those who join to work on health problems. Such ideas cannot be taught directly through "patient education," but they are always learned through relationships with health care providers. Significant learning is always the by-product—the residue—of the doctor-patient relationship. Balint's brilliant book (1957) is ample documentation of this effect. But we can move ahead now, adding concepts and techniques learned from 25 years of family therapy. By opening up the once-invisible doctor-patient exchange to include other persons on both sides of this relationship, both a more comprehensive approach to assessing problems and initiating change and a redistribution of control and responsibility are achieved. The family focus expands the ordinary view to identify ways that health is affected by our relations with others and *includes them* in the process of creating change.

Unfortunately, the new emphasis on holistic medicine, while carrying the banners of "the whole person" and "humanism," does not relinquish the convenience of conventional, reified individual approaches, including the hope that large numbers of persons can be significantly changed without having to change the circumstances of their lives. When personal consciousness, individual responsibility, and the human will are made into principal sources of focused intervention without engaging the context of significant relationships, work, and person-*plus*-environment systems, we have once again failed to grasp the greater half of our existence. It is not difficult to perceive that many of the new individual-centered technologies in health care, while potentially useful in their own right, are also symptoms of a widespread societal defense against what Shands called "the master problem, human relatedness" (1970, 1971).

Family medicine and family therapy represent an alternative approach to the universal problems of health and well-being. At a time of great loss of confidence in human relationships and "the social," family systems medicine confronts realities that conventional medical care seems to avoid or deny—not on grounds of moral necessity or by appeals to faith, but by establishing useful concepts and effective methods of intervention that derive from a systematic body of contextual thought and research.

REFERENCES

Alpert J.D., & Charney, E. (1973, Autumn). The education of physicians for primary care. *U.S. Department of Health, Education and Welfare DHEW*. Pub. No. (HRA) 74-3113.

Balint, M. (1957). *The doctor, his patient, and the illness*. New York: International Universities Press.

Barlow, K. *The Peckham Experiment*. Unpublished manuscript, 1983. (Available from the Pioneer Health Centre, Maddox Farm, Little Bookham Street, Little Bookham, Surrey, England.)

Bateson, G. (1942). Social planning and the concept of deutero-learning. In L. Bryson & L. Finklestein, (Eds.), *Science, philosophy and religion; Second symposium* (pp. 81-97). New York, Conference on Science, Philosophy and Religion and their Relation to the Democratic Way of Life. Reprinted in Bateson, G. (1972). *Steps to an ecology of mind*. New York: Ballantine.

Bertalanffy, L. von (1968). *General systems theory*. New York: Braziller.

Black, P. McL. (1976, January). Must physicians treat the "whole man" for proper medical care? *Pharos*, 8-11.

Bloch, D. (1983). Under two paradigms: The sun also rises. *Family Systems Medicine*, *1*(3), 3-4.

Bowen, M. (1978). *Family therapy in clinical practice*. New York: Jason Aronson.

Carmichael, L. (1983). Forty families—A search for the family in family medicine. *Family Systems Medicine, 1*, 12-16.

Clyne, M.D. (1961). *Night calls: A study in general practice*. London: Tavistock.

Cogswell, B.E. (1981). Family physician: A new role in process of development. *Marriage and Family Review, 4*, (1/2), 1-30.

Doherty, W.J., & Baird, M.A. (1983). *Family therapy and family medicine: Toward the primary care of families*. New York: Guilford.

Foucault, M. (1975). *The birth of the clinic: An archaeology of medical perception*. New York: Vintage Books.

Frank, L.K. (1948). *Society as the patient*. New Brunswick: Rutgers University Press.

Geyman, J.P. (1971). *The modern family doctor and changing medical practice*. New York: Appleton-Century-Crofts.

Haley, J. (1977). Toward a theory of pathological systems. In P. Watzlawick & J. Weakland (Eds.), *The interactional view*. New York: Norton.

Huygen, F.J.A. (1982). *Family medicine: The medical life history of families*. New York: Brunner/Mazel.
Jackson, D.D. (1957). The question of family homeostasis. *Psychiatric Quarterly Supplement, 31* (Part 1), 79-90.
Jackson, D.D. (1965). Family homeostasis and the physician. *California Medicine, 103*, 239-242.
Jackson, D.D. (1966). Family practice: A comprehensive medical approach. *Comprehensive Psychiatry, 7*, 338-44.
Kellner, R. (1963). *Family ill health: An investigation in general practice*. Springfield, IL: Charles C Thomas.
Laing, R.D., & Esterson, A. (1964). *Sanity, madness, and the family*. New York: Basic Books.
Litman, T.J. (1974). The family as a basic unit in health and medical care: The socio-behavioral overview. *Social Science and Medicine, 8*(9/10), 405-520.
Marinker, M. (1976). The family in medicine. *Proceedings of the Royal Society of Medicine, 69*, 115-124.
Mauksch, H.O. (1974). A social science basis for conceptualizing family health. *Social Science and Medicine, 8*(9/10), 521-528.
McEwan, P.J.M. (1974). The social approach to family health studies. *Social Science and Medicine, 8*(9/10), 487-494.
McWhinney, I.R. (1981). *An introduction to family medicine*. New York: Oxford University Press.
Mead, M. (1947). The concept of culture and the psychosomatic approach. *Psychiatry, 10*, 57-76.
Minuchin, S., Baker, L., Rosman, B.L., Liebman, R., Milman, L., & Todd, T.C. (1975). A conceptual model of psychosomatic illness in children. *Archives of General Psychiatry, 32*, 1031-1038.
Minuchin, S., Rosman, B.L., & Baker, L. (1978). *Psychosomatic families: Anorexia nervosa in context*. Cambridge, MA: Harvard University Press.
Pearse, I.H. (1980). *The quality of life: The Peckham approach to human ethology*. Edinburgh: Scottish Academic Press.
Pearse, I.H., & Crocker, L. (1943). *The Peckham Experiment: A study of the living structure of society*. London: Allen and Unwin.
Pearse, I.H., & Williamson, G.S. (1931). *The case for action*. London: Faber & Faber.
Ransom, D.C. (1983a). On why it is useful to say that "the family is a unit of care" in family medicine. *Family Systems Medicine, 1*, 17-22.
Ransom, D.C. (1983b). Random notes: The family as patient—What does this mean? *Family Systems Medicine, 1*, 99-103.
Ransom, D.C., & Vandervoort, H.E. (1973). The development of family medicine: Problematic trends. *Journal of the American Medical Association, 225*(9), 1098-1102.
Richardson, H.B. (1945). *Patients have families*. New York: Commonwealth Fund.
Shands, H.C. (1970). *Semiotic approaches to psychiatry*. The Hague: Moulton.
Shands, H.C. (1971). *The war with words: Structure and transcendence*. The Hague: Mouton.
Silver, G.A. (1963). *Family medical care: A report on the family health maintenance demonstration*. Cambridge, MA: Harvard University Press.
Silver, G.A. (1974). *Family medical care: A design for health maintenance*. Cambridge, MA: Ballinger.
Sluzki, C.E. (1974). On training to "think interactionally." *Social Science and Medicine, 8*(9/10), 483-485.
Weakland, J.H. (1977). Family somatics—A neglected edge. In P. Watzlawick & J.D. Weakland (Eds.), *The interactional view* (pp. 357-487). New York: Norton.
Williamson, G.S., & Pearse, I.H. (1938). *Biologists in search of material*. London: Faber & Faber.
Williamson, G.S., & Pearse, I.H. (1980). *Science synthesis and sanity* (2nd ed.). Edinburgh: Scottish Academic Press.

2

A SYSTEMS APPROACH TO FAMILY MEDICINE

SERGIO HENAO, M.D.

The approach to patient care I shall describe has been called a systems approach, holistic medicine, or the biopsychosocial model, among others. These names refer basically to a way of treating patients by considering the multiple systems that contribute to the development of illnesses and influence the outcome of treatment. Different writers on this subject emphasize different aspects of such a systemic perspective.

The holistic medicine model (Gordon, 1982) attempts to integrate the various aspects of medical practice including the spiritual dimensions of health and disease. This kind of comprehensiveness makes the model unique among systemic approaches. At the same time, Gordon points out (1982), "The holistic medical movement must address itself to its own blind spots, that is, the emphasis on individual responsibility at the expense of therapeutic effort and social concern, the tendency toward faddishness and uncritical embrace of the unconventional . . ." (p. 551). Holistic medicine has not produced the coherent conceptual system necessary to integrate the multiple domains of which the individual patient is a part. Some of these domains, such as the family system, have been almost completely ignored.

The holistic approach to medicine is not really new:

> Hippocrates and the tradition out of which modern biomedicine has grown emphasized the environmental causes and treatment of illness; the etiologic and therapeutic importance of psychological factors, nutrition and life style; the interdependence of mind, body and spirit and the need for harmony between an individual and his social milieu. (Gordon, 1982, p.547)

Yet systemic models and concepts are relatively new. Some of the first and most authoritative contributions came from two biologists, Weiss (1967, 1969, 1977) and von Bertalanffy (1952, 1968). Subsequent systemic models are based on their ideas.

The biopsychosocial approach, originally described by Engel (1977, 1980), represents, in my judgment, the best effort at integrating the present biomedical model of medicine, with its emphasis on science and technology, and the psychosocial model more prevalent in psychiatry, with its emphasis on humanistic and social values. Engel's biopsychosocial model, however, maintains the emphasis on the individual: "In scientific work the investigator generally is obliged to select one system level on which to concentrate, or at least at which to begin, his efforts. For the physician that system level is always a *person*, i.e., a patient" (Engel, 1980, p. 537).

Engel's model, although clearly a systemic one, fails to emphasize the essential quality of a systemic approach, namely, the quality of *interaction* between systems or systems components, which is a major contribution of the family systems approach to health and disease. Engel draws a critical boundary around the person who may be the patient, or even the physician, rather than their interaction. For example, he sees responsibility for the treating of the patient's illness entirely in the physician's hands instead of as a *joint* responsibility influenced by other complex systems like the workplace, the legal system, and so forth. As he wrote, "It is the doctor's not the patient's responsibility to establish the nature of the problem and to decide whether or not it is best handled in a medical framework" (Engel, 1977, p. 133).

This approach, although it reflects traditional psychiatric thought, represents a major advance toward an integrated systems point of view. Unlike the holistic health model, the biopsychosocial model does not encompass the spiritual/religious experience of the patient and the impact it has on the healing process. In some ways the traditional medicine men of Indian cultures are the only ones to use a systemic model in the sense that they consider the biological, psychological, familial, cultural, and spiritual dimensions of illness.

In theory, medicine is supposed to integrate all of these in a comprehensive approach to the patient. In practice, medicine as a whole has drifted into an exaggerated emphasis on science and technology with the corresponding dehumanization of practice. This has become more obvious in the modern meccas, the sophisticated medical centers of major cities throughout the country. The dilemmas of artificially maintaining life, when nature or even the family has long ago given up, are a particularly poignant example of this polarization. Irreparably brain-damaged patients are kept alive for long periods while legal and emotional arguments rage. On the other hand, psychiatry, a medical specialty, has become so involved in the psychosocial elements of human functioning that it has often lost touch with the rest of medicine. At times this has tragic consequences for the patient whose organic illnesses may remain undiagnosed or be treated as if they had been caused by psychological conflicts or troubled social interaction.

One case in point is schizophrenia which at various times has been considered the fault of a "schizophrenogenic mother" (Fromm-Reichmann, 1948) or, more recently, the result of pathological family interaction (Bowen, 1960; Lidz, Cornelison, Terry, & Fleck, 1958; Bateson, Jackson, Haley, & Weakland, 1956, among others). Many psychiatrists are now strongly advocating a return to medicine, and there is even a name for this emphasis: biological psychiatry. Is there such a thing as nonbiological psychiatry? All aspects of patient care—biological, psychosocial, and social—are within medicine, but they are, unfortunately, split one from the other. Attempts to integrate them, like the psychiatric profession's effort to bring back into relevance the biological basis of mental illness has led, more often than not, to throwing away the baby with the bathwater instead of leading to integration.

The Systems Approach to Biological Medicine

In family medicine the systems approach is in essence an extension of the systemic model medicine has applied to the biological study of the individual. Clearly, medicine has had no difficulty looking at an individual human being as a complex biological system that incorporates other systems, like the cardiovascular, gastrointestinal, immunological, and neurological. These subsystems are called open systems, meaning they interact with each other and with the outside environment. Their boundaries are arbitrary theoretical separations, for in practice they function as a whole with no clear demarcations; their interrelatedness is evident from terms like "neuroendocrine," "cardiopulmonary," and "genitourinary." Differentiating and analyzing these multiple subsystems reduces complex problems to more manageable units.

A physician examining a patient ordinarily goes through a review of systems to obtain a picture of the whole organism. Only later will the physician focus on the organ or system that seems to rank higher in a mental rating of priorities.

For example, a patient may come to the physician's office complaining of blurred vision. The physician will have to determine which system or systems are causing the problem by checking each possibility to rule out different abnormalities or illnesses. In this case, the physician will check whether the patient needs glasses (eye disturbance), has a brain tumor with increased intracranial pressure (central nervous system), has a vitamin A deficiency (nutritional system), or perhaps a metastasis from skin cancer or even a side effect from an atropine-like medication. These conditions represent possibilities, some of them clearly fitting the label of diseases (i.e., brain tumor), others being more in the category of deficiencies, or simple problems like an anticholinergic side effect.

Even if the patient's visual disturbance is evaluated and treated properly the physician will still have to evaluate the other body systems because an abnormality in one does not necessarily preclude abnormalities in others. The presence of astigmatism does not, for example, preclude a brain tumor or a vitamin deficiency.

Physicians are trained to think and operate systemically when dealing with biological disturbances. This is true not only when they examine the human body, but also when they explore the relation between the human organism and his or her physical and biological ecology, as in the case of infectious or occupation-related diseases. The investigation of malaria is a classic paradigm of systems-oriented medicine in which diverse connections between environment, parasite, insect, human being, and therapeutic measures have been carefully and systematically studied.

It is clear that a systemic approach to medicine is nothing new. What is new is the expansion of the systemic concept to other levels of human functioning in areas related to maintenance and promotion of health. Figure 1 illustrates the idea of a continuum of biopsychosocial systems or domains in which each system is in turn a subsystem of larger systems.

Medicine has for the most part concentrated on the physical and biological levels of human organisms, what we call the biological system or domain. This study has included a systemic analysis and understanding from the individual cellular system to the large and complex systems studied in public health research. More recently, medicine reached even deeper by exploring the molecular basis of disease and treatment, establishing such new disciplines as nuclear medicine, molecular biology, and orthomolecular psychiatry.

Exploration of the psychological aspects of human beings requires a significant change in method. Psychiatrists and others in mental health have attempted to do this, but because their methods differ so radically from those of others in medicine, they are perceived by the rest as unscientific. Lewis Thomas, president of the Sloan-Kettering Institute for Cancer Research and a prominent medical writer, believes that "we have greatly exaggerated the emotional content of organic medicine. Psychosomatic medicine is on the way out" (*Rockefeller Foundation Illustrated*, 1976, p. 5).

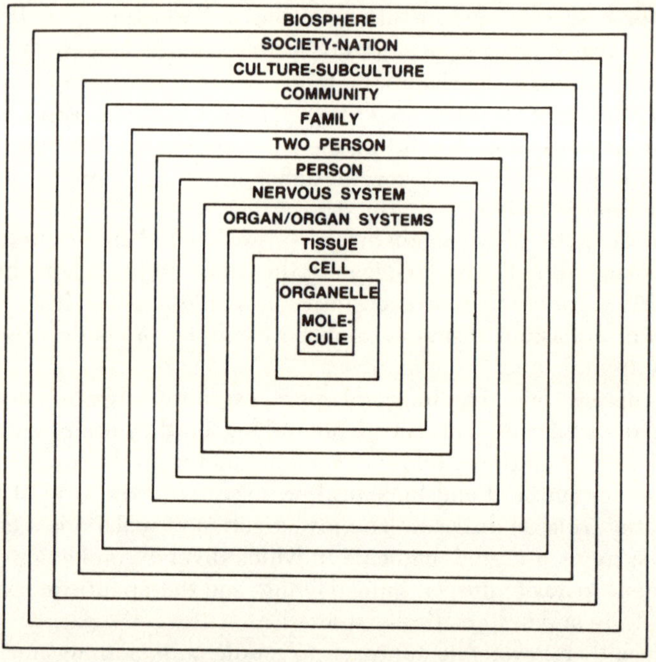

Figure 1. The clinical application of the biopsychosocial model. From G.L. Engel, 1980, *American Journal of Psychiatry, 137(5)*, p. 537. Copyright 1980 by the American Psychiatric Association. Reprinted by permission.

A Human Science

One great obstacle to integrating psychosocial data in the mainstream of science is their unpredictability. While the physical laws of nature seem formidably predictable, the formulations of the psychological and social sciences seem no more than educated guesses. The success of the physical sciences has been due, as Weaver (1955) put it, to the possibility of studying their data "bit by bit, two or three variables at a time, and treating these bits as isolated" (p. 1256). Biology, on the other hand, he continued, "presents highly complex and coupled systems. . . . It takes a lot of variables to describe a man or for that matter a virus; and you cannot often usefully study these variables two at a time" (p. 1256). Franz Boas, in his inaugural speech as president of the American Association for the Advancement of Science (1932), said he believed that fundamental differences between biological and cultural data make it impossible to transfer the methods of the one science to the other.

Both Boas in 1932 and Weaver in 1955 suggested the biological field as the human domain in which the methods of science can be applied, but only within limits. Speaking of anthropology, Boas said:

> . . . the phenomena of our science are so individualized, so exposed to outer accident that no set of laws could explain them. For each individual case we can arrive at an understanding of its relation to inner and outer forces, but we cannot explain its individuality in the form of laws. (p. 612)

In 1976 Margaret Mead's comment on this was that "both men placed the study of man in a context which to a degree is outside the domain of science in its more usual sense as a pursuit in which the aim is to establish regularities" (p. 904). These statements are to a great extent, I believe, applicable to the relationship of psychiatry, the psychological and social sciences, and the rest of medicine.

In biomedicine there is no difficulty in accepting that the various specialists use different methodologies to collect their data and different intellectual paradigms to organize these data in a manner that generates different therapeutic strategies. The methods of public health specialists, for example, in tracking and treating smallpox patients are quite different from the approach used by cardiovascular surgeons to treat the effects of arteriosclerosis, or by pediatricians in treating genetic abnormalities. Yet all these strategies are fully acknowledged as being part of the art and science of medicine.

The methods and assumptions underlying evaluation and treatment approaches to psychological problems and illnesses have for the most part been considered unscientific and only peripherally related to medical practice. This is in spite of the growing evidence that psychosocial factors lead to mental and probably to organic illnesses as well (Holmes & Masuda, 1974; Huygen, 1982; Selye, 1970).

The scientific investigation of psychological phenomena is relatively new in the centuries-old history of medicine. In the Western world, the systemic study of psychological processes really began with Freud at the beginning of this century, which may be one reason why psychological data have not been fully incorporated in the scientific study of illness.

Another obstacle to seeing psychosocial data as scientific is the idea that the study of psychological processes introduces an element of subjectivity which threatens the so-called scientific objectivity of medicine. Moreover, psychosocial data challenge the dearly held illusion that the emotional processes of physicians have nothing to do with the problems and illnesses they study in their patients. Galileo said it first: "The conclusions of natural science are true and necessary, and the judgment of men has nothing to do with them" (trans. 1953, p. 53).

This book makes the major point that medical practitioners need a high degree of self-knowledge and awareness to be truly healing and humane. Not only is this a desirable characteristic of a good physician, but it is also the only scientific attitude possible for a logically consistent systems approach to medicine, especially given the new concepts of undisputably scientific disciplines like physics, as I shall discuss later.

A systemic approach that incorporates the psychosocial elements of illness and therapy is often criticized on another ground. The argument goes that physicians should concentrate on what is properly in the domain of medicine, which in this case means biomedicine, because physicians cannot be everything to everybody. Psychological and social issues are perceived as complicating the purely scientific aspects of medicine, but even if they are considered a valid scientific endeavor they are seen as expanding the object of study to such an extent as to make the actual practice of medicine impossible.

In practice, however, this argument is spurious because patients themselves are aware of their physicians' limitations. Patients do not expect their physicians to be sociologists, psychiatrists, or ministers, any more than they expect them to be epidemiologists, radiologists, or brain surgeons. Appropriately, patients expect physicians to be aware of and sensitive to the multiple biopsychosocial systems that affect prevention, illness, and treatment outcome, although the physicians are not expected to be experts in each of these domains.

Sometimes physicians claim there is no time to assess all these additional systems. But this, I believe, reflects ignorance of the impact of psychosocial systems and the accompanying uneasiness of dealing with concepts with which one is not well acquainted. In other areas of medicine equally complex, lack of time is not accepted as an excuse. It is helpful to remember here that the now very complex and advanced specialty of surgery was once performed by barbers, not physicians. Fortunately, medicine and surgery have been fully integrated. The mental health sciences are only beginning this process.

A New Perspective from Quantum Physics

New developments in theoretical physics, specifically in quantum physics, provide a perspective on scientific thinking that is radically different from that of classic scientific models.

Concepts of linear causality, objectivity, and predictability that were the foundation of classic science are no longer applicable at the atomic particle level. New, puzzling concepts such as "complementarity," "observer-determined reality," and "probability waves" are emerging. These concepts create a picture of reality quite different from the one built on the rational models of Newtonian physics. Even Einstein could not accept that causality and certainty, as previously understood, did not exist in the physical universe that emerged from quantum physics (Pagels, 1982). Reflecting on this, he remarked that God could not play dice with the universe.

A new concept in physics is Heisenberg's Uncertainty Principle (Zukov, 1979), which asserts that at any given time we cannot measure accurately both the position and momentum of a moving particle. Mere observation of the particle will disturb it, making it impossible to observe or measure it without changing it. To illustrate this idea Heisenberg proposed imagining a superpowerful microscope that would allow us to "see" electrons. Unfortunately, if we use ordinary light, the wavelength will be too long to register the electron, in the same way that long sea waves are barely influenced by a pole sticking out of the water. In other words, to see something we have to illuminate (hit) it with wavelengths smaller than the thing we are looking at. If we then replace visible light in our imaginary microscope with gamma rays which have the shortest wavelength known, the electron will be large enough to be detected by the tiny wavelength of gamma rays. The only problem is that the smaller the wavelength the higher the energy. When gamma rays strike our imaginary electron to illuminate it, they knock it out of its orbit and change its direction and momentum in unpredictable and uncontrollable ways. In effect, at the subatomic level, nothing can be observed without changing it, so that "objective," independent observation is impossible.

Another concept of physics applicable to this discussion is Niels Bohr's "complementarity." Experiments by Arthur Coupton in 1923 had demonstrated that light can behave as both a particle and an electromagnetic wave; the results apparently depend on what we choose to demonstrate. If we choose to show light as an electromagnetic wave, it will have the properties of waves like wave diffraction. If we choose to prove that light is a particle, then it will show the properties of colliding particles.

According to the concept of complementarity, wave- and particle-like characteristics are mutually exclusive but "complementary" aspects of light. Although one always excludes the other, both are necessary to understanding light. They "are not properties of light: They are properties of *our interaction* with light. In short, what we experience is not external reality, but our *interaction* with it" (Zukov, 1979, p. 116). The concept of interactive reality rather than isolated, "objective" reality is an essential point of view of the new physics. As Bohr (1934) wrote, "An independent reality in the ordinary physical sense can be ascribed neither to the phenomena nor to the agencies of observation" (p. 53). The wave-particle duality ended the "either-or" way of looking at the world.

Are these concepts relevant to medicine, and more specifically, to understanding and integrating physical and psychological domains? Bohr answered this question himself, in a 1939 speech to anthropologists and ethnographers.

> However this development may appear in the domain of physics, I am sure that many of you will have recognized the close analogy between the situation as regards the analysis of atomic phenomena, which I have described, and characteristic features of the problem of observation in human psychology. (p. 269)

Clearly the classic scientific view of objectivity and of an objective reality independent of the scientific observer is no longer true of the investigations of subatomic and quantum physics. This simply implies that our concept of what is scientific and valid investigation needs to be expanded.

In the study and observation of human beings, and specifically in the study of psychological processes, the physician is not an objective observer but part of the process itself, part of the many systems involving him or her, the patient, the hospital, the profession, the community. To a significant degree, the result of observation will be colored by what the physician is looking for (e.g., illness, personal satisfaction, money, prestige, legal protection, and so on). The very process of conducting a psychological assessment, which is an interactive process, creates a context that inescapably influences the individual or the family being assessed, and absolute objectivity is impossible. In many ways, then, we could say that psychological health or illness is in the eye of the beholder. The more psychological the phenomenon observed, the less objectivity will there be; the more organic or concrete the phenomenon, the more classic scientific objectivity will be possible.

Social scientists have had a major theoretical problem in integrating individual psychodynamic and developmental theories (exemplified by psychoanalytic principles) with more interpersonal and social theories (exemplified by group and family therapy).

For the most part these theories are mutually exclusive and to some extent contradictory. From a systems point of view, for example, the issue of dependence may be conceptualized as residing in interaction, not individual personalities: A dominant wife and a dependent husband both depend on each other. The individual point of view, in contrast, characterized dependency as a personality manifestation not influenced, for the most part, by personal interactions. Theories that are focused on the individual highlight personality characteristics, while social systems-oriented theories blur individual characteristics in a picture of social interaction. This kind of mutual exclusion is easily dealt with if we borrow the concept of complementarity from physics. Theories of human behavior may be contradictory and in some aspects mutually exclusive, but both represent valid ways of looking at human behavior. What we see depends on the context and on what the observer, in this case the physician, is trying to investigate. In the psychological domain, reality does not exist independent of the observer, and the observer integrates the seemingly contradictory aspects of the patient's psychological reality. The physician chooses how to *organize* the psychological process being observed.

This can be illustrated by an old experiment on visual perception in which an observer will "see" different figures depending on whether he or she chooses foreground or background (Figure 2). If you choose the vase, glass,

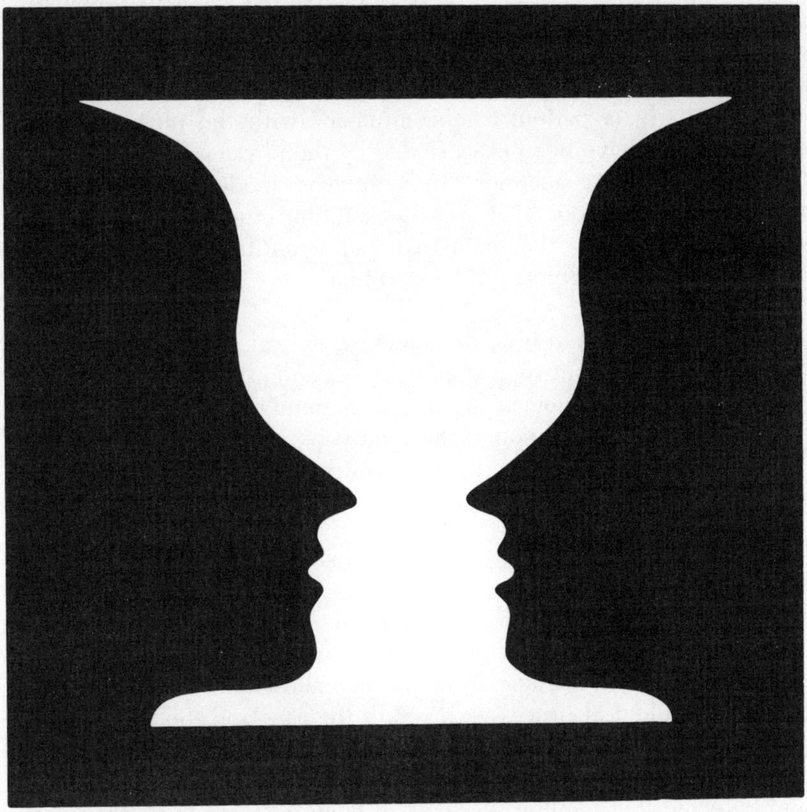

Figure 2. Ambiguous figure seen as either white vase or two black profiles. From *Encyclopedia Britannica*, 15th edition, 1974, p. 241. Reprinted by permission.

the faces in the background are blocked out; if you choose the background the vase disappears and the patterns that do not fit the faces are discarded as visual "noise" (Walter & Walter, 1971).

A similar illustration is the mental image of the half-empty glass which, by a flip of language magic, may also be described as a half-full glass. Both descriptions are accurate but the punctuation (perspective, emphasis) is different. In the scientific process of observing such phenomena as psychological processes, the observer has an impact on the observed process. It may even be said that the observer has a choice in how to organize, define, and punctuate the process. Differing aspects or perspectives of a particular phenomenon, though apparently contradictory or mutually exclusive, may be "complementary."

This complementarity is inextricably linked to the observer. When a physician describes a patient as being too dependent or too reluctant to follow instructions, he or she may not know how his or her own behavior has influenced the patient. Patients who develop extreme dependence on the physician with endless requests for advice and support may be reacting in part to the physician's excessive assumption of responsibility for the patient's health. Similarly, a patient's noncompliance with the physician's recommendations may have been exacerbated by the physician's (perhaps unconscious) guilt-inducing manner. In summary, modern quantum physics provides conceptual tools that may be useful for integrating theories of psychosocial systems into the mainstream of scientific medicine. We must, however, remember Bohr's (1939) warning:

> By such a comparison it is, of course, in no way intended to suggest any closer relation between atomic physics and psychology, but merely to stress an epistemological argument common to both fields, and thus to see how far the solution of the relatively simple physical problems may be helpful in clarifying the more intricate psychological questions with which human life confronts us. (p. 270)

A Systems Approach to Psychological Medicine

Although medicine has indeed used a systemic approach to the biological levels of human beings, medicine and psychiatry have until recently focused exclusively and at times tragically on individual psychodynamics when dealing with psychological processes. Freud's theories and the therapeutic approaches derived from them emphasized psychological development and psychological conflict almost in isolation from interpersonal and social forces. Freud believed that families were an obstacle to treatment: "In psychoanalytic treatments the intervention of relatives is a routine danger and a danger one does not know how to meet" (Freud, 1916-17). Even if this makes sense within the boundaries of the psychoanalytic process, the idea that psychological treatment can take place outside of the familial or social context is analogous to treating a patient for tuberculosis without checking whether or not family or living partners also have tuberculosis.

Even the less orthodox forms of psychotherapy have long preserved an individual or psychodynamic approach that ignores familial and social contexts. The writings of the so-called neo-Freudians like Harry Stack Sullivan (1953) brought forth a more socially oriented theory of psychology and psychiatry. Today family therapists are articulating a more systemic view of interpersonal and social psychology. Social context is highlighted by Minuchin's quote from the noted neurologist Delgado: "We cannot be free from parents, teachers, and society because they are the extracerebral sources of our minds" (1974, p. 6). The main subject of our book evolved from this view, that the psychosocial context of the family and of social relations is an essential element in understanding psychological functioning in health and illness.

Yet the political battles that were necessary to establish family therapy as an acceptable therapeutic modality, based on a social way of understanding the person, led to a rigid and exaggerated interpretation of family therapy theory that parallels the evolution of psychoanalysis. Family therapists, especially those not trained in medicine, are at times blind, on one side, to the realities of biology and individual psychological development and, on the other, to the larger social context (Taggart, 1985).

From a systems perspective, however, the family is only one of several systems to be considered in evaluating or trying to prevent a patient's problems. To look at the family as the only or "best" target for all evaluations or therapeutic interventions is therefore as narrow and inaccurate as seeing biology (biomedical technology) or the spiritual dimension (faith healing) as the only appropriate one.

The best approach does not exist in isolation, and it is contingent on the purpose or context of the problem at hand (best for what purpose? under what circumstances?). One contribution of the family therapy approach is the long overdue attention to the role of the family in illness and health, yet its most important ingredient is its emphasis on a systemic understanding which should, by definition, include not only the biological but also the psychological, social, and even the spiritual domains.

A Clinical Case Example

The following vignette illustrates some of the ideas of a systems approach in family medicine.

Mrs. E., a 45-year-old married woman who lived with her husband and four children, was strong and somewhat domineering, but the family was not aware of any significant problem. One night, Mrs. E. collapsed with what later turned out to be a massive brain hemorrhage caused by a ruptured aneurysm. After a long time in the hospital, she returned home paralyzed on one side, could barely talk, and her mental condition showed a mixture of brain damage and depression. During her absence her family's functioning had deteriorated to the point of chaos; she had been the central figure in the family. The father, diagnosed some years back as "schizophrenic," had lost his only part-time job because of frequent absences from work to visit the hospital. Two of the younger children had stopped attending school and the family was on welfare. Facing this situation, the mother became progressively more depressed, started refusing food, and said she wanted to die. She was admitted to a general medical hospital several times and received medical treatment that included forced feeding and antidepressant medication. Eventually she was referred to our family psychiatric clinic for evaluation, from which the following picture emerged.

Mrs. E. was emaciated and she could hardly sit up—most of the time she lay in bed demanding that someone stay with her constantly. She particularly wanted her husband with her and so he was unable to work. The oldest daughter needed to stay at home because Mrs. E. was unable to move by herself, and had to be carried to a wheelchair, the bathroom, and elsewhere. The daughter had to do this because her father complained of a "bad back." She did not work, go to school, or socialize with anyone outside the family. Her main role in life was to help move her mother around the house. In therapy sessions she said she was extremely angry about this.

Mrs. E., who before her illness had been the family leader, attempted to maintain that role despite her handicaps. She gave orders from her bed and demanded constant attention. Naturally, her manipulative and guilt-inducing behavior generated a tremendous amount of resentment, which the family members, for obvious reasons, did not express fully. Mrs. E., who was quite aware of it, reacted with depression, suicidal thoughts like wanting to starve to death, and more guilt-inducing statements like "nobody wants me because of my illness." The family was surrounded by a cloud of fear and anger—fear that she might die if another cerebral aneurysm ruptured, as she had been told by her neurologist, anger because of the frustration of caring for her. As if this were not enough, nobody was working and two children were not going to school.

The last time we saw this family their old car had finally given up and they had no transportation. They were looking for a new apartment because they were on the verge of eviction. The electricity had been cut off and they had little money. During their last visit, family members reported that they had been eating cold sandwiches because they had no other food. Mrs. E. was doing much better, had stopped her constant demands and accusations, and was accepting whatever food was offered to her.

Despite the sad and painful aspects of this case, it is an excellent illustration of the multiple, overlapping and interacting systems that impinge on a patient at any given time.

Discussion

Let's look at some of the systems that influenced the patient and her family.

The biological system. The patient had a clearly defined biomedical illness with clearly understood pathophysiological causes. She had suffered brain damage from a massive intracerebral hemorrhage in which a congenitally malformed brain artery had ruptured.

The psychological system. Mrs. E.'s mental status was abnormal, partly because of the brain damage and partly because of her own emotional response to a catastrophic illness that caused serious physical handicaps and a radical change in her leadership role in the family.

The family system. The differentiation between psychological and familial systems becomes blurred if one looks at psychological processes as inescapably embedded in a network of social interactions. To distinguish between the two systems has mostly heuristic value, but it helps to highlight the issues involved.

Mrs. E.'s attempts to maintain her control of the family were, given her handicaps, totally inappropriate. But they were understandable if one considers her former role and the fact that she was extremely afraid of having another stroke while alone in the house.

The family reacted to her behavior with anger and frustration. She, in turn, resorted to guilt-inducing maneuvers and unreasonable and changing demands on the family members in a desperate effort to remain in control. She was also testing whether or not her family loved her in spite of the burden she had become. The father and oldest daughter used the mother's behavior to justify their own behavior, claiming, for instance, that neither could work or leave the house for extended periods because of her demands.

Our family sessions revealed that the oldest daughter, in her early twenties, was a socially isolated person who had never worked. The father worked sporadically, often explaining his problems by saying he had been diagnosed schizophrenic in the past and that he had a bad back. We learned also that the father demanded the company of one of his two young daughters whenever he went anywhere, even for brief shopping trips. If they refused to accompany him, he would say he might have a heart attack or faint! The daughters clearly said they felt blackmailed and controlled by this kind of threat and identified it as the same kind of approach the mother was taking with the rest of the family.

The social system. Obviously, the family's poverty became the overriding issue at the end. Faced with these basic survival issues, the family was unable to continue coming to the clinic, even though the biological and psychological issues of Mrs. E.'s illnesses had become stabilized and even her attitude and behavior toward the family had improved. She was no longer depressed or suicidal and was eating whatever was prepared for her.

Another aspect of the social system was this family's contacts with the health care delivery system. In this case, the physician in charge of treating Mrs. E. originally had warned the family to be careful not to upset her because an arteriogram had revealed another cerebral aneurysm that might also rupture. (See Williamson and Bray's chapter on the impact of the language physicians use when talking to their patients.) In this family, in which the mother played such a crucial role, the impact of the physician's warning is obvious. After her initial treatment, she was discharged to her family without any assessment of the family and its social situation. The patient would improve in the hospital but, as soon as she was discharged, she would go back to not eating. Because of this situation, Mrs. E. and her family were referred to us by her physician.

The multiple systems that affected the development of symptoms in this patient, the repercussions throughout the family, and the eventual outcome are relatively easy to understand, at least in theory. In practice, however, this knowledge is difficult to apply, partly because the narrowness of the biomedical model does not allow us to become aware of these multiple systems, and partly because of the economic factors that have led to specialization in the practice of medicine.

I shall end this chapter with an old Sufi story that illustrates beautifully the inherent logic of a systems approach.

Once upon a time a crowd was watching a hanging. One person in the crowd said: "I know *why* they are hanging that man." Someone responded, "Well, if you know *why*, tell us." "Because," said the first one, "he stole some money." "No, that's not true," said another. "The reason *why* is because he is a sick person." "No, that's not the reason," said someone else, "the real reason is because the police caught him." Another bystander insisted that the psychological reason was that the man's mother had not taught him to respect people's property. Finally, someone said they were all wrong, and the only and real reason was that there is a law in the country that says if you get caught stealing people's property, you get hanged.

Is there any one real reason?

REFERENCES

Bateson, G., Jackson, D.D., Haley, J., & Weakland, J.H. (1956). Toward a theory of schizophrenia. *Behavioral Science, 1*, 251-264.

Bertalanffy, L. von (1952). *Problems of life*. New York: John Wiley & Sons.

Bertalanffy, L. von (1968). *General system theory*. New York: Braziller.

Bertalanffy, L. von (1969). Chance or law. In A. Koestler & J.R. Smythies (Eds.), *Beyond reductionism*. New York: Macmillan.

Boas, F. (1932). The aims of anthropological research. *Science, 76*, 605-613.

Bohr, N. (1934). *Atomic theory and the description of nature*. Cambridge, England: Cambridge University Press, p. 53.

Bohr, N. (1939). Natural philosophy and human cultures. *Nature, 143*, 268-272.

Bowen, M. (1960). A family concept of schizophrenia. In D.D. Jackson (Ed.), *Etiology of schizophrenia*. New York: Basic Books, pp. 346-372.

Engel, G.L. (1977). The need for a new medical model: A challenge for biomedicine. *Science, 196*, 129-136.

Engel, G.L. (1980). The clinical application of the biopsychosocial model. *American Journal of Psychiatry, 137*, 535-544.

Frank, P. (1947). *Einstein, his life and times*. New York: Knopf.

Freud, S. (1916-17). Introductory lectures on psychoanalysis, lecture 28: Analytic theory. In J. Strachey (Ed.), *The standard edition of the complete psychological works of Sigmund Freud*. London: Hogarth, p. 459.

Fromm-Reichmann, F. (1948). Notes on the development of treatment of schizophrenia by psychoanalytic psychotherapy. *Psychiatry, 11*, 267-277.

Galileo, G. (1953). Dialogue on the great world systems. G. de Santillana (Ed.) (trans. T. Salisbury). Chicago: University of Chicago Press, p. 53.

Gordon, J. (1982). Holistic medicine: Advances and shortcomings (special essay). *Western Journal of Medicine, 136*(6), 546-551.

Holmes, T.H., & Masuda, M. (1974). Life change and illness susceptibility. In B.S. Dohrenwend & B.P. Dohrenwend (Eds.), *Stressful life events: Their nature and effects*. New York: Wiley.

Huygen, F.J.A. (1982). *Family medicine: The medical life history of families*. New York: Brunner/Mazel.

Lidz, T., Cornelison, A., Terry, D., & Fleck, S. (1958). Intrafamilial environment of the schizophrenic patient: VI. The transmission of irrationality. *A.M.A. Archives of Neurological Psychiatry, 79*, 305-316.

Mead, M. (1976). Towards a human science. *Science, 191*, 903-909.

Minuchin, S. (1974). *Families and family therapy*. Cambridge, MA: Harvard University Press.

Pagels, H.R. (1982). *The cosmic code: Quantum physics as the language of nature*. New York: Simon & Schuster.

Perls, F.S., Hefferline, R.F., & Goodman, P. (1951). *Gestalt therapy: Excitement and growth in the human personality*. New York: Julian Press, p. 26.

Selye, H. (1970). *The stress of life* (rev. ed.). New York: McGraw-Hill.

Sullivan, H.S. (1953). *Interpersonal theory of psychiatry*. New York: W.W. Norton.

Taggart, M. (1985). The feminist critique in epistemological perspective: Questions of context in family therapy. *Journal of Marital and Family Therapy, 11*, 113-126.

Thomas, L. (1976). Doing better and feeling worse: Some dilemmas of American doctors and patients. *Rockefeller Foundation Illustrated, 3*(1), 5.

Walter, R., & Walter, N. (1971). The equivocal principle in systems thinking. *General Systems, 16*, 3-11.

Weaver, W. (1955). Science and people. *Science, 122*, 1255-1259.

Weiss, P. (1967). 1+1=2: When one plus one does not equal two. In G.C. Quarton, T. Melnechuk, & F.O. Schmidt (Eds.), *The neurosciences: A study program*. New York: Rockefeller University Press.

Weiss, P. (1969). The living system: Determinism stratified. In A. Koestler & J.R. Smythies (Eds.), *Beyond reductionism*. New York: Macmillan.

Weiss, P. (1977). The system of nature and the nature of systems: Empirical holism and practical reductionism harmonized. In K.E. Schaefer, H. Hensel, & R. Brody (Eds.), *Toward a man-centered medical science*. Mt. Kisco, NY: Futura.

Zukov, G. (1979). *The dancing Wu Li masters: An overview of the new physics*. New York: William Morrow.

3

THE FAMILY AS A PSYCHOSOCIAL SYSTEM

DONALD A. BLOCH, M.D.

Family systems are basic. None of us lives alone. We are born into a social context, a seamless web that stretches back into the mists of antiquity and forward to the unknowable future. Any significant event in our lives is, among other things, a social event with consequences for those to whom we are most closely bound, and which is affected by them as well. This is part of the age-old wisdom of human beings revealed again and again by artists. During the last four decades, clinicians have found tools for directly intervening in families and, by changing some of the families' patterns of behavior, they have been better able to relieve some human misery. In active association with this, researchers and theoreticians have been building models that fit the newly generated empirical data.

Physicians meet families under a wide variety of circumstances. No single definition or model of family will be completely appropriate to all those circumstances. What is shared by all who adopt a systemic concept of the family is the view that this natural group functions, not simply as a collection of individuals, but as an autonomous organism with its own rules and roles, its own structures and processes.

Specific models of family therapy—structural, strategic, and others—have emerged and are discussed in other chapters. A concept they all share is the view of the family as a psychosocial system. This is the model I shall present here. I hope to make clear the properties and consequences of this approach and the benefits to physicians of thinking about families in this way.

Selecting a Relevant Context

If by family we mean the proximate emotional and social context of the individual, then physicians think about families a good deal. In almost all instances, physicians meet the "leading edge" of a family when they treat physical or emotional malfunction in a single individual. Often it is necessary to map the patient's physical condition and behavior onto some model of the patient's family or intimate social network.

The intimate social network, or surround, is relevant to the problem the patient brings to the physician in varying ways and to differing degrees.

Only a small fraction of the surround is attended to; most of the events and materials in it are of no consequence, that is, do not have *meaning* for the system. We would say that they are not information.

When a diabetic patient, for example, is brought into the emergency room because of ketoacidosis, the physician's first task is to control the condition and at the same time find out what precipitated it. The immediate cause may be an infection, hence the patient's biological system is the only system of concern at that time. Perhaps the acidosis occurred because the patient, an adolescent, was locked in a power struggle with parents, or he could not afford to buy insulin. Here the system to be considered enlarges—family and social welfare have contextual relevance.

As a convention, let us call "context" all events in the surround that have actual or potential information or energy value for the target system. Since the system is, in turn, context for *its* environment (physicians and patients, for example, co-determine each other), let us think of this mutually defining, interacting set of systems as an ecological unit.

We speak of families as open systems, as indeed all living systems are. We mean by this that their boundaries are selectively permeable with a constant exchange of matter and information across the boundaries. Truly closed systems, except for the universe, do not exist in nature, but they can be imagined and approximated so far as nonliving systems are concerned. Living systems are always in active, selective exchange with their surround.

Physicians are familiar with this open systems orientation. We speak of the cardiovascular system, the renal system, the respiratory system, recognizing that they are in continuous, selective exchange of information and energy with their environments. The boundaries of these systems are defined in ways that depend on the situation at hand. It is appropriate, for example, to speak of the cardiovascular-respiratory system when we are concerned with a patient whose pneumonia reduces blood oxygen levels and puts an additional burden on her impaired heart. Similarly, the extended kin network is significant for some life and death problems of the nuclear family. The surround is everything that exists in the immediate environment outside of the system boundary. Energy and information are constantly being exchanged across the boundary, in both directions; the integrity of the system depends on this being carried out successfully.

The cardiovascular-respiratory system mentioned would be one such ecological unit; patient and family make up another; patient and physician (or health care team) are still another. In all instances we are speaking of elements in a mutually regulatory, patterned relation. All of them—family, cardiovascular system, health care system—share certain formal properties. They are all open systems; they are all in states of dynamic equilibrium. They are also, as is true of all living systems, hierarchically arranged, that is, in levels of increasing complexity from cell to organ to organism, family, community, nation, and earth ecosystem.

How does the physician know what part of the surround is relevant? There are, after all, innumerable ways to delimit it. The best definition of relevance will come from questions related to the presenting symptom: What other systems are involved in this? What are the relevant social networks of which this person is a part?

These questions are most easily illustrated in relation to such matters as:

- *Etiology:* Was the gonorrhea contracted from this partner or that? Who is at risk of infection?
- *Public health:* Are other children in the family endangered by eating the paint whose ingestion led to this child's lead poisoning?
- *Preventive medicine:* Can work with this person's family improve compliance with the effort to reduce cardiac risk factors?
- *Treatment:* Can a working mother care for her 10-year-old child during a course of chemotherapy for the child's malignancy?

The Physician and Models of the Family

The perspective of the family as a system is useful for understanding the family's social and emotional organization; it is the theoretical basis for direct clinical intervention into the organization of the family, the method known as family therapy. Other models have utility as well, depending on the circumstances. Many debates, ostensibly about what family *is*, are really disagreements about which model of family is being used.

The word "family" is deceptive. We seem to know what we mean by it, yet, on closer examination, it slips away from us. Who is in our family? When we think of a patient's family, just who belongs to the system?

The answer in a particular situation depends on the professional task of the moment. Consider this example: Our patient is a pregnant 15-year-old girl, physically healthy although possibly retarded; her parents are divorced; the boy involved indicates an interest in the unborn child. A decision must be reached whether to terminate the pregnancy or continue it. If the decision is to keep the baby, with whom shall the child live? Shall the young couple marry and create a new family? Several "families" are involved, or, in the language we are using here, we have a choice of several relevant contexts:

- *Legal*: The law in many localities determines who must be informed and whose consent is needed for each of the possible courses of action. Is parental consent required and for which procedures? Given the divorce of the girl's parents, what is her legal family? What rights does the unborn child's father have? Family is a legal entity.
- *Economic*: What are the economic consequences of each course of action? If the young couple marry, how will they earn their daily bread? If the girl alone keeps the child, will her parents help support her, or will she and her infant go on welfare? Family is an economic entity.
- *Cultural*: What cultural values in relation to abortion, early marriage, and adoption prevail in the families of the pregnant girl and the young father? Are they the same in both families, and in the culture at large? Family is a cultural entity.
- *Psychosocial*: What are the emotional and psychological relationship structures of the family? How does the pregnancy change these structures? Does it weaken or reinforce them? How is the pregnant girl linked emotionally to her mother, her grandmother? What interpersonal coalitions or other alliances are created or changed by the pregnancy? Family is a psychosocial entity.
- *Biological*: Are there hereditary or constitutional factors in the boy, the girl, or either of their families that need attention? What is the nature of her suspected retardation? Family is a biological entity.

Each of these "entities" has different contexts, and obviously none is "correct" or appropriate to all circumstances. It also seems evident that the physician, attending to a primary concern with a physical event such as a pregnancy, is inevitably required to give meaning to that event by selecting one or more family contexts and mapping the event onto it. Indeed, the event has no meaning, is not even an event, without this process going on. Moreover, the physician's actions, indeed the very choices made about which models are appropriate, have an unavoidable effect on the family system.

The Family as a Psychosocial System

The systems perspective in science has been developing over the last hundred years; family systems theory and family therapy have come to represent the projection of this paradigm into the world of the clinician. Perhaps best known as general systems theory, but appearing under numerous other names according to the emphases of various authors, this perspective is most profoundly an expression of a systemic and relativistic epistemology. There is a substantial literature. The perspective or orientation that is most satisfactory to me braids three principal strands: general systems theory (Bertalanffy, 1968; Miller, 1978); cybernetics and artificial intelligence (Hofstader, 1979; Weiner, 1948); and evolutionary anthropology (Bateson, 1972, 1979).

The term "system" is used so widely and carelessly these days that one worries for its fate. As used here, it means—with deceptive simplicity—elements in a patterned relation to each other. Our concern, of course, is with living systems, but a quick sense of the word can be had from considering such nonliving systems as the solar system in which the elements are the sun and the planets and the pattern of their movements in relation to one another.

All living things can be similarly thought of: A cell is something other than a heap of chemicals in the right proportion; these elements are organized in a pattern of relation in such structures as a nucleus, mitochondria, cell membrane and the like, and these in turn are in a patterned relation to each other that makes up the cell. In the same fashion, a forest is a living system in which the elements—trees and plants, mosses and lichens, as well as animals, birds, and insects, soil and meteorological conditions—form a complex whole whose parts are interrelated and co-determine each other.

In exactly this spirit we describe family as a living system. It is an organized, durable, self-producing, slowly evolving pattern of human behaviors grouped together as roles (child, grandparent), structures (the parental dyad, sibling set), and functions (decision-making, affect management).

Until one has come to think automatically in relational terms, many of the concepts with which family therapists concern themselves may seem insubstantial—in some way unreal, like subatomic particles. After all, we can pierce the boundary of a cell with a micropipette; what instrument is analogous when it comes to a family boundary? The instrument, of course, is the human observer. Our task, in the words of Peggy Papp, is "to make the invisible visible" (Papp, 1979).

Before we turn to specific characteristics of systems as they apply to families, we should attend to the overall aspect that is most important: A system is an organized whole. The parts of a system are continuously interconnected; they extend in spacetime, and a change in one component is inevitably associated with changes in the other components with which it is in relation. Indeed, it is in this most primary sense that the family is a system.

The clinician is at a considerable disadvantage if the problem dealt with is not understood in its appropriate context. Taking a systemic perspective often makes sense of the otherwise unintelligible. The following personal example depends on a simple but profound notion: Elements in a system co-determine each other; this is how they make up a coherent whole. In this instance, the proper context for understanding a physical disease (diabetes) and a treatment event (insulin reaction) must include a psychosocial phenomenon (hypoglycemic irritability) and a family pattern (spousal relationship).

My wife is an insulin-dependent diabetic and, as all familiar with this disease know, one hazard is the possibility of insulin reactions. On several occasions the difficulty of establishing the diagnosis of an insulin reaction was complicated by two psychological factors: my increased anxiety when I believed my wife was about to have a reaction (experiences with inadequately treated reactions had been very unsettling), and her increasing irritability and clouded sensorium as her blood glucose level fell. It was difficult at times to know if she was irritable for some interpersonal reason (most often her view) or because of hypoglycemia (most often my view). The linchpin in the system was the not uncommon denial—as is the wont of many diabetics in similar situations—that anything was wrong. Thus, we have a system in a positive (deviation-amplifying) feedback condition as my efforts to press my point of view generated more resistance, which in turn made me more apprehensive and my wife more irritable. Not a good state of affairs.

This problem was partially solved by a change in our marital pattern. We made an agreement that I had the right to decide she take some sugar whenever I felt it appropriate, and that she would comply even if she disagreed completely. That solution rocked along fairly well but was superseded by a better one, that she would comply with my suggestion that we test her blood glucose level—a possibility that depended on the only recently available technology for such determinations at home. My apprehension dissipated; the problem was solved and has stayed solved.

Diabetes is a disease with manifestations at all levels of organization in which changes at one level, glucose metabolism, are associated with shifts at other levels, the psychological and familial as in my example. As is well known, these are not unidirectional changes because emotions have metabolic effects as well. The physician treating this condition must be aware of these complex feedback loops. Educating the individual patient as to proper care often will not be enough to produce therapeutic change when the system is malfunctioning. Indeed, chronic conditions of all kinds must be thought of as the disease-in-the-patient-in-a-context if the promise of the technical advances of biomedicine are to be realized in patient care. The relevant context most often is that intimate network, the family.

Systemic Properties of the Family

Let us turn now to a consideration of some of the specific characteristics of systems that have been useful in understanding families, disease, and the health care processes.

Boundaries

Characteristic of any system is that it has a boundary; the elements of the system exist within that boundary and everything else is external to it. Thus a cell has a boundary, an organ like the liver has a boundary, and a family has a boundary. Depending on one's purposes in defining them, a system has many boundaries.

Thus, families and persons as systems have boundaries that physicians are required to cross all the time. The converse is, of course, true as well: The patient coming to our office or being admitted to the hospital is crossing the boundary of the health care system. Every time a physician touches the body of a patient a boundary of personal space is crossed by virtue of society's and the patient's special permission to do so. When the physician makes a house call, he or she must cross the psychosocial boundary of the family in addition to entering its physical space. At times this is easy to do, when the family is eager for the visit and welcoming in its attitude; at times it is difficult, when the family is guarded and restrictive, limiting information and perhaps even physical access.

A systemic perspective would lead us to ask such questions as: Given the boundary-maintaining characteristics of a particular family, what methods of joining the family, of gaining access to needed information, for example, can be devised? How can a family practice be structured so that patients and their families can join most appropriately to optimize the joint work of health care?

The components (subsystems) of a system can be considered as systems in their own right. The systems review that physicians automatically conduct when they interview a patient acknowledges this. The family therapist is interested in such subsystems as the marital dyad or sibling set.

Dynamic Equilibrium

The concept of dynamic equilibrium first found expression in physiology. Such notions as Claude Bernard's (1957) *le milieu intérieur* or homeostatic equilibrium (Cannon, 1932) developed from physiological studies that aimed to understand variation around a constant: temperature, blood pressure, blood-gas level. For a long period the preferred term was "homeostatic equilibrium," but this has fallen into disfavor for the good reason that it seems to emphasize stasis rather than drawing attention to the constantly fluctuating interaction of equilibrating and disequilibrating forces that, through their dance, generate the patterns we call equilibrium or stability.

Equilibrium is the most useful of all the concepts the newer theories have generated. Consider, as an example, a tightrope walker. For her to be in equilibrium means to be constantly in motion with body position and weight distribution varying around an imaginary comparison point: a center of gravity line vertical to the tightrope. As she strays, deliberately or otherwise, from the comparison point, inpouring information is generated to tell her that this is so, and she makes corrective, equilibrating moves to restore her balance.

The information is multichannel in nature, generated from within the system through vestibular and proprioceptive reflex arcs, and, externally, from pressure on the pads of the feet, weight shifts in the balancing pole, and the audible response of the circus audience. To make matters more interesting, the skilled performer will generate disequilibrating moves to involve and please the audience; another comparison standard is superimposed on the primary one of maintaining balance, what might be called the optimal performance of staying erect while appearing to be in constant jeopardy. These are feedback loops in operation.

Families, too, are in constant motion around comparison points. While our concern is with how they do this in behavioral terms, it is instructive to think for a moment about one of the famous families who perform on the high wire, the Flying Giacondas, known throughout the circus world for the enigmatic smiles that play over their faces as they perform their daring acts. Father and an uncle ride unicycles; a pole on their shoulders connects them. On the pole stands older son, carrying another pole at the ends of which his mother and older sister hang by their teeth while younger sister stands on her brother's shoulders. The delicacy and complexity of family equilibrium can be understood by contemplating this kind of situation.

Physical disease and other changes in life circumstances may act as disequilibrators for families. Let us look at some examples:

- The sexual adjustment of a young couple was satisfactory until the birth of their first child.
- Depression in a middle-aged wife appeared after her husband received a promotion at work that required a shift in residence.

- Four months after his father had a coronary episode a 14-year-old boy began failing in school.
- Persistent and bitter disputes erupt in a couple as the Alzheimer's disease of the man's mother becomes more obvious.
- Hypertensive episodes in a 40-year-old woman become more frequent and severe in the six months following her youngest child's departure for college; the child, who is scholastically capable, has an unexpectedly bad academic year.

These vignettes highlight the connection between disequilibrating force and symptom. It is useful to think of the symptom as having a rebalancing effect but it should be emphasized that we are *not* saying that the disequilibrating event *causes* the symptom. More properly, we would say that the system adjusts to a new set of conditions—the symptom is part of the adjustment. In the last instance, the mother's hypertension may call the child home to care for her; the child's school difficulties may lead her to return home.

Hierarchy

Hierarchical organization is one characteristic of living systems that is of great importance to physicians and to family theorists. This means that a system at any level is made up of component subsystems on one hand, and is itself, in turn, a component subsystem of suprasystems. The events with which we are concerned take place at multiple levels: molecular, biochemical, cellular, organic, organic systemic, psychological, familial, institutional, and societal.

Physicians and most professionals are required to attend to phenomena at multiple levels. It is manifestly impossible for any single one of us to stretch knowledge and treatment techniques all the way from molecular-biological to societal levels, yet it is helpful to recognize this dimension of our task. At the very least, we may avoid the political turf wars that seek to establish primacy for one or another level of conceptualization and organization.

The Giacondas on the high wire are organized into subunits that together make up the whole: The two unicyclists, the four-person team balancing on the pole between them, mother and older daughter at the ends of the pole brother carries, and so on. For some analytic purposes differing levels of the hierarchy should be scrutinized. Should the Giacondas complain that a family fight is ruining their act, we would approach the matter differently than if a Ménière's syndrome appeared in a family member.

Thus it is accurate to say of our high-wire family that their performance depends *only* on their family social organization. Indeed, the actual group on the high wire depends on a support system that includes those other family members (probably part of the extended kin network) that help them on and off the wire, sew costumes, book the act, and so on.

Replication and Historical Continuity

Living systems have histories; the past is stored in such a fashion that it becomes part of the goal-directedness of the organism. This is true at all systemic levels of organization. Genetic codes in the nucleus of cells are, among other things, self-reproducing. At the psychological level, memories provide templates that organize new experiences so as to replicate themselves. Similarly, families store experience in their roles and rules, myths and aspirations so as to organize their relation to new events in a fashion that strengthens the already established patterns.

The Giacondas place themselves in—that is, self-select for—environments (circuses, in their case) that favor certain kinds of transactions with the surround. In those environments they elicit self-confirming responses that further strengthen a family identity. The smell of the grease paint and the roar of the crowd all contribute.

The relevant family system extends in both space and time, in both a biological and social-historical context. The Giaconda family has, over generations, been biologically selected for certain aptitudes, and socially selected by developing traditions that both motivate them to perform and equip them with the needed know-how.

Family therapists working in medical settings have learned to pay attention to kin other than those in the immediate nuclear family. This is particularly important in regard to assembling additional support for a harassed family group struggling to deal with such problems as cancer in a child. At times, the effects of such an illness reverberate through the generations.

For example, a woman sought consultation for her problems in her relationship with her new husband. In her early sixties, she had been widowed a few years before. The new marriage had gone well for awhile but had recently deteriorated. Everyone agreed that the deterioration was related to a grandchild's increasingly grave illness. The 11-year-old boy had developed a brain abscess that required multiple operations, and he was recovering from severe neurological deficits slowly and uncertainly. The child's mother, the grandmother's only daughter, had, because of her own anxiety and guilt, excluded the grandmother from direct care for the youngster. The daughter's marriage was languishing as well as she obsessively clung to the child's bedside. Both the grandmother's new husband and the child's father were neglected and excluded by their wives. Both marriages were maintained by therapy directed to a revision of the response to the child's illness. This, in turn, had positive benefits for the future of the entire family.

Unlike other important social groups, family exists in unbroken continuity of membership with its own past and its own future. That lineage may or may not be known directly to the members of any given generation; so many of us come from immigrant families that the latter is most often true. The larger culture may be inclined to look backward, or, as in modern times, favor only future-gazing. Despite this considerable variation, family is, by its very nature, a historical event. It may not know its history, but it *is* its history.

The Giacondas exemplify this. It took hundreds of years of Italian and Russian circus history to develop the two lines which then blended together with the marriage of mother Nadia and father Nico. It was truly what Napier (1971) has called a "marriage of families."

From this perspective how are we to understand new family formation, the process by which a young couple locate each other and form an attachment strong enough for the formation of a new family? Since so many of the difficulties that families experience can be traced to the conditions under which the new family originated, to unrealistic expectations and conflicted motivations, it may be useful to discuss this briefly. Connecting the process of family formation to the emotional and psychological place of the young couple in his and her family of origin is an enlightening notion. The underlying concept is that a person chooses a mate in some measure based on a calculation, usually unconscious, of his or her own position in the family. An interesting instance of this concept at work can be found in Walter Toman's charming book, *Family Constellations* (1976). Toman considers the place of the individual in a sibling set as this relates to choice of mate. Older siblings who marry younger siblings are apt to have more stable relationships; this is particularly true if an older son marries a younger daughter, and even more so if an older brother of a younger sister marries a younger sister of an older brother. These threads can be spun out in a variety of ways. Sibling position is only one of many factors that determine the choice of a marriage partner and the fate of that relationship. We grow up and live in a family context of roles and relationships, conflicts and resolutions, which, on the personal level, are experienced as our personal selves, our motivations and needs. Not surprisingly, as we form a new family, these earlier contexts serve as models—to be sought after in some instances, or avoided in others. It is perhaps excessively simplistic to say that, under these conditions, we marry our spouses to solve unresolved issues in the families in which we grew up. Yet that insight has been a potent tool in the hands of family therapists working with troubled families.

Physicians, for instance, often have to deal with marital pairs who have organized their relationship around a rescuer-rescued axis (Penn, 1983). When this pattern is examined from a multigenerational perspective, it turns out to have a history in each of the marital partners' families of origin and to be related to their choosing each other as mates. When a severe physical illness occurs in such a family it tends to have (a) a powerful *disequilibrating effect*, if the illness occurs in the traditional rescuer, and (b) a powerful *stabilizing effect* if it occurs in the traditionally rescued partner. The physician may be faced with unexpected responses to the illness—in the second case, sometimes, with excessive clinging to and overfocusing on the illness. The line of reasoning that follows the trail of the illness back to the "reason" for the marriage, in terms of the partners' place in their family of origin, helps to make all of this understandable and provides a rationale for appropriate referral and treatment.

Summary

The family has been presented from a systemic perspective with particular attention to the ways in which this paradigm is of importance to the practicing physician. Certain aspects of the family have been emphasized: that it operates as a whole, that it is hierarchically organized, that it is in homeodynamic equilibrium, that it is a boundaried open system in constant interchange with its surround, and that it is self-reproducing in endless and meaningful connection with its own past and future.

REFERENCES

Bateson, G. (1972). *Steps to an ecology of mind*. New York: Ballantine.

Bateson, G. (1979). *Mind and nature: A necessary unity*. New York: Dutton.

Bernard, C. (1957). *Introduction to the study of experimental medicine*. New York: Dover.

Bertalanffy, L. von. (1968). *General systems theory*. New York: Braziller.

Cannon, W.B. (1932). *The wisdom of the body*. New York: Norton.

Hofstader, D. (1979). *Godel, Escher, Bach: An eternal golden braid*. New York: Basic Books.

Miller, J.G. (1978). *Living systems*. New York: McGraw-Hill.

Napier, A. (1971). The marriage of families: Cross-generational complementarity. *Family Process, 10*(4), 373.

Papp, P. (1979). *Making the invisible visible*. (Videotape). New York: Ackerman Institute.

Penn, P. (1983). Coalitions and binding interactions in families with chronic illness. *Family Systems Medicine, 1*(2), 16.

Toman, W. (1976). *Family constellations*. New York: Springer.

Weiner, N. (1948). *Cybernetics*. New York: John Wiley & Sons.

4

STRUCTURAL FAMILY THERAPY

SALVADOR MINUCHIN, M. D.

The body of theory and the interventive techniques labeled "family therapy" are concerned, fundamentally, with changing dysfunctional aspects of a family system. The goal of therapy is a more adequate family organization, one that will maximize the growth potential of each member of that family.

A family is a natural social system that has evolved ways of organizing and transacting that are economical and effective for that particular group. It comes into therapy when some stress overloads the system's adaptive and coping mechanisms, thus handicapping the optimal functioning of its members.

The family's diagnosis of the problem is usually that one of their members is behaving in ways that are stressful for the family. They want the therapist to change the member who is having or causing difficulties. The family therapist, however, focuses on the whole group. One of the members may be expressing the family stress in ways that are clearly visible, but the problem is not confined to the identified patient. The whole family is responding to a stressful situation.

The source of family stress may be internal or external. It may spring from internal problems around a transitional stage in the family's development, such as the emergence of a child into adolescence, the inclusion of a new family member, or the separation of a member. It may spring from idiosyncratic problems, such as a child's retardation or physical handicap. Or family stress may spring from one member's stressful contact with the extrafamilial world, for example, a child's having problems in school or a father at his job. It may come from total family contact with the extrafamilial world. The

Reprinted from *American Handbook of Psychiatry, Second Edition* (1974), Vol. 2, with permission of the publisher, Basic Books.

family may be pressured by poverty, discrimination, separation from natural systems of support, and so on.

In any case, when the family comes into therapy, the therapist will enter the family, buttress or change the system in whatever ways seem necessary, and then leave the family to continue its own enhanced growth-encouraging, supportive, and reparative functions. Therapy is a transitional process that can be schematized as: 1) [family] + [therapist]; 2) [family + therapist]; 3) [family + therapist's ghost] − [therapist].

Concepts of Family Therapy

The Prospective Approach

Family therapy is prospective; its orientation is to the present and future. This is one of the aspects that distinguishes it from dynamic theory, which is retrospective. In dynamic theory the patient's present transactions are seen as a projection of the past, and growth is defined as casting loose from this past. Understanding the past is seen as necessary for changing the present. In family therapy, the tool of therapy is not the exploration and understanding of the past but the manipulation of the present. The past history of the family was instrumental in the creation of the family's present organization and functioning; it is, therefore, manifest in the present and available to change-producing interventions. Manipulation of the present is the tool for changing the present and the future.

The Scope of the Therapist

The family is a socializing, educational, and reparative unit. In family therapy, therefore, the family itself is seen as performing many of the functions that in individual dynamic theory are the functions of the therapist.

The family therapist does not join the family to educate or socialize. His function is to be the enabler of the family's own functioning, so that it can perform these tasks. Many of his transactions will have educational input, and this may sometimes be essential for family functioning. But his main input will be in terms of the family's structure and organization.

The scope of the therapist is also affected by reliance on the systemic properties of the family. In dynamic theory, change is seen as having to occur in the interaction between the therapist and patient. As in the traditional healing by the laying on of hands, the therapist must be present for change to occur. By contrast, in family therapy, the family is recognized as a self-perpetuating system. The processes the therapist has initiated with the family may be perpetuated in his absence. In other words, when family change has been effected, the system properties of the family will preserve that change; the input of the therapist will affect family members even in his absence.

This quality of therapy makes new ways of using time in therapy possible. For example, the therapist can spend the initial phases of therapy in intensive work with the family. At the point at which dysfunctional sets begin to change, he can recess the family and reconvene later to see if the family is continuing the new organization. He can then continue therapy or recess again, with the understanding that he is available for problems that may arise. Like a general practitioner, the therapist brings the family to a level of health and then stands ready to be called in if necessary. The advantages of brief and prolonged therapy are thus combined.

Orientation Toward Sets

Family sets are patterned sequences of interaction among family members. Family pathology can be conceived of as the development of dysfunctional sets. These are nonproblem-solving reactions of family members as the result of stress, reactions that repeat in the family without modification when there is conflict. Changes that could restore a functional equilibrium—a realignment of family members, adaptations of rules, and so on—become blocked. For example, the father experiences stress at work. He comes home and attacks the mother. She counterattacks, and symmetrical or escalating non-stress-resolving interactions develop, continue without change, and finish when one member of the dyad abandons the field. Each member suffers from the sense of nonresolution. A similar situation can involve a triad. The mother and father attack each other, then both become concerned with controlling a misbehaving child. Or the father, under stress, attacks the mother and the mother seeks a coalition with the son against the father. The father counters by seeking coalition with the son against the mother.

Dysfunctional sets can also involve the entire family group. For example, a child emerges into adolescence. His participation and status in the extra-familial world increase. Problems around control and autonomy develop within the family. The relationship between the adolescent and the mother resists the changes necessary for adaptation. The mother attacks the adolescent, the father enters the conflict on the adolescent's side, and younger children enter the conflict, attacking the adolescent. When all family members participate in dysfunctional sequences, a variety of groupings and coalitions can occur. The situation generalizes. All family members become involved in the conflict, but the family organization does not change. The dysfunctional sets will, therefore, repeat in the next stressful situation.

Sets may also be functional. For example, a man experiencing stress at work comes home and attacks his wife. She withdraws and a few moments later returns to support him. Or there may be a fight, but it finishes with closure in spite of escalation and increased level of attacks. The field is not abandoned with a sense of lack of resolution.

Functional sets can change. Realignment, changes in rules, and other conflict-resolution sequences are possible. They tend to resolve or diminish stress for family members. Dysfunctional sets do not change; they repeat when stress occurs, and they tend to maintain stress. Or if stress in one subsystem is alleviated, it is at the expense of another subsystem in which stress is maintained or increased (see the example of the T family on p. 59).

Dysfunctional sets can assume a salience in family life that obfuscates functional sets that are supportive and encourage growth. The therapist scans family structure to pinpoint salient sets. He will explore functional sets and search for steps to buttress them. He will emphasize family strengths, mobilizing supportive mechanisms to enhance what is functional. Change-producing interventions will be directed toward the dysfunctional sets.

Points of Entry

The common mode of describing an interaction is like stopping a motion picture. We say, "father provoked mother," excluding the factors that the mother provoked the father to provoke her and that the sequence has impact on the father, mother, and other family members.

The family therapist sees individuals as subsystems of larger systems; these individuals initiate processes that have impact on the system, and they react to system processes. The therapist deals with the sequences of interpersonal interaction which broaden possible points of entry. He can work with individuals as subsystems of the family. He can work with dyadic family subsystems, that is, helping parents strengthen interactions as adults so as to strengthen the boundary between adults and children in the family. He can work at the interface of the family system and societal systems. In other words, the therapist can direct interventions to any promising point in a sequence. When working with a child's problem, the family therapist can enter to utilize any useful part of that child's ecosystem.

Implications for Therapy

Theoretically, child psychiatry encompasses an understanding of the importance of the child's ecosystem; but for therapeutic purposes, the child may be conceptualized as an intrapsychic entity preserved unchanged through the vicissitudes of an average environment. This retrospective approach minimizes exploration and manipulation of the present life context. The Group for the Advancement of Psychiatry's 1966 Report contains innumerable examples of this point of view.

The boundaries imposed by the artificial dichotomy between internal and external processes and influences limit the child therapist. If a child is referred to treatment because of a school phobia, the GAP Report says: "the child has unconsciously displaced the content of his original conflict onto . . . a situation in the external environment that has symbolic significance for him. . . . Thus the child avoids those . . . situations that revive or intensify his displaced conflict. . . ." (p. 232). The focus of this diagnosis does not take into account the environment of the child or the target of the phobia. But looking at the child with school phobia in his current life contexts broadens possible points of entry. The problem and/or area available to therapeutic intervention might be found in the school, the home, or at the interface between school and home.

In exploring the school context for possible points of entry, the therapist looks at the child's performance as a student. He explores the child's position in the peer group and his self-perception as a member of this peer group, his relationship with the teacher and the ways he perceives the teacher as similar to or different from other significant adults, the teacher's view of the child and how correct and differentiated that view is, and how the child and the teacher work together (Minuchin, Biber, Shapiro, & Zimiles, 1969).

Both home and school have, in a broad sense, an educational style and expectations of the child. The child can be seen as operating at the interface of the two socializing institutions. Are the two syntonic, or do they interact with him in conflicting ways (Minuchin, Chamberlain, & Graubard, 1967)?

Exploring the family context, the therapist looks for the possibility that dysfunctional sets in the family are rewarding the child's phobia. The needs of the mother might be creating dysfunctional sets in the mother-child dyad and keeping the child at home. Or there might be a conflict between the parents in which the child's symptoms are useful; if so, dysfunctional sets in the triad might be reinforcing his not going to school. Or the school phobia could be supporting the child in a position of strength in his sibling group. Or the siblings might be supporting his symptoms as part of a scapegoating process (Ackerman, 1961, 1970; Vogel & Bell, 1960).

Given this expanded focus of observation, the family therapist can look at the multiple forces impinging on the child in his current contexts and select areas for intervention that his analysis and goals have highlighted as promising.

These concepts could only be a product of twentieth-century philosophy and technology. The old idea of the individual acting on his environment becomes the concept of the individual interacting in his environment. As Bateson (1971) writes:

> Consider a man felling a tree with an axe. Each stroke of the axe is modified or corrected, according to the shape of the cut . . . left by the previous stroke. This self-corrective . . . process is brought about by a total system, tree-eyes-brain-muscles-axe-stroke-tree; and it is this total system that has the characteristics of immanent mind. (p. 6)

In nineteenth-century thought, actions were expressed simply: "The boy chopped the tree down." But twentieth-century cybernetic thought recognizes that a human being is controlled, in Bateson's words, "by information from the system and must adapt his own actions to its time characteristics and to the effects of his own past action. Thus in no system . . . can any part have unilateral control over the whole" (Bateson, 1971, p. 5). The individual influences his context and is influenced by it in constantly recurring sequences of interactions.

The broadening of focus implied by this approach affects every aspect of therapy, including its diagnostic categories. A diagnosis is no longer a nonevolving label pasted on a contextless intrapsychic entity. It is an evolving, broader description of relevant sequences. Furthermore, it includes implications for therapeutic interventions. The diagnosis of encopresis implies only that the child should be cleaned up. The diagnosis of a child's responding to unresolved conflict in the family's spouse subsystem, or the diagnosis of sequences of enmeshed interactions between mother and child that isolate the husband-father, contain the germ of possible therapeutic interventions.

Another implication of this broadened theory is the recognition of diagnosis as something achieved by therapeutic strategy. In a system-oriented framework, the entrance of the therapist into the family group is recognized as a massive intervention in itself. He becomes part of a new system—the therapeutic unit [family + therapist]—and he acts and reacts as a subsystem of that system.

His diagnosis is an evolving analysis (Minuchin, 1970). For example, a family comes into therapy with a teenage girl who is shy and withdrawn, and having difficulties in her social life. The therapist notices that when the family enters the therapy room, the girl moves quickly to sit next to her mother and pushes the two chairs close. The therapist asks what the problem is, and the mother responds. When the daughter tries to add something, the mother continues talking about her as though she had not spoken. There is a great deal of noise and confusion in the family, with the girl's siblings talking while the mother talks. The mother's knowledge of her daughter's life is intimate, going far beyond material usually shared by adolescent girls.

Four minutes after the beginning of the session, the therapist makes his first intervention, asking the mother and father to change chairs. This intervention tests the flexibility of the family, suggests to the family an interpretation of pathology in the mother-child dyad, and brings the father into the picture, providing a general reframing of the problem with a larger focus.

The idea that the child responds to stresses that affect the family, which is accepted by both child and family psychiatry, is the basic tenet of family therapy (Ackerman, 1961, 1966, 1970; Boszormenyi-Nagy & Framo, 1965; Haley & Hoffman, 1967; Hoffman, 1971; Hoffman & Long, 1969; Jackson, 1968a, 1968b; Minuchin, 1969; Minuchin, Montalvo, Gurney, Rosman, & Schumer, 1967; Spiegel & Bell, 1959; Zuk & Boszormenyi-Nagy, 1967). This response has largely been a clinical supposition, based on observation, but recent family research gives it experimental grounding.

For example, in one psychophysiological research project (Minuchin, Rosman, & Baker, 1978) parents are subjected to a stress interview while their children observe them through a one-way mirror. Blood samples are taken from all family members at 15-minute intervals for later analysis of the free fatty acid level changes at different times in the interview.* The children can see and hear their parents, but they are physically unable to take part in the conflict situation. Nevertheless, their free fatty acid levels rise as they observe their parents under stress. The cumulative impact of current psychological stress is powerful enough to cause physiological changes, even in children who are not directly involved.

This experiment also shows the utilization of a child in dysfunctional sets. In the T family interview, for instance, the parents were engaged in their usual spiral of nonresolving conflicts, with the wife blaming her husband and her husband apologizing but indicating no intention of changing. During this period the parents' free fatty acid levels increased significantly. The identified patient, a 9-year-old diabetic boy who was having trouble in school, observed their bickering. His free fatty acid level rose almost twice as much as those of his parents.**

When this boy was brought into the therapy room, each parent tried to entice him into a coalition against the other parent. The spouse conflicts were submerged in the sequences of triangulating the child. In the half hour of this situation the parents' free fatty acid levels returned to their basal levels. The child's increased and remained high.

The stress associated with chronic nonresolved spouse conflicts was lessened for the parents by the possibility of triangulating the child. The stress

---

*Free fatty acid level is a biochemical variable that rises within five to 15 minutes in response to stress. It is used in this study as a physiological indicator of emotional arousal.

**In a nonstressful control period his free fatty acid level remained close to his basal level.

associated with this type of position in the family system is shown by the child's large rise in free fatty acid, poignantly demonstrating the price paid by what Ackerman (1961) calls the "family healer." The family healer's instability is necessary to lessen the stress in another subsystem. The triadic dysfunctional set operates at his expense.

Techniques of Family Therapy

Family therapy is not a technique to be defined by the number of people in a therapy room during a session. It is an interactional theory, which encompasses any number of techniques.

Bell (1961) is generally considered the therapist who first treated families as a group. He originated a distinct procedure for treating disturbed children, seeing first the parents, and then the parents and the child, emphasizing the refocusing of the problem from the child's behavior to parental conflict.

As the concept of family therapy began to gain currency in the 1960s, interventions directed toward every conceivable unit were tried (Boszormenyi-Nagy & Framo, 1965; Bowen, 1967; Haley & Glick, 1971; Laqueur, Laburt, & Morong, 1964; Minuchin, Montalvo et al., 1967; Satir, 1964; Speck, 1967; Taber, 1970; Watzlawick, Beavin, & Jackson, 1967). There have been experiments with different locations (Friedman et al., 1965; Minuchin & Barcai, 1969). Different time units have been used (Barcai, 1967; MacGregor, Ritchie, Serrano, Schuster, & McDonald, 1964). Different cotherapists have been utilized (Landes & Winter, 1966; Minuchin, 1970; Minuchin, Montalvo et al., 1967). Various mechanical devices have been used, and total-family diagnostic tools have been developed (Winter & Ferreira, 1969).

When a child is brought into therapy by his family, he has already been diagnosed by the school, his pediatrician, the court, the police, or his peers. This diagnosis reinforces the family's labeling of the child as a problem.

The family therapist's initial objective is to transform this individual label into a diagnosis that includes the family. For example, if the child is caught in enmeshed interactions between his parents, either trapped in the position of a go-between, as in the previous example, or used as the battleground, the diagnosis will reflect this dysfunctional set. The therapeutic goal will be to achieve a family organization in which the spouse dyad can function without triangulating the child.

In order to work toward this goal, the therapist will look at the sets of spouse interactions, pinpointing the ones that seem to have to utilize the child's symptoms. These will be the targets of his change-producing interventions.

Therapeutic Tactics

Therapeutic tactics will, in general, fall into two categories: coupling and change production. Coupling can be defined as everything the therapist does to enhance his therapeutic leverage within the therapeutic unit. Change production is the stratagems directed toward changing dysfunctional sets.

Coupling

When two different systems adjust themselves in terms of direction and become one system, this is coupling, a label coined by Braulio Montalvo. The union in space of a lunar module and the command ship is an example. The therapist, one system, joins the family system, and the two become one therapeutic system. The therapist facilitates his entrance into the family by accepting the family organization. Coupling operations are obviously vital to therapy. If the family drops out or the therapist loses the leadership of the therapeutic unit, nothing can be accomplished. There are three types of coupling interventions:

1) *Maintenance* involves supporting the family structures. A family system is governed by rules that regulate the behavior of its members. The therapist joining the family feels the pressure to behave according to these rules. He may accept them, in the beginning, as a way of gaining entrance to the system. For example, if the mother is the central pathway by which family communication is routed, the therapist also talks to her and allows her to mediate his communications to the family. The therapist must be aware of the family's threshold of stress. When family members need support, he will provide it. When change-producing stratagems are pushing the family toward its threshold, he will use maintenance techniques to move back to a point where the family is more comfortable. Other examples of maintenance operations are supporting areas of family strength, rewarding or affiliating with a family member, supporting an individual member who feels threatened by therapy, and explaining a problem.

2) *Tracking** is a method of adopting the content of family communications. As a phonograph follows a record's grooves, producing sound, the therapist takes over the family content and uses it in a therapeutic maneuver. For example, a family may be complaining about the father's authoritarian

*I am indebted to Mariano Barragan for labeling this operation and for the example.

stance. The father says, "I want to be a leader, but I want to be a democratic leader. I want to be the president of this family." The therapist says, "OK, if you want to be a democratic leader, let's hold an election." In tracking, the therapist does not challenge the family. It is a method that has its roots in hypnotic suggestion, in which the patient is never confronted. If the patient refuses a suggestion, the hypnotist accepts his refusal but manipulates the situation so that the refusal is a form of obeying the hypnotist's command. As in the technique of jujitsu, one uses the opponent's own movement to propel him. With a family, the therapist utilizes the family's movement to propel it. But he maintains the framework so that he is propelling it in the direction it wants to go. He seems to enter the family as a supporter of family rules. But he makes the family rules work in the direction of his goals for it.

3) *Mimesis* is a coupling technique aimed at the family's style and affect, as reflected in the members' activities and moods. The therapist may use the tempo of family communications. If the family is restricted, his communications may be sparse. He may adopt the family's affective style. In a jovial, expansive family he may use expansive body movements. He pays attention to their language and begins to use some of their terms. If they discuss a bar mitzvah, he may use a Yiddish word. If a Puerto Rican family is urging a daughter to find a husband, he may suggest that she turn St. Anthony's statue upside down. Mimetic operations are mostly explicit and quite spontaneous. Experienced therapists perform them without realizing it. In one family, a father who was derogating himself took his coat off. Immediately, the therapist took his own coat off, but did not recognize this as an intervention until an observer pointed it out in a postsession discussion.

Change Production

Unlike coupling, change production involves some form of challenge to the family's natural style in order to change dysfunctional sets. It is helpful in conveying this to picture the family as a jazz group. Music is produced by improvisation, but the tempo, the order in which the instruments play solo, and sometimes the key are firmly predetermined. The many improvisations open to the individual player are chosen according to his mood and the possibilities of his instrument. There are areas of great flexibility within a strictly patterned organization, but they are governed by the sets.

Change-producing interventions will be directed toward the sets, or the system "memory," which dictates the repetition of accustomed interactional patterns. Coupling operations will continue throughout, but they are not to be confused with the change-producing operations that will be directed toward pathogenic sets. Therapy is often unnecessarily long because therapists waste their efforts on areas in which flexibility is already possible, instead of identifying and concentrating on pathogenic sets.

The following example may help present some of the clinical consequences of family therapy theory. The presenting problem was a serious case of anorexia nervosa in a 10-year-old girl. The priority of intervention was, obviously, the abandonment of the symptoms in the child. Once this had been accomplished (Minuchin, 1978), we embarked on a nine-month course of family therapy, which was vital to the continued change of the family patterns that had generated and supported the anorexia nervosa.

The following data are presented in terms of an analytic schema, rather than in process-recording form. When one thinks of therapy as a process involving a system's needs, interventions oriented toward a goal, and outcome, this organization of data becomes cogent. It is not sequential. Much of the material in the diagnostic formulation, for instance, was explored only after the anorexia symptoms had been abandoned. But it is a logical course of phases that the family therapist must think through.

The schema divides therapy into four phases:

1) Determination of family structure, areas of strength, and dysfunctional sets. Assignment of priorities for intervention (diagnosis).
2) Determination of objectives, or goals for change. This will be closely related to the diagnostic assessment, but will evolve through therapy.
3) Assessment of therapeutic options and selection of strategies. Given a diagnostic assessment that includes objectives, there are many possible strategies. The therapist must assess the potential impact of each option in terms of its power, its type, and its cost. In terms of power, does it mainly affect the individual, another subsystem such as the spouses, the entire family, two interlocked subsystems such as family and classroom, and so on? In terms of its type, is it change production or prevention? What will it cost in therapeutic time and input, psychological pain and financial burden to the family? Stratagem selection takes into account the family's assessment of priority, the pathways open within the limitations imposed by the family's style, and the therapist's style and capability.
4) Periodic evaluation of the results of stratagems leads to the reassessment of priorities, new evaluation of therapeutic alternatives, the selection of further stratagems, and further evaluation of implementation.

Case Example

The Smith family is composed of the father, a successful architect in his mid-forties, the mother, and four daughters: Helen, 14 1/2; Barbara, 12; Sally, 10; and Jane, 8. The family was referred to family therapy by their pediatrician. Sally had been hospitalized, and diagnosed as suffering from anorexia nervosa after losing 15 pounds during a two-and-a-half month period. On her arrival in the hospital she had weighed 42 pounds; after a week in the hospital, she weighed 40 pounds. The family assessed itself as a "normal American family." Its goal was that Sally eat.

Diagnostic Formulation

The priority of therapy was obvious—the abandonment of the anorexia symptomatology. In priority, the therapist's assessment coincided with the family's. But because he saw the anorexia syndrome as a response to family organization, rather than as an individual's illness, his diagnostic formulation of needs was much broader than the family's perceived needs. Both the immediate and long-term objectives depended on a broader diagnostic formulation.

The therapist's assessment of the family was that they were operating in a tight, enmeshed system (Minuchin, Montalvo et al., 1967). Dyadic transactions rarely occurred; they became triadic or group transactions. These interactions were characterized by a rigid sequence that promoted a sense of vagueness and confusion in all family members. A parent criticized one of the girls; the other parent or a sibling joined in to protect the child; another family member joined the critic or the criticized; the original issue would be diffused, to start again through a similar sequence, to be similarly unresolved. There was a helpful, protective quality to the enmeshed interactions. The avoidance of aggression or even disagreement was striking. The family described all interactions as harmonious.

In the therapist's assessment, there were many unnegotiated husband-wife conflicts. Such conflicts were submerged and never allowed to become explicit. They were expressed in a family organization in which the mother joined the daughters in a coalition of females that left the husband-father trapped in a position of helpless isolation. He was perceived by the women as an absolute despot. In reality, his power within the family was negligible. The mother parented the daughters; the husband-father was disengaged and peripheral. Only in the area of parenting were spouse disagreements expressed: The father felt the mother was too lenient with the girls.

Another expression of disagreement that might have been related to the selection of the anorexia symptom was the mother's constant attempts to improve the father's table manners. This was a disagreement that had run throughout the 20 years of the marriage and was now discussed with bantering by all the family members, particularly at mealtime.

The boundaries of the spouse subsystem were very weak. The peripheral husband-father had strong ties to extrafamilial systems, particularly his business and his own family of origin. The mother was firmly bound in the female subsystem, which was an enmeshed, high-resonance system. Small movements by members of this system brought countermovement from the other members. The mother was the main point of contact between this system and others. The father communicated with the girls through the mother. Therefore, the mother controlled the nature of their communication, screening out nurturant elements of the interactions but letting controlling elements pass, thus strengthening the coalition of the girls with her against their father. Her relationship with her daughters was overcontrolling, intrusive, and overnurturing. The close communication, appropriate with younger children, had led to difficulties beginning a number of years before when the oldest daughter, emerging into adolescence, had begun to make demands for age-appropriate increased autonomy. At this point, the relationship of mother and oldest daughter was fraught with demands for autonomy, countered by the mother's demands for obedience. Barbara, the second oldest daughter, was allied with her older sister, Helen, in this conflict.

The family malfunctioning was affecting all the family members. The symptomatology of anorexia nervosa overshadowed the symptomatology of the parents and the "well" siblings, but clinical scrutiny of the total group showed each member responding to the family stress in idiosyncratic ways. The anorexia nervosa syndrome was deeply embedded in the family's pathogenic sets.

The Smiths, like other pathologically enmeshed families, were highly resistant to change. When a situation that required family change occurred, they typically insisted on retaining their accustomed methods of interaction. Consequently, situations of chronic imbalance were maintained for long periods.

When significant members of a pathologically enmeshed family system feel that the family can neither withstand change nor adapt to it, the system demands that particular family members change in a way that will maintain the malfunctioning homeostasis. A symptom bearer is selected (and self-selected) as a conflict-avoidance circuit. Whenever the rather low perceived danger point of family stress is approached, the symptom bearer will be activated for use in conflict-detouring sequences. The family system reinforces the development of symptomatology and rewards its continuance because the symptomatology is necessary to the conflict-detouring sequences that maintain the status quo of the family system.

In the Smith family, Sally was functioning as the chief conflict-detouring pathway. Her most important use and source of reinforcement was in the spouse subsystem, but the symptomatology was, of course, multideterminate.

Spouse subsystem. The never negotiated conflicts between the parents were perceived as a particular danger area. All the children were involved in keeping these submerged, but when one arose, it was most often Sally who crossed the generational boundary to diffuse the parental conflict. Her function was to allow her parents to detour their conflict via concern for her.

Furthermore, the symptom defined one safe area in which spouse conflicts could surface. The father thought the mother should make Sally eat. The mother, though very worried, thought that Sally should not be forced to eat. The coalition of the mother and daughter against the father was explicitly manifested in the mother's protecting Sally against the father's assertion that she should eat. At the same time, the selection of the symptom was an implicit coalition with the father, whose fight with the mother had also been allowed to surface in the area of eating.

Sibling subsystem. Sally was the least powerful member of the rather undifferentiated group. She was isolated and excluded. The sibling subgroup, of course, conformed to the family style. Whenever conflict arose, there was immediate bunching into coalitions. Sally was always excluded from these coalitions, and was often their target. Since open disagreement was to be avoided, her isolation took the form of tomboy interests. The girls said Sally did not want to play with them because she preferred boys' games, and Sally agreed. The anorexia nervosa kept the structure of the sibling subgroup intact, but it improved Sally's position. She was still isolated, but the coalitions against her became coalitions of concern and protectiveness.

Individual subsystem. The anorexia syndrome was a means of self-assertion. By not eating, Sally was asserting herself in a way that was permissible within the value system of the family. She was disagreeing, but not openly. The family's priority of avoidance of conflict was maintained because her not eating was not an explicit confrontation or rule breaking.

The symptom, then, was being reinforced by the spouses as a conflict-avoidance circuit, by one spouse in coalition against the other, by Sally's experience of "legal" self-assertion, and by Sally's being able to protect her family and even ally herself, on an implicit level, with her father. The siblings also reinforced the symptom as part of a protective and scapegoating system.

Objectives posed by diagnostic formulation were:

1) The disappearance of the anorexia nervosa symptomatology.
2) A change in the spouse subsystem. Supportive, complementary transactions between the spouses must increase. A strongly bounded subsystem of mother and father, parenting their children in a mutually supportive relationship, must appear. The mother must be disengaged from parenting to give her more space for spouse subsystem operations and for clear supportive parenting operations. The father must be more engaged in parenting, able to contact his daughters directly without going through the mother; the mother's function as contact must disappear.
3) A change in the sibling subsystem. The enmeshed functioning of the subsystem must decrease. The boundaries must be weakened so that the daughters can interact with their parents and with the extrafamilial world without choosing a representative of their needs. There must be clear differentiation with clear age-appropriate increased autonomy for the adolescents, and a change in Sally's powerless, scapegoated position.
4) Effective dyads and triads in the total family system must be possible. The degree of flexibility must increase, and enmeshment must decrease. Flexible alliances and coalitions, capable of shifting, must be possible.
5) Clear communication among all family members. This must be fostered, so that the real nature of transactions can be recognized.

It will be obvious that these objectives are mutually interdependent. All changes are predicated on generic change in the family's enmeshed style and the degree of flexibility possible. Furthermore, the goals are interlocked within the system just as the pathology is. The older daughters cannot become adolescents until the mother becomes a wife. The mother cannot be a wife until her husband pulls her away from her daughters. The daughters will not let their mother go until the mother has some support from the father as a husband in the areas of spouse support and tenderness. As long as contact between the father and daughters has to go via sequences that include the mother, the father cannot get his wife into his own orbit. While the mother and father are divided, the girls will have to struggle with the mother's intrusive overnurturance and overcontrol. As long as the girls remain part of an undifferentiated, highly enmeshed sibling subgroup, they will struggle through the use of the anorectic sibling, further reinforcing the symptomatology.

Assessment of Therapeutic Options and Stratagem Selection

It is clear from the diagnostic formulation that only an approach to the whole family system will respond to family needs. If an option directed toward only part of the family system, such as individual therapy, were selected, this would still be an intervention affecting the total family (whether or not the therapist recognized and utilized this impact). Working with the child on an outpatient basis brings the therapist into the family system. He uses the therapeutic relationship to block the child's participation in the family interactions as a conflict-avoidance circuit, and he attempts to use the changes in the child as modifiers of family transactions. Furthermore, in working with the parents as part of the treatment of the child, the therapist has another handle on changing family organization. When the child is hospitalized, the forced separation of the child from the family joins the factors that can help mobilize family conflicts that will have to be dealt with in the absence of the anorectic child.

But therapeutic interventions directed toward an anorectic child without explicit attempts at changing the family organization of which she is a subsystem would be expensive. Even if they were successful, they would be costly in terms of psychological pain for the identified patient, the pain of duration of the anorexia symptomatology, financial burden on the family, and lack of preventive qualities for siblings and parents. The family therapist is particularly aware of the parents and three siblings, each of whom is currently showing responses to family stress and might become the new scapegoat if the presenting problem were dealt with without change in the family system.

Accordingly, the option chosen for the Smith family was family therapy. Sally had already been hospitalized prior to referral. The therapist's preference was to work with the child in her family, shortening the period of hospitalization insofar as this was consistent with medical needs. The pediatrician and family therapist collaborated in a strategy of iatrogenic family crisis designed to break the symptomatology, so that Sally could return home quickly.*

Change-producing strategies are always predicated on the therapist's opening up repetitive vicious pathogenic sets as he joins the family system. Though he does not have absolute freedom to manipulate the system in the

*A pediatrician may be reluctant to allow an anorectic child to return home to the family, fearing the medical consequences. The family therapist may find himself in the position of having to educate both the family and the pediatrician, so that the pediatrician does not unwittingly reinforce the family's labeling of their symptom bearer.

ways he wants, he does have several options within the mode of family therapy. He can, for instance, elect to defuse the stress that brought the family into therapy, returning the family to a sort of status quo ante, and continue long-term therapy to change the pathological sets. But in working with a rigidly dysfunctional family system such as the Smiths, this approach would only reinforce the dysfunctional organization. A return to the status quo ante would not be even an interim solution.

When working with pathologically enmeshed families with psychosomatically ill children, it is preferable to work in the development of crises, organizing the family transactions in such a way that the family is forced to deal with the stresses it has been submerging. The therapist monitors the resulting crises, creating experiential situations in which the family members can and must learn to deal with one another in new and different ways. In a family that insists on defining itself as perfectly normal, except for one member's medical problem, a medically induced crisis opens up the significance of family sets which have created and supported the symptom. The symptom area offers the obvious route to this crisis.

During the first session with the Smith family, the signs of pathological enmeshment were obvious. Since the first step in iatrogenic crisis is to observe the family's reaction to and handling of conflict, the therapist searched for an area in which a conflict could be framed. But the family was extremely resistant to attempts to elicit conflict. Only after an hour and a half of probing was an area of difficulty brought out—the mother's constant attempts to nag her husband into improving his table manners. This provided a cue for asking the family to order lunch (initial sessions with anorectic cases start at 11 A.M.). The session stopped while sandwiches were brought in and a lunch table was set up in the therapy room.

The technique of having lunch with an anorectic family is valuable for several reasons. For one thing, it makes things happen in the session with the therapist. When a conflict around eating can be enacted in the session, talking about anorexia nervosa would be a waste of time. Furthermore, organizing a family crisis around the anorexia symptom makes it available to direct intervention. Interventions on an individual level directed at the anorexia symptomatology, such as exploration of the anorectic's ideation about food and the like, might only serve to reinforce and further crystallize the symptom. But when a family crisis is organized around the syndrome, it is the interpersonal negotiation of parents and child around the eating that gains salience, rather than the symptom itself. Not eating becomes the "ground" instead of the "figure" because of the dramatic emergence of interactional factors, which then become available for change-producing interventions.

Evaluation of Implementation

The strategy of increasing stress between parents and daughter around the anorexia syndrome yielded immediate results. Sally started eating during the session, continued to eat during two more days in the hospital, and kept eating after her return home. In a month her weight returned to normal.

Once the dramatic presenting symptom had disappeared, the needs of other family members came more sharply into focus, forcing a reassessment of therapeutic goals. Since the core of the problem was the inability of the spouses to negotiate together, the next therapeutic priority became change in the spouse subsystem.

Sessions with the spouse subsystem were interspersed with total family sessions. Once the facade of mutual agreement was broken, the spouse sessions dealt with the wife's sense of being unacceptable to her husband, her sense of being in competition with her mother-in-law, her complaints of her husband's not supporting her in parenting and not respecting her as an adult. The husband brought up issues of being isolated in the family, being needed to intervene with his daughters only when the wife failed, and feeling that his wife was not interested in him as a sexual partner. Therapeutic interventions in these subsystem sessions were addressed to facilitating the negotiation and resolution of disagreements and encouraging the experience of mutually supportive and pleasurable nonparenting interactions.

Meanwhile, total family sessions continued. Various stratagems were utilized in the intrafamilial sphere. During total family sessions, communication style was challenged. When a conflict between two members developed, the therapist made them continue until they achieved a resolution or until a third member could join in explicit form, either asking to be included or being invited by the original dyad. Members of the family changed chairs so that the two or three people involved in a discussion sat next to each other; the others moved out of the circle and observed.

This technique was particularly useful in differentiating the siblings. For example, as the oldest girl's conflicts with her mother became prominent, the father was requested to intervene. The three brought their chairs to the center of the room while the other girls moved out. With the mother strongly supported by her husband, negotiations ensued that gave Helen much more autonomy, explicitly related to her status as the oldest. The therapist increased this differentiation by treating her as an adult. He also assigned a task (Haley, 1963) to the mother. She was to watch for actions Helen performed that deserved her approval and reward them. This was directed to a double audience. Helen heard the task assignment and increased the type of actions that her mother could reward. Helen began to emerge as a teenager.

The individuation and disengagement of Helen from the sibling subsystem left Barbara as Jane's playmate; Sally was excluded. Now the three girls occupied the center of the room, with the mother and father helping them from outside the circle. Jane and Barbara were directed to play with Sally. The three played a board game together, and the game became enmeshed and chaotic. Therefore, the girls were assigned the task of playing board games at home. The parents bought the games, helped select them, and saw that the rules were followed.

Barbara, the brightest and most psychologically minded of the family, began to ally with the therapist, sitting near him and commenting on family functioning. She began to have more school friends, spending more time with them in an age-appropriate process of contacting the extrafamilial. Sally and Jane became closer.

In one session, Jane complained that Sally played roughly and threatened her with frightening fury. Now Jane and Sally took the center, with Helen asked to act as the mediator, helping Jane to understand Sally's explanation. Her role as oldest sister was buttressed by participation in a play that differentiated her two youngest siblings.

In all these sessions, the clear demarcation of the parties in a negotiation and the resolution of clearly stated conflicts were emphasized. This use of space to create explicit proximity and distance, delimit subgroups (actors and observers), intensify affect, potentialize the enactments of fantasies or roles, and so on is useful in rigid, deeply enmeshed, undifferentiated families. It enables the therapist to function like the director of a play, setting the stage, creating a scenario, assigning a task, and requiring the family members to function within the new sets that he has imposed.

Therapy with this family terminated successfully after nine months.

Conclusion

The Smith family case demonstrates that a child presenting a symptom is presenting a symptom of family stress. If one broadens the focus, the forces within the family that maintain the symptom will appear and can be dealt with.

It will be obvious that the case example concentrates on the change-producing interventions done with this family. Change-producing stratagems can best be conveyed by describing family members and the therapist as though they were cybernated robots. The inaccuracies of this approach in describing human beings and describing therapy with human beings are too obvious to need elaboration. But coupling operations are so idiosyncratic to a therapist's style, a family's style, and the way the two interact that a description of them would simply be case recording. Change-producing interventions can be described in more generic fashion.

In conclusion, an orientation that takes the child's ecosystem into account will combine the possibility of maximally potent interventions with preventive operations. This approach involves the least possible psychological pain for the people involved and, therefore, becomes the most humanitarian as well as the most effective way of approaching a problem.

REFERENCES

Ackerman, N.W. (1961). Prejudicial scapegoating and neutralizing forces in the family group, with special reference to the role of family healer. *International Journal of Social Psychiatry*, [Special issue], (2), 90-96.

Ackerman, N.W. (1966). *Treating the troubled family*. New York: Basic Books.

Ackerman, N.W. (Ed.). (1970). *Family therapy in transition*. Boston: Little, Brown.

Barcai, A. (1967). From the individual to the family and a step beyond. Paper presented to the American Orthopsychiatric Association, Washington, D.C.

Bateson, G. (1971). The cybernetics of self: A theory of alcoholism. *Psychiatry, 34*, 1-18.

Bell, J.E. (1961). *Family group therapy*. [Public Health Monograph, No. 64.] Washington, DC: U.S. Government Printing Office.

Boszormenyi-Nagy, I., & Framo, J.L. (Eds.). (1965). *Intensive family therapy*. New York: Harper & Row.

Bowen, M. (1967). Presentation of a family experience. Paper presented to the Conference on Systemic Research in Family Interaction, Philadelphia, PA.

Friedman, A.S. et al. (1965). *Family treatment of schizophrenics in the home*. New York: Springer.

Group for the Advancement of Psychiatry (1966). *Psychopathological disorders in childhood: Theoretical considerations and a proposed classification*. Report No. 62. New York: Mental Health Materials Center.

Haley, J. (1963). *Strategies of psychotherapy*. New York: Grune & Stratton.

Haley, J., & Glick, I.D. (1971). *Family therapy and research: An annotated bibliography of articles and books 1950-1971*. New York: Grune & Stratton.

Haley, J., & Hoffman L. (1967). *Techniques of family therapy*. New York: Basic Books.

Hoffman, L. (1971). Deviation-amplifying processes in natural groups. In J. Haley (Ed.), *Changing families* (pp. 285-310). New York: Grune & Stratton.

Hoffman, L., & Long, L. (1969). A systems dilemma. *Family Process, 8*, 211-234.

Jackson, D.D. (Ed.). (1968a). *Communication, family and marriage*. Palo Alto: Science and Behavior Books.

Jackson, D.D. (Ed.). (1968b). *Therapy, communication and change*. Palo Alto: Science and Behavior Books.

Landes, J., & Winter, W.D. (1966). A new strategy for treating disintegrating families. *Family Process, 5*, 1-20.

Laqueur, H.P., Laburt, H.A., & Morong, E. (1964). Multiple family therapy: Further developments. *International Journal of Social Psychiatry* [Special issue], Section K, (2), 69-80.

MacGregor, R., Ritchie, A., Serrano, A., Schuster, F., & McDonald, E. (1964). *Multiple impact therapy with families*. New York: McGraw-Hill.

Minuchin, P., Biber. B., Shapiro, E., & Zimiles, H. (1969). *The psychological impact of school experience*, New York: Basic Books.

Minuchin, S. (1969). Family therapy: Technique or theory? In J. H. Masserman (Ed.), *Science and psychoanalysis, Vol 14*. New York: Grune & Stratton.

Minuchin, S. (1970). The use of an ecological framework in child psychiatry. In E. J. Anthony & C. Koupernik (Eds.), *The child in his family*. New York: Wiley.

Minuchin, S., & Barcai, A. (1969). Therapeutically induced family crisis. In J. H. Masserman (Ed.), *Science and psychoanalysis. Vol. 14*. New York: Grune & Stratton.

Minuchin, S., Chamberlain, P., & Graubard, P. (1967). A project to teach learning skills to disturbed delinquent children. *American Journal of Orthopsychiatry, 37*, 558-567.

Minuchin, S., Montalvo, B., Gurney, Jr., B.G., Rosman, B.L., & Schumer, F. (1967). *Families of the slums: An exploration of their structure and treatment*. New York: Basic Books.

Minuchin, S. Rosman, B.L., & Baker, L. (1978). *Psychosomatic families: Anorexia nervosa in context*. Cambridge, MA: Harvard University Press.

Satir, V. (1964). *Conjoint family therapy*. Palo Alto: Science and Behavior Books.

Speck, R.V. (1967). Psychotherapy and the social network of a schizophrenic family. *Family Process, 6*, 208-214.

Spiegel, J., & Bell, N. (1959). The family of the psychiatric patient. In S. Arieti (Ed.), *American handbook of psychiatry, Vol. 1* (pp. 114-149). New York: Basic Books.

Taber, R.H. (1970). A systems approach to the delivery of mental health services in black ghettos. *American Journal of Orthopsychiatry, 40*, 702-709.

Vogel, E.S., & Bell, N.W. (1960). The emotionally disturbed child as the family scapegoat. *Psychoanalysis and Psychoanalytic Review, 47*, 21-42.

Watzlawick, P., Beavin, J.H., & Jackson, D.D. (1967). *Pragmatics of human communication: A study of interactional patterns, pathologies, and paradoxes*. New York: Norton.

Winter, W.D., & Ferreira, A.J. (Eds.). (1969). *Research in family interaction: Readings and commentary*. Palo Alto: Science and Behavior Books.

Zuk, G.H., & Boszormenyi-Nagy, I. (Eds.). (1967). *Family therapy and disturbed families*. Palo Alto: Science and Behavior Books.

5

THE STRATEGIC APPROACH

JOHN H. WEAKLAND and RICHARD FISCH, M.D.

As they should be, physicians in family practice are usually the first professional recourse for most families who encounter somatic—and many psychosomatic—difficulties. In the course of this, however, primary-care physicians are often presented with problems that "don't make sense" as standard medical problems, and in ways that make diagnosis and treatment puzzling and difficult.

To take a somewhat extreme example, an obese mother brings an obviously overweight child to the doctor with the complaint that "he doesn't eat," and she insists that this is the problem, brushing aside the doctor's attempts to suggest that, if anything, the child must be overeating. Or a mother brings her child because he is passing black stools. On careful examination the physician finds that the child is basically quite healthy, but this does not allay the mother's concern, and the symptom persists (S. Henao, personal communication, 1982).

Other examples, although less blatantly confusing, still involve situations difficult to understand and deal with effectively: A man comes for his physical checkup accompanied by his wife. She expresses marked concern about his physical condition, but the patient himself seems strangely passive, unconcerned, and uncooperative—he gives minimal information and discounts the seriousness of any findings. Or a young man comes in complaining of vague symptoms and, despite negative physical findings and reassurance by the physician, remains uneasy and insists on further tests.

Without claiming to be exhaustive, we can list several kinds of puzzling and difficult situations the family practitioner is apt to meet fairly often:

1) The problem seems to be an ordinary one, but the patient's (or concerned relative's) complaint persists after standard treatment is applied. Either

the signs and symptoms continue, or the complaint persists despite objective evidence of amelioration or resolution of the physical problem.

2) The complaint does not make sense to the physician from the outset. This can occur in several ways:
   (a) Information given is so vague or inadequate that diagnosis is very difficult.
   (b) Information given by the patient and/or family members is contradictory, so that there is no clear picture of the problem.
   (c) The patient's or family's statements are clear enough, but they do not fit the physician's observations and medical knowledge; this may concern either the nature or the severity of the complaint.

Such puzzling situations, we suggest, often result from the fact that, in addition to physical factors, family factors may play a considerable part in the nature, genesis, and resolution of complaints brought to family physicians. In emphasizing the existence and importance of family factors in the practice of family medicine, we do not aim to complicate further the tasks facing the family physician. Rather, we propose that such factors simply exist. Like it or not, they are inherently involved in medical practice, and understanding them can help physicians to handle them effectively and, therefore, "uncomplicate" treatment.

The Family as Case Environment

While viewing the medical patient in the context of his or her family is not an indispensable concept for physicians in carrying out their duties to patients, it is a conceptual tool that offers interested physicians a means of expanding their range of effectiveness with patients and making their work more efficient. Moreover, this viewing of the patient-in-context-of-the-family essentially is not novel in medicine. It is, rather, an extension of the tradition of viewing the patient in his environment, with the family now seen as a significant part of that environment.

Let us use an analogy: A physician may diagnose a case of lead poisoning correctly and apply appropriate treatment to reduce lead levels in the patient's blood. But the physician will not be satisfied until the *source* of the poisoning—perhaps lead in a water pipe—is identified, because otherwise continuing contamination of the patient will make the physician's best treatment efforts futile. In similar fashion, the family of the medical patient may, in their interactions, influence one another's health and compliance with treatment for good or ill. Thus, in our first example, the patient's wife may be acting in a way that unwittingly provokes stress and anxiety in him, contributing—like the lead in the water pipe—to a continuation of the problem, so that it can be resolved only by dealing with this source of trouble.

Family factors were also involved, though in more complex ways, in the other examples. Maternal anxiety and the accompanying distorted perception or evaluation were basic to the first two cases mentioned above. In the first, the mother was so anxious that her son eat "enough" and so overcontrolling in her attempts to ensure this that she provoked some discernible resistance in her son. Although he still ate too much, his resistance then appeared to her as an unquestionable sign that he was "not eating," a sign more significant to her than his weight or appearance. In the other example, it was discovered that the mother was worried about her child's being "sickly," so she had been giving him iron pills to "build his strength"—hence the black stools.

In the next case, the husband and wife were involved in a covert, and possibly unrecognized, struggle for control, which was being played out in terms of nurturance and concern for his health by her, and passive resistance and rejection of any proposed basis for such concern by him. In the final example, it turned out that the young man's anxieties, expressed as somatic concerns, were largely based on his having doubts, which he was reluctant to face directly, about his approaching marriage.

When Family Factors Matter

While the family is relevant for all patients a family physician sees, there are, of course, many instances in which this presents no treatment problem. When the patient and family members are reasonably informative and cooperative, and there is a clear physical problem, family factors need no special attention. Several common sorts of situations can be identified, however, in which deliberate attention to family interaction is likely to be important, or even crucial. In the first place, it is well known that many of the common miseries for which the family physician is usually the first recourse—for example, anxiety, tension, depression, insomnia—are likely to be psychological or behavior problems as much as strictly physiological ones. In all such cases the family is highly pertinent because it forms a major part of the environment in which the individual patient is functioning poorly.

Next are the many problems now classified as "psychosomatic," which indicates that a relationship between evident physiological dysfunction and psychological state is highly dependent on family interaction—an obvious potential source of stress as well as support—and that the family situation needs to be taken into account more than has been customary in such cases.

Indeed, we have proposed that this territory might better be called "family somatics" (Weakland, 1977). Conceivably, also, certain kinds of interaction may lead to, or at least potentiate, a person's susceptibility to infectious agents or physiological abnormality; we do not yet know how strongly such interactions may influence physiological functioning. That is, family interaction may have relevance even for clearly physical, not only psychological, problems. This is, however, more a matter for future research than for current medical practice.

An apparently physical problem may be a direct, although unanticipated and unrecognized, consequence of family behavior. The example of the young child passing black stools is one case in point. More commonly, family concern about an aging member's infirmities may lead to that person's taking too much medication, or too many kinds, until he or she becomes confused, which then is interpreted as senile dementia. This example also suggests that, by withholding relevant information and applying direct or subtle pressure for inappropriate treatment, the family as well as the physician may play a significant role even in some apparently "iatrogenic" disorders.

Thus family interaction may be important in the origin of a problem brought to a physician's attention. It is certainly significant for the medical handling of any case. When family interaction is helpful there is no problem, but the physician should be alert because it often may be harmful: Family factors may profoundly influence the initiation or delay of treatment, how seriously a symptom is regarded, how well the patient cooperates with the physician and the treatment program, and how satisfied the patient is with the outcome of treatment.

None of this is really new information. Practicing family physicians have long known that anxiety and tension may be rooted in a family or marital relationship, that some patients or family members minimize problems while others exaggerate them, and that patients and their family members—who are inescapably involved in any illness and treatment—may be uncooperative, cooperative, or even overly cooperative. Physicians once absorbed knowledge about the medical significance of the family, and about how to deal with this aspect of practice, by prolonged direct contact with whole families. Today this is seldom feasible.

Meanwhile, however, family therapists and associated family systems researchers have been accumulating knowledge about family interaction and its powerful influence in determining the behavior and functioning of individual members that can usefully be extended and applied in the practice of family medicine.

In short, we are only proposing to outline and exemplify how family physicians can take family factors which are inherent in their practice into account more systematically and effectively—much as physical factors are explored and dealt with systematically rather than piecemeal and ad hoc in modern medicine.

From the contents of this book alone, it is plain that family therapists vary considerably in their emphases and approaches. We believe the strategic approach developed at the Brief Therapy Center of the Mental Research Institute (Fisch, Weakland, & Segal, 1982; Herr & Weakland, 1979; Watzlawick, Weakland, & Fisch, 1974; Weakland, Fisch, Watzlawick, & Bodin, 1974) is especially relevant for wider application to family practice. Some approaches to the family are so broad or comprehensive that, although they may be useful in obtaining an overall view of family functioning, they are very time-consuming for a busy practitioner, and much of the information gathered may be irrelevant to the particular medical complaint at hand. In contrast, our approach focuses more narrowly on how the family is involved in the current problem and its treatment. Although an adequate medical history is of course necessary, our approach does not require gathering all family members to seek an overall view of family structure and functioning, or family history. Nor do we see either general family reorganization or basic personality change of individuals as needed for successful treatment. Only certain limited information needs to be gathered and limited behavioral changes encouraged.

Focal Aspects of the Strategic Approach

Our approach focuses explicitly on: 1) clarifying the presenting complaint; 2) investigating in what ways the patient and family may be promoting the persistence of the complaint, especially by attempted "solutions" that only keep things bad or even worsen them; 3) identifying changes that seem needed to resolve the complaint; and 4) determining effective means of promoting these changes. These foci are important not only in family psychotherapy, but they apply equally and similarly to family medical practice, in which puzzling cases are likely to present difficulties as follows: in diagnosis (forming a clear picture of the presenting problem); in formulating what needs to be done to resolve or ameliorate the problem, either by direct treatment or appropriate referral; and in obtaining the patient's and family's cooperation to ensure that this *is* done.

Diagnosis

The presenting complaint is, of course, not everything, either in strategic family therapy or in family practice, and it is not necessarily to be taken at face value. It may also be a sign of an underlying problem that needs alteration or correction. It may, as some of the earlier examples illustrate, be a cover or substitute for a problem of a different sort. In addition, there may be little correlation between the "seriousness" of someone's complaint and the related physiological, psychosomatic, or behavioral problems as judged from a detached, objective viewpoint. A patient or family member may not show appropriate concern about a serious health problem or may conversely show excessive concern about something minor. Any of these situations pose complexities and obstacles to effective diagnosis and treatment, and they may, understandably, irritate a concerned and busy practitioner.

Yet the presenting complaint is highly important in several respects. It is the starting point, the matter that brings the patient to treatment, and the center of the patient's (or the family's) interest and concern. It must therefore be accepted and taken seriously, at least overtly, to begin that cooperative relationship between physician and patient on which any effective treatment depends. Similarly, the status of the presenting complaint is crucial for termination of treatment and evaluation of its outcome. No matter what has been accomplished objectively in regard to the patient's health and functioning, the patient or family will usually not be *satisfied* unless the complaint has been resolved somehow. If it has not, demands for treatment are likely to continue, even though the physician deems this unnecessary from a strictly medical standpoint.

In all difficult or confusing cases—even those in which a medical diagnosis is clear from physical examination and history—it is therefore important to get a clear, specific, concrete statement of the complaint. Here again, we simply emphasize and spell out what experienced physicians have long known: "Even in this age of medical technology it is well to remember the words of the nineteenth-century French clinician Laënnec, who would tell his assistants and students, 'Listen, listen to your patient, he is giving you the diagnosis' " (Niederland, 1983, p. 163). Information about the complaint should include *what* is being complained of, *who* is mainly concerned (as the examples indicated, this may not be the patient but another member of the family), and just *how* the matter complained of is a source of concern—this last point may not be self-evident, and inquiring about it may clarify just why the patient has come for treatment. In addition, particularly when a symptom complained of has had some duration, it is useful to ask what led the patient to come in *at this particular time*. Often, general questions like "Why have you come to see me?" elicit only vague or general answers, which need to be followed up more specifically. In this situation, the information gained by inquiring about the particular precipitating circumstances may help to reveal a hidden agenda: for instance, that the patient has come under duress from another family member rather than voluntarily, or that the problem complained of is not the patient's main concern but only, so to speak, his ticket of admission.

Ordinarily this information about the presenting complaint is best obtained by direct questions. Asking for examples is often helpful in getting specific and concrete information from patients and family members. If a patient is stressing what seems to be a minor problem, asking how it affects the person's daily life may bring an enlightening answer. A man might, for example, show the physician a minor lesion of the penis, a small abrasion or heat rash. Yet his concern seems excessive and he does not seem relieved when told, "It's not much of anything." If asked then how this condition worries him, he might say, "I just wondered if I had contracted something more serious." If asked, "Serious, how?" he might explain that he thought it could be a venereal disease, that for some time he has suspected his wife of having an affair but has been afraid to confront her about it. Thus, not the lesion itself but what it represented was the significant problem for him.

Physicians are likely to have difficulties with patients who give vague, general, or tangential responses. Persistence in posing specific questions will often resolve these problems; the main danger is to assume one understands what the complaint is when the patient has not stated it clearly. While this may appear to save time, it is likely to lead to more time lost in fruitless or misdirected effort.

Formulating What Needs to Be Done

It is important to determine what the patient and family members are doing that may be promoting the persistence of the problem or hindering its resolution. In family therapy most complaints are reducible to problems of troublesome but persistent behavior, and the therapist accordingly looks for other behaviors which may be provoking the problem behavior, or at least blocking change. Such unwitting "maintenance" behaviors may be significant in family practice as well. The wife of a patient who complains of anxiety and apprehension may, for example, be telling him there is nothing to be worried about. The patient takes this as an indication that she doesn't understand the seriousness of his situation, and this increases his anxiety. In family practice this kind of information may also be relevant in two other respects. First, patient or family actions may strongly influence evaluation of the importance or significance of any given symptom or problem and, as noted, either under- or overconcern will present special obstacles to resolving the complaint. Second, even when a problem is strictly physiological, what the patient and family members are doing about it may obstruct effective cooperation with the medical treatment plan. For instance, a man diagnosed to have diabetes needs to follow a restrictive diet, which he is willing to undertake. However, his wife, overly concerned about his welfare and wanting to "make it easier for him to do without forbidden foods," puts the whole family on the restricted diet. Now the husband feels that the whole family is suffering because of his health needs. He tries to resolve that problem by making light of his illness and departing from his own diet to show his wife that such restrictions are not all that necessary. With little time and effort, the physician can help the patient avoid diabetic incidents by telling the wife she can be most helpful to her husband by not rearranging the whole family's routines and diet. Concentrating only on the patient and constantly urging him to be "more careful" is not likely to be useful.

In our experience, the best way to obtain information about possible problem-maintaining behaviors is to ask the patient and closely involved family members what they have been doing in their attempts to resolve or ameliorate the problem complained of. The inquiry is logical and legitimate, as it is explicitly aimed at behavior closely related to the matter of primary concern. Like the investigation of the complaint itself, the questions should be directed to eliciting clear, specific, concrete answers: *Who* is doing *what* (including *saying* what) in attempting to improve this situation? When this kind of information is reviewed with a deliberately critical eye—in effect, asking oneself, "Can I see any way in which these actions might actually be making matters worse?"—it will often appear that the patient's or family members' "solutions" may well be part of the problem: The iron pills mother gave to strengthen a child she saw as being in frail health led directly to his symptoms. Though this may seem ironic, it should not be surprising. People often try to cope with problems themselves before they seek professional help and, with the best intentions, they may—especially when anxiously concerned—readily make errors in judging the nature of the problem and inappropriately apply conventional "remedies" and so on.

Even if it turns out that the patient's and family members' attempted remedies are not maintaining the problem in any discernible way, such an inquiry lays a foundation for any necessary further exploration; at the same time, the information gathered helps clarify how the patient and family view the problem—its nature, origin, and severity. Getting the family members' views can be critically important for obtaining their cooperation in treatment, as we will discuss later, *especially* when their views differ, perhaps widely, from those of the physician.

Resolving the Problem

Resolution of a presenting complaint, in either family therapy or family medical practice, may occur in one of two general ways. First, of course, the problem complained about may be modified or eliminated, thus removing the grounds for the complaint. Sometimes, a problem may be resolved by simple reassurance and a little time for this to take effect, like the prescription, "Take two aspirins and call me in the morning" when a patient is anxious about a minor or self-limiting physical problem. If such simple measures do not work, however, it is not wise to repeat or increase them, any more than it is wise to continue treating an infection with the same antibiotic that has already been tried without positive results.

Those difficult problems that have no discernible physical basis, or that persist after a physical basis has been identified and treated appropriately, are likely to have a behavioral basis, probably centered on the patient's or family's ameliorative efforts. Once such a complaint-reinforcing behavior has been identified, one must get the patient or the family member to stop doing it; ordinarily, the problem will then disappear. But, because it is difficult or impossible simply to stop doing something, a new behavior, one that is incompatible with the one that reinforced the symptom, needs to be substituted. This might be an activity that is useful or healthy in itself—for example, an anxious or depressed patient might be encouraged to take long walks instead of sitting and ruminating about his condition. But this is not essential; engaging the patient in any action that blocks the undesirable behavior is useful, even if the new activity is otherwise trivial or neutral.

Another way of resolving a complaint is to change the patient's or family's interpretation of it. This does not, of course, mean false reassurance in the case of a serious behavioral or medical problem. But two common situations call for the promotion of reevaluation. In the first, the patient or family may be making a "federal case" of a basically normal situation: Parents may be too anxious about a child's minor misbehaviors, or someone may interpret ordinary bodily sensations as symptoms of some serious disease. Reassurance is the main treatment required in these instances, though giving it effectively may require indirect or strategic means. For instance, a patient who is apprehensive about her coughing may well remain anxious if her physician, after examining her, simply says, "It's nothing serious, don't worry about it," but be calmed if instead the physician says, "I'm going to order a chest X ray, but I expect it will be negative."

The second situation involves complaints for which the best or only answer is to bring about a different sort of interpretation—getting those concerned to accept a problem as being something that must be accepted and lived with, because it cannot be changed. In such cases, efforts to produce an impossible change are very likely to make things worse. Again, this is not a counsel of inaction, but of recognizing realities and adapting to them once reasonable attempts at change have been tried without significant results.

An aging person's social functioning, for example, need not be seriously affected by a moderate degree of memory loss. But if the person or family members see any loss as an alarming sign of "senility" and try anxiously to improve things, the pressure to perform better is likely to make primary functioning worse and worse. The situation is similar for physical disabilities of almost any kind and degree—after a certain point, further treatment efforts may not only be useless but may interfere with the patient's getting on with life to whatever extent is still possible.

In some cases, both reevaluation and behavioral change may be needed to resolve a complaint.

Obtaining Cooperation

How can the physician gain and maintain the cooperation of the patient and family members? This may be crucial even for gathering basic information at the outset of treatment; certainly it is critical for effectively promoting necessary actions and changes. "Good patients" and sensible cooperative families present no problem; they will recognize the physician's knowledge and authority and accordingly will give information, take medication, institute actions, and accept reassurances as the physician proposes. But many patients and families are balky and noncompliant, some are overly compliant (twice the prescribed dose must be twice as good), and some are overly dependent on the physician to do everything while they sit passively by. And, unless the way is well prepared, almost anyone may be difficult when it is proposed that one should change a view or an action that, even though mistakenly, is firmly held as *the* right and proper stance toward a problem.

Similar to our emphasis on getting clear what the patient's complaint is, we suggest that the key to gaining effective cooperation in difficult cases is to recognize the patient's and family member's own views of the problem and treatment, then using these in the service of whatever changes are essential for effective treatment. It is natural for the patient and family members to have views of the problem that differ, often considerably, from the physician's professional observations. They are lay people, and they are personally involved and therefore highly subjective. The latter factor can at best be moderated, not basically changed. Concerning the former, although certain explanations are appropriate and essential, in a busy medical practice (as in brief family therapy, only more so) there is no time to reeducate the clients to any level of understanding comparable to the physician's own. To attempt this is likely only to provoke dissatisfaction and resistance by patients and family members who are attached to their own views and mainly want to get on with resolving their complaint. The physician need only obtain cooperation and compliance with the views and actions that appear critical for resolving the problem. These usually will be limited to specific matters such as adherence to a treatment regimen, reevaluation of the seriousness of a complaint, or changing certain specific behaviors that reinforce the problem.

In our experience, patients go along with treatment best if the physician does not argue with their views. Where a change of stance or action is essential, this principle can still be utilized. There are two main types of such situations. First, a patient or family member may concede that an action is perhaps needed but hesitate to get on with it. If this ambivalence persists after the physician has explained the need for action, it usually is helpful not to pursue the matter. Instead, the physician may find it useful to side with the patient's doubts explicitly for a while: "On second thought, I must agree with you that although the operation is likely to be helpful, there always is some risk, so think it over carefully before deciding." Such overt recognitions of and joining with the patient's doubts and fears, by assuring him that he is not alone with them, can be reassuring and thus lead to the desired action.

As suggested earlier, however, in many difficult cases the task is greater. It involves getting the patient to stop doing something that is reinforcing the problem, or even to do the opposite, when he or she is viewing the present behavior as helpful or essential. Here the same principle, avoiding argument and resistance by accepting and joining with the patient's views as much as possible, is applied by "reframing" the situation so as to lead to a change of stance and behavior. That is, the point in question is presented at first in terms of the patient's own views and language—the way he or she sees and describes it. Then, rather than arguing with this view, something is added—more information or another perspective—so that the situation's significance and implications for action, in the patient's own eyes, are now altered or even reversed. A patient might balk stubbornly at following a medical regimen (medications, rest, dietary changes), insisting that she has never been one to pamper herself. Since her frame of reference is that she wants to be regarded as a "strong" person, the physician can use that frame of reference to gain cooperation. The physician might frame the situation as one "that requires extraordinary strength of character and self-discipline to make the sacrifices necessary to take care of one's body when it has special needs."

Some of these points are illustrated in the following example. A patient recovering from myocardial infarction reveals that he has not followed his physician's advice to eat more sensibly and not to "push" himself. The patient explains he has never pampered himself nor does he see himself as a "cripple." Besides, he has a lot of work to do taking care of the animals on his ranch, and their care and welfare come first. The physician is not likely to gain the patient's cooperation by reiterating that he has a serious and potentially lethal medical condition and has to take it easy. The patient will hear this as insistence that he must see himself as crippled. Instead, the physician can appeal to another value important to the patient, that he is a caretaker of others. Thus, he can use an analogy and say: "Look, you respect your horse. He'll take you wherever you want him to go, and all day if necessary. When you bring him back to the corral, you're not going to throw him some moldy hay. And when he's put in a good day's work for you, you're not going to take him out again all sweaty and wet. I'm only asking that you have the same respect for *your* body. It needs taking care of too, and only you can do it. Do you have enough self-discipline to do that?" Of course, similar analogies can be used for patients engaged in many other kinds of work in which a high value is placed on respect for and judicious care of the tools and materials of one's trade.

Application of the Approach to the Examples

We have described briefly the main foci and principles of our approach as it can apply to family practice, but this sort of statement is a long way from the specific realities of daily practice. To move at least a step closer, we will conclude by returning to our original examples, outlining how these cases might be handled in actual practice.

In the case of the hypertensive patient, assuming that the medication is appropriate for his type of hypertension and that serial blood pressure readings show a sustained elevation, further information must be gathered. To start with, the patient needs to be asked to describe more explicitly *exactly how* he is "faithfully" following the physician's directives. It is always possible that the patient believes that what he is doing is what the physician asked, when, in reality, it is a significant departure. If he is actually following instructions, then other kinds of information need to be elicited. Mainly, is he experiencing some significant psychosocial stress at home or at work? Depending on the information gathered, the appropriate treatment might not be a matter of changing dosages or medications but, rather, one of getting the patient to adhere more accurately to the regimen, or one of helping him deal more effectively with the stresses he is facing.

With the mother who complains that her overweight child is not eating enough, the key is for the physician to recognize that her complaint, though misguided, reflects her basic concern to ensure her child's health and welfare. To argue with her that, if anything, the child needs to lose weight is not likely to be successful, since this appears contrary to her own values and perceptions. She may even interpret this as an accusation of failure to be a duly protective mother. Instead, she needs to be reassured effectively about her motherhood, so that she can relax about the child's eating. This can be accomplished if her "protectiveness" is supported, but in a different direction:

> It might be better if he ate more, but after careful examination it seems that the food you give him is remarkably nutritious so that, even though he could be eating more, he is in good health. Thanks to the care you put into the selection and preparation of his food he is a healthy child. Moreover, every child wants some distinction from other members of the family, and I believe his thin image is important to him for his own identity. It may require a sacrifice on your part to allow him to hang on to that identity for as long as he needs it.

Successfully reassured that she is a good mother, she probably will lessen her pressure on the child to eat, and the weight problem will gradually resolve itself.

Another general point is also illustrated by this extreme case of overconcern. The more usual situation is excessive worry based on scanty evidence, but this mother's concern is so great that it overwhelms and inverts the evidence. In either situation, discrepancy between the patient's position and the physician's observations is so great that there is a strong tendency simply to state the professional view as a means of clarification and reassurance. The danger is that the patient will not respond reasonably to this but will restate the original concern, perhaps more strongly. If the physician is drawn into reiterating his or her statement, a covert or overt argument has begun, which will probably lead to a stalemate unsatisfactory to everyone. If the physician can keep in mind that such excessive concern is itself a prime indicator that a patient is thinking illogically (in this one area), he or she will be warned to avoid the trap of attempting logical persuasion with an illogical person. Instead, the physician might test the waters by one, preferably tentative, direct statement of clarification and reassurance. For example, "I imagine some people have said that he seems to be eating enough and that his weight looks OK. Have you been told that and, if so, what do you think of that kind of comment?" In this way, the physician is not committed to that comment but feeling out the mother's commitment to her own view. If this does not go well, the physician can shift to meeting the patient's emotional need and concern on her own ground, as illustrated earlier. This will also lay the foundation for cooperation in any medically necessary actions.

Resolving the problem of the child who has been passing black stools depends primarily on adequate inquiry, to discover the mother's concern about "sickliness" and her giving the child rather large doses of iron pills, which she had not associated with the symptom. Thus, she is appropriately alarmed at what seems to her to be a worsening of a mysterious illness. In this case, a simple explanation might suffice to reassure her and cause her to stop giving the pills. If not, the "symptom" could be redefined as the body's normal and healthy signal that the iron pills are no longer needed and that it was fortunate she paid attention to this signal.

The unconcerned husband coming in for a physical is likely to be there under duress from his concerned wife. Thus he will be resistant because he regards the examination as an unnecessary nuisance. He simply wants to get through with it as fast as possible to pacify his wife, which neglects the fact that she is quite unlikely to be pacified unless he cooperates and takes the examination seriously. The physician is unlikely to succeed by appealing to ordinary reason, by saying that the wife may have legitimate reason for concern, or that it is important for everyone, including the husband, to have a routine physical examination. The husband, believing that there is nothing really wrong with him and that his wife is therefore silly in her concern and urging, is very likely to view any such statements as joining with the wife's position and he will therefore resist them.

The physician may increase the chances of cooperation, however, by using the patient's own position. He can frame the examination as a challenge to the husband's own certainty or judgment:

> All right. Your wife is concerned and it may well be an unnecessary concern. Perhaps you should not allow yourself to be examined, because you might not want to take any risk that she could be proved right. By not being examined and not giving me the information I need for your history, you can avoid bringing this issue to the mat to see just who is right about the state of your health.

This framing avoids getting involved in the counterproductive argument of "You could be sick"—"No I'm not" and implies the question, "Are you a big enough man to put your money where your mouth is?" Then the husband is more likely to cooperate and the wife more likely to be satisfied, whatever the outcome of the examination.

For the apprehensive young man who keeps insisting on further tests, the first requisite is an adequate inquiry into his complaint and its circumstances, a history taking that includes attention to the interpersonal context in which the symptoms are occurring. This will disclose the pending marriage; its possible connection with the patient's vague but persistent physical complaints is not hard (for the physician) to see. It should be assumed, however, that the patient resists considering this rather obvious connection, or he would have done so already. Therefore, any direct or forceful approach to this possibility is likely to increase the patient's resistance and his insistence on the physical nature of the problem.

Handling this difficult situation more strategically has two aspects. First, the physical: The apprehensive young man, insisting on further tests, will not be reassured if the physician tries to persuade him that the tests are unnecessary or performs them begrudgingly, even if further tests prove "negative." More likely, the patient will insist on yet other tests, or seek other physicians and go through the same routine. The physician stands a better chance of blocking this inappropriate path if, rather than resisting, he or she will say: "I would like to do another test. I don't think it is necessary, but I would rather be absolutely sure. I don't expect the test to show anything wrong, but I would prefer to err on the side of overcaution." If, as anticipated, the test turns out "negative," the patient has been prepared for it, and this confirmation of the physician's prediction heightens the credibility of any further judgments of the patient's status, even more so because the physician, not the patient, suggested the test. In a moderate case of this kind, this may be sufficient to reduce the patient's concerns to a normal level, or at least enough so that he will be able to express his underlying anxieties about the marriage.

If not, the physician is still in a position to initiate some consideration of the interpersonal and psychological aspects of the patient's situation, because the physical aspects have been dealt with at length and in a way that is acceptable to the patient. This can usually be accomplished best by suggesting that, *in addition* to physical factors, some psychological ones *might* be relevant to the patient's symptoms, in part because everything in life has both physical and psychological aspects. Such phrasing makes it much easier for the patient to be in agreement than any statement that implies, "It's all in your head." Acceptance of this possibility, limited as it seems, opens the door sufficiently to begin whatever discussion of the patient's life situation seems necessary to relieve his anxiety—perhaps just characterizing it as normal: "Every man is nervous before marriage; it's a very big step." This in turn may end the demand for more and more physical tests.

In concluding, we would like to emphasize that, although this approach to observing and dealing with family factors in medical practice is simple in principle, its application to practice is a different and more complex matter, as indeed the application of principles to the variability and individuality of specific cases always is. On this matter we have offered only some brief illustrative examples here, and ultimately, of course, practice can only be learned by practice. Nevertheless, we hope that this chapter provides stimulation and guidance toward taking that next step.

REFERENCES

Fisch, R., Weakland, J.H., & Segal, L. (1982). *The tactics of change: Doing therapy briefly*. San Francisco: Jossey-Bass.

Herr, J.J., & Weakland, J.H. (1979). *Counselling elders and their families: Practical techniques for applied gerontology*. New York: Springer.

Niederland, W.G. (1983). Importance of case history. *Psychosomatics, 24*, 163.

Watzlawick, P., Weakland, J.H., & Fisch, R. (1974). *Change: Principles of problem formation and problem resolution*. New York: Norton.

Weakland, J.H. (1977). Family somatics—A neglected edge. *Family Process, 16*, 263-272.

Weakland, J.H., Fisch, R., Watzlawick, P., & Bodin, A.M. (1974). Brief therapy: Focused problem resolution. *Family Process, 13*, 141-168.

6

THE INTERGENERATIONAL POINT OF VIEW

DONALD S. WILLIAMSON, PH.D. and JAMES H. BRAY, PH.D.

> The universe is a single organism. When a human being is wounded, the universe is wounded. When the individual abuses nature, he wounds himself.
>
> Rolling Thunder, 1981

Intergenerational family systems theory offers some ideas that are useful for understanding individual and family health (Boszormenyi-Nagy & Ulrich, 1981; Bowen, 1978; Framo, 1981; Williamson, 1981, 1982b). This systemic point of view makes both distinctions and assumptions about human behavior that can enrich an otherwise exclusively physical perspective. Before discussing these further, it is important to consider the overall *role of assumptions* in the treatment of human health problems.

The Importance of Assumptions

It is readily acknowledged, and not only by family systems theorists, that what the physician (or any healer) does about a presenting health problem is largely determined by how the problem is assimilated and conceptualized, that is, how one "makes sense of it." In professional education, techniques and procedures often are taught and learned without much exploration of or reflection about the assumptions that underlie these methods.

We assume that in medicine, as in the world of psychotherapy, the quality of the relationship between physician and patient will influence considerably the effectiveness of the treatment in general, and the degree of compliance with the treatment in particular. The quality of this relationship will be largely defined by the physician's ability (or lack of it) to identify and address key social and psychological aspects of the patient's current life, going beyond the physical manifestations of the presenting problem.

This fact has two important implications for family practice. First, the family physician can broaden the usual medical view of health and disease as being invariably the result of purely or predominantly physical processes. It is valuable to do this to put the presenting health problem into a *richer systemic framework*. Secondly, the physician can, with great benefit, use his or her own emotional life, including personal marital and family experiences, for reflection and subsequent therapeutic use. Without this process he or she may not be emotionally able to acknowledge and address these same matters in the lives of patients.

The healer must be readily available in the healing process. If the physician can identify with the patient, he or she is more likely to penetrate through to the driving force behind the illness. This may be threatening and psychologically uncomfortable for some practitioners, and quite exciting for others. In addition, it may be experienced as contrary to the usual theory and ethos of contemporary medical education. But that is just the point! Intergenerational family theory encourages family medicine to take a broader systemic view of human behavior, particularly of that frequent family systemic creation known as "physical illness."

Systemic Family Thinking

Obviously, even as a single entity, the individual human being is a complex system or, more accurately, a system of systems. The various systems within the individual include the social, emotional, intellectual, and spiritual processes, as well as the biological-physical ones. Together these create the continuing patterns and levels of consciousness that constitute the self-system. Even the physical processes, taken alone and as a whole, constitute a system of systems (e.g., circulatory system, nervous system, endocrine system). A combination of intellectual agility and emotional flexibility will permit a simultaneous appreciation for the multiple systems of the individual self, as well as the individual self in the context of the extended family culture. This in turn will provide a rich opportunity to understand healthy and troubled human behavior from a multidimensional rather than an exclusively physical perspective. This is to take a step beyond simply a systemic understanding of the self in isolation, to a systemic view of the self in the transgenerational family system.

To fully understand an individual patient's behavior or dysfunction, it is essential to understand the overall context, or system of systems, in which it occurs. Our view of the treatment context is the intergenerational family system. Patterns of interactions develop in the family which help family members grow and cope with life stresses. However, these patterns readily become dysfunctional. Both functional and dysfunctional patterns are passed on to individuals across the generations, hence the need for an intergenerational diagnostic focus.

While illness often expresses itself in physical and chemical imbalance, it is common to find its prior stimulus in the context of marital and family conflict, as experienced in both observable social behavior and inward fantasy life (Bowen, 1978; Coyne & Holroyd, 1982). In fact, there is now considerable evidence that psychological conflict and stress often precede physical symptomatology (Coyne & Holroyd, 1982; Dohrenwend & Dohrenwend, 1982; Holmes & Masuda, 1974; Sarason, Levine, & Sarason, 1982; Selye, 1976). There is also evidence that improvement in family life is likely to be followed by improvement in individual well-being at every level, including physical health (Coyne & Holroyd, 1982; Williamson, Bray, & Malone, 1984).

The important point, then, is that to think and practice "systemically" means to have a "both- and" rather than an "either- or" attitude to human behavior and problems (Taggart, 1983). This means that one need not get caught in a "psychological versus physiological" polarization, or any similar dilemma. To think systemically means to think "both- and" to the point that the recursiveness of the behavior of all living systems becomes evident. This is a powerful vantage point from which to understand the phenomenon of human "illness."

Admittedly, each individual and individual family will have a rich and idiosyncratic biological and psychosocial history. Consequently, there will be individual and family patterns of both biological and psychological predisposition and vulnerability (Bowen, 1978; Kerr, 1981; Sarason & Sarason, 1980). However, there is one transcending implication in the fact that all human behavior occurs in a biopsychosociocultural context, composed of elements ranging from the larger culture to the individual's personal social network, with the intergenerational family at its center. The implication is that individual human behavior, whether characterized by wellness or disease, expresses a self-system that exists within a family system, interacting within a community system within a cultural system, and continuing on and on in ever-increasing and more complex circles. For such is the complexity of living systems. The consequences for treatment of this systemic perspective are far-reaching. And the underlying question is now explicit.

Who and Where Is The Patient?

The crucial and overarching question now becomes clear: Who and where is the patient? Who is to be treated? What is the most valuable information to be used to create a diagnosis and treatment program? Where is the appropriate professional and treatment boundary to be drawn? Should it be with the individual, or the marriage, or the nuclear family, or the transgenerational and extended family, or the larger culture, or just where?

Arguably, a world dominated by two superpowers, each surrounding the territorial boundaries of the other with a superabundance of life-destroying missiles, can be seen as dysfunctional or diseased (and so by implication are those who live in it). But, just as obviously, this broad conclusion does not instruct the physician how to respond to the individual patient now sitting in his or her office and presenting symptoms of physical distress and expecting some early relief.

Intergenerational family theory holds, in general, that it is both essential and adequate to examine and interview the individual patient in the context of his or her three-generational family life. (This will involve the use of a genogram to be described later.) In this view, this is the discriminating dynamic boundary to be drawn. Less would be too little and more would be too much. It will narrow the scope of the inquiry adequately. It will at the same time widen it beyond an exclusively individual and physical view, to include what is regarded here as a powerful influence on health and well-being in the individual's life. This element is, of course, the present and continuing marital and intergenerational family experience of the patient. Most significant in this family experience are the highly emotional relationships between the adult patient and his or her spouse and, secondly, between the patient and his or her parents, whether alive or deceased (Williamson, 1978, 1981). The character, quality, and dynamics of these relationships are a significant influence in the creation of individual well-being or disease.

Symptom Development in Families

Symptoms frequently develop as a result of stress and anxiety in the family system. The stress may be caused by external pressures of living, predictable family life-cycle changes, biological imbalances, or dysfunctional patterns of living passed from one generation to the next (Carter & McGoldrick, 1980). It is assumed that individuals and families have a basic capacity and set of skills to deal with stress and anxiety. The interaction of this capacity with the level of stress and anxiety in the family will determine whether or not an individual or particular family will develop symptoms at any given time.

This basic capacity, referred to as the level of differentiation of self (Bowen, 1978; Kerr, 1981), is the degree to which an individual operates in an individuated and autonomous manner in his or her current relational contexts. At the other end of the continuum is fusion of the individual in relational contexts. Bowen (1978) has found that more differentiated persons are able to function in an autonomous manner around significant others, even in the face of stress; more undifferentiated or fused individuals are usually more dependent and emotionally reflexive in relationships with significant others. In addition, and of particular relevance here, the more undifferentiated people are more likely to develop physical symptoms in the face of stressful experience.

When two people form an intimate relationship and get married, the form of this relationship and new family is a major issue to be negotiated. People bring ideas and learnings from the significant family relationships in which they have grown up. The form their new relationship takes is highly influenced by these previous learnings. It will also activate the emotional system inherited from unresolved emotional patterns of the parental marriages, as well as from one's family of origin in general (Bowen, 1978; Kerr, 1981).

When anxiety and stress occur, increased emotional fusion is activated as the couple seeks solutions to cope with the stress. If the stress reaches too high a level, symptoms will develop in the family. This stress is generally handled in one of three ways (Bowen, 1978).

First, *marital conflict* may occur. Typically this is characterized by fighting and bickering within the marital dyad. This usually happens in symmetrical relationships, i.e., relationships in which each spouse is perceived as "equal."

Second, *dysfunction in a spouse* may occur. This tends to happen in complementary relationships, i.e., those in which one spouse is perceived as dominant and the other submissive. Dysfunction in a spouse may take on any one of the following three patterns:

Physical illness. Acute or chronic illnesses develop in which the dysfunctional spouse is responding to the stress and anxiety in the relationship.

Psychological dysfunction. This may be manifested as acute or chronic problems such as depression, anxiety, phobias, or psychosis.

Social problems. These may occur in the relational patterns between people rather than "within" the individuals. Examples include alcohol abuse, drug abuse, and behavior problems.

Finally, *dysfunction may occur in one child or several children*. This is hypothesized to be a result of drawing—triangulating—children into the marital problems. This process may appear as relational conflict with a child or as dysfunction in a child's behavior. The child's dysfunction may follow any one of the three patterns described for dysfunction in a spouse.

Triangulating is defined as a method of dealing with stress in dyadic relationships by bringing in a third person to deflect the anxiety and stress (Bowen, 1978). This serves to stabilize the dyadic relationship. The process is a major coping mechanism in families, if not in all human relationships.

A recent case exemplifies these processes. An 11-year-old boy who had severe headaches was brought by his mother to see the family physician. The initial evaluation indicated migraine headaches. The boy was prescribed medication and sent home. He soon returned, complaining he had even more severe headaches and that the medication was not effective. After an extensive medical evaluation in which all findings were negative, the physician discovered that the headaches had begun soon after the parents separated, and increased after the parents divorced. The boy was then referred for psychotherapy. The first psychotherapeutic interview revealed that the boy had a special attachment to his father and identified with him strongly. The father also had a history of headaches when under stress. So the boy seemed to be continuing a pattern learned from the father.

Two important points should be noted. First, families may use one or all of these symptom patterns in coping with stress and anxiety. Therefore, a patient may present with a physical complaint, while the spouse may have a history of alcoholism, and a child may have chronic health and behavior problems. Second, dysfunction may occur in one child or several children. This is why one child may be disabled while the others function relatively symptom-free. Either a parent or a child may show the symptoms of acute or chronic physical illness in response to family stress.

Other Possible Inferences from Intergenerational Family Theory

We make several more inferences about individual health and its relationship to intergenerational learning.

Attitude to Existence in the World

First, we propose that the individual's deeper and most persistent emotional attitude to his or her personal existence in the world is the fundamental context for and source of health or disease. Except for unusual biological predeterminants, the positive or negative character of this personal attitude may be the single most powerful source of the consistent presence or absence of personal well-being. This deeply emotional attitude toward one's own life is developed during the growing-up years in the family of origin, through social learning with parents and grandparents as models and teachers (Bandura, 1977; Wrightsman & Deaux, 1981). By participating fully in the family emotional system (Bowen, 1978), the individual learns an attitude about the world and his or her own being-in-the-world, which is consistent with and loyal to the ambience of the family of origin and the individual's place in it. Basically this attitude comes down to the decision to believe (or not believe) that the world is benevolent, rather than malevolent.

Personal Lifestyle

Another inference dynamically related to the first has to do with personal lifestyle. Lifestyle is also acquired by the individual in the family of origin, and it is transmitted in striking ways from generation to generation, usually with minimal conscious awareness that it is happening (Paul, 1981). Lifestyle has four elements. Diet and physical activity are the first two. Next is relaxation-meditation or rebalancing of all systems of the self—chemical, emotional, and spiritual. At the heart of this process is the ongoing dialogue with the self, that is, the cognitions that make up the self-image, including expectations for one's personal future. This dialogue includes dreams and daydreams which may have an enormous influence on physiological processes and so can direct a healing attention and energy wherever there is distress and disarray in the body. The fourth aspect is the general focus of this paper and consists of marital and intergenerational family experiences, which have been discussed above. *Personal lifestyle expresses a particular way of coping with stress in life*, physical and chemical as well as psychological stress. Coping well with stress in all its dimensions is of first importance for the creation and maintenance of good health and personal well-being.

During the developmental years in the family of origin, the individual will have learned more (or less) skill in dealing with tension and the various kinds of stress that occur in normal human life. Persons who have spent long periods in highly stressful situations, especially if they have acquired little skill in adapting well, are likely to exhaust their life-supply of "adaptation energy" when coping with stress over long periods. These people may experience early burnout and will be at risk of disease (Selye, 1976). On the other hand, we propose that individuals who have developed skill and discipline in the practice of good diet, adequate physical exercise, a positive self-image with hopeful expectations, and open and negotiable family relationships can use this pattern of life skills to create and recreate new and additional adaptive energy. A "systemic medical practice" will certainly, therefore, address these various levels which together create the overall pattern for a healthy personal lifestyle.

Transmitted Family Emotional System

Our next inference is that the family emotional system (Bowen, 1978), which is a rich patterning of predictable emotional responses to all kinds of stimuli and situations that have developed over time and which is transmitted across the generations, teaches the individual family member, at least in broad detail, when and where and how to be well or ill. In some families illness is simply "unthinkable" and seldom occurs. In others, illness and the expectation of illness shadow the family as constant companions. Members of these families are seen repeatedly in the doctor's office. In these families the patient may think of himself or herself, consciously or covertly, as a third-generation heart or cancer candidate. The patient may do so years before any supporting evidence appears. Once again, family history "is gathered up in both arms and thrown out in front of the individual and labeled the future," with the implicit challenge to live up (or live down) to it (Shaw, 1983).

Because the physician's very language may unwittingly encourage or reinforce this expectation, the family physician will be wise to be careful in the use of language and to be selective with images and expectations projected or incited (King, Novik, & Citrenbaum, 1983). Well-intentioned comments like "we'll watch this," or "keep an eye on that," or "we can expect this in six to 12 months," or "well, that frequently accompanies this," or "well, you are this age and we know what that means," or "after all, your parents had this" may create an effective and pervasive pattern of negative suggestion and expectation and also encourage dependency. Obviously, the physician has legal and ethical duties to inform the patient about current or potential problems (Oppenheim, 1966). But the manner in which this information is presented influences the way the patient processes and subsequently uses it. Language and nuance as commonly used in medical practice, with the clear intent of being helpful, may often be a remarkable instance of "the solution becoming the problem" (Watzlawick, Weakland, & Fisch, 1974).

In some families the fears and expectations of illness may be communicated from generation to generation until they actually take on the character of a covert and subtle encouragement. Thus, an individual family member may examine his or her body expectantly and constantly entertain a mental image of "the problem" as though it were already present. This type of imaging unwittingly welcomes the problem and holds it in the mind, and so is the healing intent *in reverse*.

If a problem does occur, it may be seen as "biological destiny" or bad luck. Rarely is it considered, even in part, as the creation of the family or the individual over time. Sometimes, when there is a tragic final outcome, it will be received with muted and grief-laden "celebration" as "destiny fulfilled." A powerful identification with and dependence on one or the other parent may result in a son's or daughter's uncanny recreation of that particular parent's experience in physical as well as psychological ways.

The following example illustrates this process. Approaching his fortieth birthday, one of us (Williamson) "just knew" he had developed a gall-bladder problem. He did not know how he knew; he just knew that he knew. As it turned out there was no problem at all. Although his father knew nothing of the incident, a few weeks later a letter from him noted: "Now you're 40. That's the age when your mother first started her gall-bladder trouble." This anecdote illustrates intergenerational learning and identification and the way in which patterns and timing of illness may be transmitted across generations. Such is the power of the biopsychosocial loyalty and commitment to the faithful discharging of intergenerational mandates and legacies (Boszormenyi-Nagy & Ulrich, 1981) about the course of health and disease.

Focusing Family Distress on One Person

Another notion about intergenerational behavioral patterns is that diffuse anxiety and distress felt throughout a family system may become focused on and primarily expressed in the life of one family member. This person has been "selected" for this office and serves as the "scapegoat," taking on the anxiety of the whole family (Whitaker & Keith, 1981). The anxiety may be expressed in the individual member's life by repeated failure in educational or vocational goals and/or intimate relationships. Or it may be expressed by chemical addiction of one kind or another, by socially delinquent behavior, or by psychological dysfunction. Yet another and frequent alternative is for the distress to evolve instead into a pattern of physical symptomatology and illness, either as a chronic disease or repeated acute illnesses. Thus, physical symptoms in a child or adult may reflect a more basic disturbance in the balance of the family emotional system. It is possible to bind the anxiety in a family by physical illness, a kind of "somatic psychosis," just as easily as by psychiatric problems.

Bodily Focusing of Unresolved Family Conflict

A fifth inference from intergenerational family theory is the idea that frequently the emotionality of unresolved family conflicts will be located oppressively somewhere in the individual's body. All life experience is grounded in the person's physicalness. Cumulatively, this may be enough to depress the spirit and produce a "heavy body" weighted with sighs and frozen emotion as readily as with body weight. We hypothesize that this in turn encourages susceptibility to disease. An ongoing dialogue and a caring relationship with one's own body is mandatory for good health. For a problem may express itself in an "unclear bodily discomfort" (Gendlin, 1978) before it finds its way into consciousness or words. Through the inner dialogue with the self, the individual discovers the ways in which personal problems have come to exist concretely in the body—and often these can be changed.

By constrast, simply to view the body in neutral or indifferent fashion as a "bag of red sawdust" (Green, 1978), and so be out of touch with the body organs, bodily processes, and key bodily systems is to be in a potentially lethal situation. To *reject* one's body is to be even worse off. To be cut off from unconscious psychological processes, even in symbolic form, may produce irrational thinking and craziness. However, life is likely to continue and to present another chance. But not to be in a listening and responsive dialogue with one's body may lead to the end of life itself. The individual will have lost contact with and therefore influence over what is happening "inside."

Personal Authority in the Family System

The last inference from intergenerational family theory to be noted here is the idea that, ultimately, the key to personal well-being is to have internalized and accepted personal responsibility for one's own good health in life at all times regardless of changing life circumstances, and so to be able to behave in a manner that produces positive growth and health (Williamson, 1981). This is a natural consequence of developing personal authority in the family system (PAFS) (Williamson, 1981, 1982a, 1982b). PAFS means that the adult has assumed an adult peer stance and has established peer relationships in the family of origin and especially in relationship to parents (Williamson, 1978, 1981). As a consequence, the adult holds himself or herself accountable for the totality of his or her experiences in life and particularly in regard to the course of health and illness. This highly differentiated posture greatly enhances the sense of personal freedom and the awareness of voluntariness and therefore of different alternatives. It proclaims the reality of different choices being available in the matter of personal health. All of this, at whatever level of awareness it occurs, prepares the way for re-creation and self-healing.

A recent study of ours offers some empirical support for this particular assumption. As part of an evaluation of the effects of an intergenerational family therapy process (c.f. Williamson, 1982b; Williamson, Bray, & Malone, 1984), former clients were asked to assess their level of personal authority on the Personal Authority in the Family System Questionnaire (Williamson, Bray & Malone, 1983) and to complete the Symptom Index (Shealy, 1982). This questionnaire assesses a comprehensive range of physical, psychosomatic, and psychological symptoms and stress indicators. We found significant correlations between reported levels of personal authority and reported symptoms and stress. The correlations indicate that people who reported higher levels of personal authority and lower levels of triangulation, particularly within the nuclear family, also reported fewer symptoms of ill health and stress.

The therapists were asked also to rate the amount of change evidenced in therapy, including estimated increases in personal authority. Next, two groups of subjects were selected from the total sample: the 20 people who were rated as changing the least in therapy, and the 20 people who were rated as changing the most. A comparison of the two subgroups indicated that subjects rated as changing most in therapy reported significantly fewer symptoms than did subjects who were rated as changing least. Taken together, these findings support the view that higher levels of personal authority in the family are associated with fewer physical symptoms and more personal good health.

What Do These Theoretical Inferences Show?

The systemic intergenerational point of view suggests that illness and accident are not nearly as involuntary nor as coincidental as is commonly assumed, and not simply a matter of fate or luck. Important choices are made at multiple levels of awareness, and since one generation may covertly make choices for the next one, or at least be believed to have done so, there is consequently much more voluntariness in most criticial life events than is usually recognized.

This same process may be illustrated in another way. Excessive sugar, salt, nicotine, caffeine, as well as chronic physical inactivity, will all contribute to the development of the longer term degenerative diseases. This much is now evident, and clearly this kind of lifestyle reflects a choice. But in like fashion, chronic conflict in the family or repeated failure in work and in love, with the subsequent loss of hope, may so neutralize and disarm the spirit and the life force that many individuals at certain times are much more likely to "choose" to get sick or to have "accidents." For such a circumstance is likely to lessen daily demands, may secure more relational and emotional support, and may even provide final escape or rest from what now seem to be the intractable problems of living.

Further, it is very valuable for the physician to acknowledge and reinforce the patient's own emotional and ethical responsibility for his or her personal health and healing. Good health or disease does not exist outside of and apart from the patient. And so the physician does well not to take over responsibility for the patient's well-being, however helplessly or seductively the latter may act, or however powerful or resourceful the former may feel. In the long run this is not a good service to the patient. For there are critical moments in a patient's life when either surgical or chemical intervention will fail to deal with the underlying nature and etiology of the problem, and will therefore be unnecessarily and unsuccessfully invasive of the human body and abusive to the spirit. On those occasions (such as depression after divorce or a child's death, or despair after loss of a job with subsequent loss of good health), and when physical symptomatology develops, these kinds of solutions are a poor substitute for an identification of the underlying life issues, mobilization of self-healing, and the acknowledgment of personal responsibility for well-being. Daily, the family physician, like no one else because of continuing contact with the individual family members, has a remarkable, indeed unique, opportunity and authority to elicit and support good health and self-healing in families.

All of this points to the central importance of an awareness, not just the responsibility for, the power of self-healing. Franz Ingelfinger, the late editor of the *New England Journal of Medicine*, recently concluded that 85% of all patients have self-limiting illnesses (Cousins, 1983). In other words, the body is capable of meeting most of its own health needs. It is the physician's primary task, therefore, to identify the other 15% and to know when it is appropriate to provide "do-nothing support." Even here, Cousins points out the important distinction between the *treating* and the *healing* processes. The purpose of treatment is to support the body's own healing abilities. But the center of the healing process remains within the individual. And the thoughtful physician knows how to summon it (Cousins, 1983), for this will mean connecting to a healing system via a belief system (or value system) that activates healing.

This view is in marked contrast to the attitude that disease comes from the outside and so it will take outside resources to deal with it. William Kroger (1982) suggested that "there is a great natural pharmaceutical storehouse in the brain if we know how to tap it," that is, if the individual knows how to release the natural "librium" and "valium" already in the brain. Because the human brain understands symbolic communication and can function by analog and image, it can also change the images. Other animals are controlled simply by what they see in the environment. But the human animal can also create alternative images to what is seen, and then use these new images to create a different personal reality and future—different, that is, from a future which even prior to social learning is biologically preprogrammed through an intergenerationally transmitted pattern. If one's theory determines what can be observed, then what is believed to be possible usually determines what can happen. There is now growing evidence that it is possible to connect consciousness with physiology and mind with body (Millon, Green, & Meagher, 1982).

The transcending personal health question then becomes, how does one get the fundamental life energy to flow? High-tech medicine often begins with chemistry and ignores the electric energy or "spirit" that produces the chemistry (admittedly the notion of spirit is a slippery concept). Family practice has the opportunity to take a richer systemic approach, leading to a change in the general orientation of modern medical practice in the direction of greater individual authority and accountability for good health, and to do so from within the system. The alternative is not attractive.

Assessing Intergenerational Relationships

Assessment of intergenerational patterns and processes is important for an accurate evaluation of the impact of family relations and stress on personal health. There are several methods of assessment. One is to take a family history that focuses on family relationships and patterns in addition to medical data, and to make an initial assessment of potential problem areas (Guerin, 1976).

The genogram or family map is a useful technique for recording data on both genetic and family relationships (Guerin, 1976; Jolly, Froom, & Rosen, 1980). From information gathered for a genogram, the physician can glean the medical and psychosocial functioning of the patient in his or her multigenerational family context. A list of important life events on the genogram (e.g., divorces, significant illnesses) and life changes (moves, new jobs) provides a concise social and psychological record of the patient and family. This technique may also save valuable time because the information needs to be accumulated only once and can then be copied for each family member's chart.

A recent study by Jolly et al. (1980) indicated that a physician can complete a genogram in about 16 minutes. Information is easily added to the genogram during subsequent visits if it is not finished during the first consultation. Jolly et al. also found that the information gathered on a genogram is very accurate and easily used by other physicians. If it is collected in a standard manner, nonmedical personnel can be trained to obtain the information.

Inspection of the genogram is a rapid means of assessing intergenerational patterns of illness and psychosocial dysfunction. A genogram replete with physical illnesses or psychological problems strongly indicates that dysfunctional intergenerational patterns are operating. Further exploration of these issues may be warranted to assess accurately the need for appropriate treatment and possible referral to a family-oriented mental health professional.

When taking a family history and/or genogram it is important to assess the individual's or family's current life-cycle stage. The transition from one family life-cycle stage to another is usually a highly stressful time that may result in symptom development (Carter & McGoldrick, 1980). Attention to these life-cycle changes further clarifies the context of the problem and may have important implications for treatment. When evaluating the family's life-cycle stage, three issues are important: the current problems and symptoms associated with this stage; how the family has coped with previous life-cycle transitions; and how the adult's family of origin coped with similar life-cycle stages.

For example, a six-year-old boy was taken to the family doctor by his mother because of repeated vomiting and soiling of his clothes. During the initial examination it was learned that these illnesses resulted in the boy's being unable to attend first grade, and the mother had to stay home with the child. The mother also expressed great anxiety about the boy's going to school and fear that he would not do well. *She said that she also had problems in her first year at school*. The physician found no medical cause for the child's behavior and, after appropriate medical treatment, he referred the family for family therapy to help them deal with this life-cycle transition.

Observing the *process* of the way the patient describes the family, rather than focusing only on content, also provides important data. If there is a history of children becoming ill during high stress periods, for example, it is evident that, in this family, triangulating is an often used strategy for dealing with stress. If the patient complains intensely about the spouse during the medical interview, the physician should be aware that he or she may easily become triangulated into the patient's marital problems. This is not to say that the physician should not be empathic to the patient, but rather that it is important to be aware of not getting emotionally hooked into the couple's problems.

Fusion, differentiation, and personal authority can also be assessed by observing the patient's language and "music" during the interview. Differentiated individuals tend to express their opinions through "I" statements ("I think," "I believe," "I want," "I intend," "I prefer") rather than "we" statements. If pushed for explanations, they tend not to argue or try to persuade others that they are right. The bottom line is that "this simply is the way I think, believe or feel" about something. Undifferentiated individuals, on the other hand, tend to blame others for their actions, do not take responsibility for their lives and physical health, and/or are frequently stuck in indecision. Low personal authority is indicated by being intimidated by significant hierarchical figures in the person's life, especially parents. Such individuals tend to be inhibited and to function at a lower level, particularly around authority figures. They tend also to have difficulties forming close, intimate relationships.

Psychological instruments are a more formal method for assessing intergenerational patterns. The Personal Authority in the Family System Questionnaire (PAFSQ) (Bray, Williamson, & Malone, 1984) is one such instrument designed to assess intergenerational processes in the three-generational family system. The PAFSQ is a self-report measure that patients can complete on their own. It is hand-scored easily and provides eight scale scores that measure these behaviors and processes. We have found the PAFSQ useful not only as an assessment device, but also as an intervention tool to help patients begin to think about the current status of their intergenerational family relationships and general well-being.

In summary, the physician develops an intergenerational understanding of personal health problems by assessing current individual and family functioning, as well as family life-cycle stage, and the patient's relevant intergenerational patterns. Use of the genogram or PAFSQ or other assessment techniques to include information about family relationships when taking a medical history will provide this type of information. By thinking about health behavior in this manner and practicing the technique, family practitioners can integrate this way of working with problems to enrich the practice of family medicine.

Conclusion

To summarize, the assumptions, implications, and methods discussed here mean that when an individual presents physical-medical complaints, the overall examination-interview process should include at least a brief and to-the-point inquiry into the patient's current marital and family experiences, including experiences within the family of origin. This information will give the physician a more complete data base from which to make sense of the illness and determine the influence of family distress on the patient's condition. This includes not only its etiology and prognosis, but also why it occurs at this time and which family circumstances will support or will be in the way of a successful and speedy recovery process. This information will help to identify the important and necessary ingredients in a successful and lasting treatment program.

This is not to say that the physician needs to offer psychotherapy in the medical office or even spend a lot of time with the patient. Rather, with a minimum of training, and assuming both some resolution and some openness in his or her own emotional and family life, the physician can learn readily how to make the patient's unresolved and current family emotional issues explicit; he or she can then, as appropriate, begin to relate these issues to the onset and behavior of the patient's illness or symptoms. Obviously, a supportive referral for family therapy will be appropriate in some cases. For example, when there is evidence of acute or chronic stress in the patient's marriage, or between the patient and older parents or with a child, a family therapy consultation should be considered, as this is likely to support and hasten the recovery process.

Systemic medical evaluation is a crucial ingredient in human health services. Most patients will enter the medical office at a time of extreme vulnerability and acute personal need. They are more open to recommendation, advice, and personal change than at most other times. The physician's words have an unusual impact on this occasion. The effect of the psychological suggestion and expectation in the physician's language, manner, and person, whether explicit or implicit, positive or negative, is powerful without peer. The simple request for personal accountability on the individual's part and the physician's suggestion and unequivocal expectation of change in the direction of health and well-being are potentially much more powerful than any other healing arts.

Here is a closing example: A few years ago a six-year-old girl began visiting the pediatrician's office biweekly because of a variety of minor complaints that began soon after her parents' divorce. Everyone involved knew this was a highly stressful time for the family. During one visit the physician lifted her up on the examination table so she would be at eye level with him. He told her quietly and confidently that he had decided that, although her illnesses had been useful so far, she did not need to be sick anymore and indeed probably would not need to come back for another office visit for a long time. There was a remarkable improvement thereafter.

The point is that technical skill alone does not create artistry in medical practice. So perhaps there is no greater opportunity going begging in contemporary medical education than to give instruction in how to relate psychologically to patients in order to use language and suggestion effectively and positively. In his or her professional person and role, a family physician embodies unparalleled psychological and moral authority. More than any other professional discipline, medicine today holds the "keys to the kingdom." If the possibility for exploitation is considerable, by the same token the potential for good is enormous.

REFERENCES

Bandura, A. (1977). *Social-learning theory*. Englewood Cliffs, NJ: Prentice-Hall.

Boszormenyi-Nagy, I., & Ulrich, D. (1981). Contextual family therapy. In A. Gurman & D. Kniskern (Eds.), *Handbook of family therapy*. New York: Brunner/Mazel.

Bowen, M. (1978). *Family therapy in clinical practice*. New York: Aronson.

Bray, J.H., Williamson, D.S., & Malone, P.E. (1984). Personal authority in the family system: Development of a questionnaire to measure personal authority in intergenerational family processes. *Journal of Marital and Family Therapy, 10*, 167-178.

Carter, E.A., & McGoldrick, M. (Eds.). (1980). *The family life cycle: A framework for family therapy*. New York: Gardner Press.

Cousins, N. (1983). *The healing heart*. New York: Norton.

Coyne, J., & Holroyd, K. (1982). Stress, coping and illness: A transactional perspective. In T. Millon, C. Green, & R. Meagher (Eds.), *Handbook of clinical health psychology*. New York: Plenum Press.

Dohrenwend, B.S., & Dohrenwend, B.P. (1982). Some issues in research on stressful life events. In T. Millon, C. Green, & R. Meagher (Eds.), *Handbook of clinical health psychology*. New York: Plenum Press.

Framo, J. (1981). The integration of marital therapy with sessions with family of origin. In A. Gurman & D. Kniskern (Eds.), *Handbook of family therapy*. New York: Brunner/Mazel.

Gendlin, E. (1978). *Focusing*. New York: Bantam Books.

Green, E. (1978, March). *Biofeedback in holistic healing*. Presentation at the Austin Area Holistic Health Meeting, Austin, Texas.

Guerin, P. (Ed.). (1976). *Family therapy: Theory and practice*. New York: Gardner Press.

Holmes, T.H., & Masuda, M. (1974). Life change and illness susceptibility. In B. S. Dohrenwend & B. P. Dohrenwend (Eds.), *Stressful life events: The nature and effects*. New York: Wiley.

Jolly, W., Froom, J. & Rosen, M.G. (1980). The genogram. *The Journal of Family Practice, 10*, 251-255.

Kerr, M. (1981). Family systems theory and therapy. In A. Gurman & D. Kniskern (Eds.), *Handbook of family therapy*. New York: Brunner/Mazel.

King, M., Novik, L., & Citrenbaum, C. (1983). *Irresistible communication: Creative skills for the health professional*. Philadelphia: Saunders.

Kroger, W. (1982, May). *Hypnosis and healing*. Paper presented at Healing Brain Conference, Houston, Texas.

Millon, T., Green, C., & Meagher, R. (Eds.). (1982). *Handbook of clinical health psychology*. New York: Plenum Press.

Oppenheim, C.D. (1966). Valid consent to medical treatment: Need the patient know? *Duquesne Law Review, 4*, 450-477.

Paul, N. (1981, September/October). *The unconscious transmission of hidden images and the schizophrenic process*. Presented at the 7th International Symposium on the Psychotherapy of Schizophrenia, University of Heidelberg, West Germany.

Rolling Thunder. (1981). Houston workshop (untitled). April, 1983.

Sarason, I.G., Levine, H.M., & Sarason, B.R. (1982). Assessing the impact of life changes. In T. Millon, C. Green, & R. Meagher (Eds.), *Handbook of clinical health psychology*. New York: Plenum Press.

Sarason, I.G., & Sarason, B.R. (1980). *Abnormal psychology, 3rd ed*. Englewood, NJ: Prentice-Hall.

Selye, H. (1976). *The stress of life* (rev. ed.). New York: McGraw Hill.

Shaw, R. (1983, June). *Mastery: A context for psychotherapy*. Seminar in Houston, Texas.

Shealy, C.N. (1982). *The symptom index*. Springfield, MO: Shealy Clinic.

Taggart, M. (1983). *Clinical epistemology and questions of context: The aesthetics/pragmatics debate*. Unpublished manuscript, Houston Family Institute.

Watzlawick, P., Weakland, J., & Fisch, R. (1974). *Change*. New York: Norton.

Whitaker, C.A., & Keith, D.V. (1981). Symbolic-experiential family therapy. In A. Gurman & D. Kniskern (Eds.), *Handbook of family therapy*. New York: Brunner/Mazel.

Williamson, D.S. (1978). New life at the graveyard: A method of therapy for individuation from a dead former parent. *Journal of Marital and Family Counseling, 1*, 93-101.

Williamson, D.S. (1981). Personal authority via termination of the intergenerational hierarchical boundary: A "new" stage in the family life cycle. *Journal of Marital and Family Therapy*, 7, 441-442.

Williamson, D.S. (1982a). Personal authority via termination of the intergenerational hierarchical boundary: Part II—The consultation process and the therapeutic method. *Journal of Marital and Family Therapy, 8*, 23-27.

Williamson, D.S. (1982b). Personal authority in family experience via termination of the intergenerational hierarchical boundary: Part III—Personal authority defined, and the power of play in the change process. *Journal of Marital and Family Therapy, 8,* 309-323.

Williamson, D.S., Bray, J.H. & Malone, P.E. (1983). The Personal Authority in the Family System Questionnaire. Houston Family Institute.

Williamson, D.S., Bray, J.H., & Malone, P.E. (1984). Personal authority in the family system: A family psychotherapy outcome study. Manuscript submitted to *Family Process*.

Wrightsman, L.S., & Deaux, K. (1981). *Social psychology in the 80s (3rd ed.)*. Monterey, CA: Brooks/Cole.

II.
THE SYSTEMIC EVOLUTION OF THE FAMILY

7

THE DOCTOR-PATIENT-FAMILY RELATIONSHIP

MICHAEL L. GLENN, M.D.

Patients come to see the doctor for different reasons. They may be suffering from a number of diseases—arthritis, cardiovascular disease, pulmonary disorders—and, frightened by the exacerbation of their symptoms, they worry that something is getting worse.

Other patients may feel basically sound but become annoyed by some physical complaint; they want the doctor to assure them that everything is all right. Some, experiencing the effects of stress, come to the physician feeling tired, run down, and irritable.

People who live alone may like the human and social contact provided by a visit to the doctor. Perhaps some of their friends are in the waiting room, and a few minutes' conversation and the warmth and bustle of the office help cheer them up.

Others come to the physician because they need welfare papers filled out, a disability certificate for an employer, a letter to their attorney, a physical examination for school or work. The visit is occasioned by the legalities of life, which require notes from the doctor.

Still others arrive in the throes of a painful family crisis. Not knowing how to proceed on their own, they wait for the doctor to pick up clues.

Finally, patients may appear as a result of many problems: physical complaints, depression or anxiety, worry about their jobs or families.

Often, patients are accompanied by family member, close friend, or relative. At times, the interaction with this person seems relevant to the illness.

Example 1

Emma B, an 84-year-old widow who is hypertensive, in heart failure, and has Parkinson's disease, is always accompanied to the doctor's office by her sister. Emma B is senile and paranoid. She thinks her neighbors plan to rob her. She looks under her bed every night and is afraid to eat or drink certain foods. When she arrives at the office, however, she nods, smiles, and says, "Everything is fine." She is pleased if her blood pressure has remained stable. In the meantime, hovering unseen behind her, her sister bobs and weaves, makes faces at the physician to qualify each phrase Emma utters, and winks knowingly whenever Emma makes a suspicious statement, shaking her head sadly when Emma denies being ill. Whenever Emma becomes too suspicious or worrisome at home, her sister gives her a sedative saying, "Here, this will be good for your pressure. This is what the doctor wants you to have."

Physicians have a choice of what problems to pursue in the limited time they spend with a patient. To choose wisely, they must understand the encounter from a broad perspective, which helps them grasp the full complexity of what is going on. The perspective chosen here views the patient, the illness, the family, and the physician as parts of a complex interactive and changing system.

An Overview

Although the doctor-patient relationship traditionally has been viewed as a dyadic encounter rather than a broader interaction, much that has been written about it can be extended to include the family as well.

The traditional approach views physicians as skilled and compassionate healers, and patients as ailing and dependent folk. "Good" patients cooperate with their doctors: They follow instructions, take their medicines, answer questions, and undergo the advised procedures. "Bad" patients do not: They ask lots of questions, defy the doctor's orders, and create problems. The inequality in the relationship is supposed to be for the patient's own good.

In fact, the relationship between doctors and their patients varies a great deal. Specialists, for example, have different kinds of relationships with patients than do generalists: The former may see the patient a few times, usually for a grave problem, and they appear as superspecialists whose words may not be challenged. Specialists are often more responsible to the generalist who provides their patients than they are to the patients themselves.

The generalist, on the other hand, is responsibile to the patient who comes to see him or her year after year. Their relationship may be more colloquial, more informal. The generalist usually has come to know the patient's family, and may even (in family practice) treat many of them. A generalist tends to be more responsive to patients' wishes. Thus the family doctor may prescribe antibiotics in the case of a cold, because the family insists on it, whereas the specialist is under no such pressure. This difference has been referred to as colleague-dependent versus client-dependent practice (Freidson, 1970).

The two categories contain far more variations, however. Physicians from different class and cultural backgrounds, for example, form different kinds of relationships with patients and their families. Patients from different cultural backgrounds come to the physician with different complaints and different expectations (Zola, 1966).

Some relationships are brief, as in an emergency room, or with a surgeon. These should more properly be called doctor-patient *encounters*. Others last a long time, as with a pediatrician or family doctor, and a genuine relationship may develop.

Some relationships are intense, as in care for a patient with myocardial infarction or cancer. Others are relatively bland, as in much routine care, and some are so bland as to be invisible, as in the case of the hospital radiologist.

Family practice is marked by a gradually evolving closeness between patients, their families, and the physician. They come to know one another over time, through the crises and sicknesses that mark the family's life. The relationship shifts and changes. Now it expands and deepens; now it contracts.

Patients begin to know a family physician at different points in their lives. Some may be born into a practice. Others approach the physician because they have just moved into town, or because they are about to get married and need a blood test, or because their previous family doctor has died.

Families may introduce their members to the physician cautiously, one at a time, checking out the physician first. Some families may bring everyone in at once for a checkup, or they may bring everyone except one or two people whom they keep hidden, secreted away. These family members frequently turn out to be "hidden patients"—people whose sickness is a family secret.

A Systems Approach to the Doctor-Patient-Family Relationship

Physicians and patients belong to large, complicated, and interacting systems whose relationships are constantly changing. Among the several different systems each group belongs to at once, those that concern us here are *the medical system* and *the family system* (Glenn, 1984). These are most involved in the usual clinical interaction of patient, family, and physician.

The relationship between the two systems may be expressed visually as two spheres, constantly moving and capable of engaging one another in a diversity of ways. At any time, the relationship between patient and physician is like the tip of the iceberg, a relationship that readily extends into other arenas as well.

Family Medicine and the Family

The physician belongs to the medical system, an enormous social subunit that involves millions of people—doctors, nurses, hospital workers, clerks, paramedics, lab technicians, radiology personnel, and so on. This aggregate devours more than 12% of the United States' gross national product.

Patients and their families come in contact with many members of this system in the course of the patient's illness, so that the interaction between the family and the medical system is exceedingly rich.

Family concerns are always present. Even in the simplest of problems, the common cold, family concerns become important issues: How will the illness upset the family's routine? Will anyone have to stay home with a sick child? Will anyone have to miss a day's work? Will people lose sleep by staying up with a sick family member? Will the cold go from one family member to another? In more serious illnesses, of course, the questions become more severe: Will the wage earner be able to continue working? Will mother have to stop nurturing others to take care of the sick family member? If mother falls ill, who will take care of her, and who will assume the tasks of caretaking? Will hoped-for plans now have to be postponed, dropped? Will there be a shared family hardship necessitating new allocation of family time and family resources? Will old fears of a family sickness come true? How will family roles have to be redefined? Will the family have to face dissolution?

Most families have patterns for coping with illness. They have rules that say when a sickness is severe enough to require a physician's attention, and they have rules that tell what the physician's appropriate response should be when he or she is called. They know who is the caretaker, who the go-between, who should notify the rest of the family, and so on. Family patterns are transmitted from generation to generation.

To appreciate the family context more fully, the physician might consider several questions: What is the patient's life stage, and how does it correspond to the family's own life cycle? What are the family's tasks, and how do they mesh with the patient's own tasks?

Other questions are: What is the family structure? Who is close to whom? How are generational images transmitted in this family? How does the identified patient model himself or herself after other family members? What is the family's image of illness? How do patients explain their illness to themselves, the physician, the family?

Bibace and Walsh (1982) have written extensively about the stages people follow in understanding their illness. Others (Stoeckle & Barsky, 1980) have described the patient's attributions of illness: what patients think their problems are, where they come from, and so on. Such views, it need hardly be pointed out, are often at variance with the views of the physician. Such divergence may reflect the gap between "educated" and "popular" views of illness, as well as differences between social classes and different cultural groups.

We are born into, grow up, live our lives, become sick, and die in families. Family life, whatever our view of this or that particular kind of family, is universal.

Illness develops in context and is treated in context. Not only does context affect the emergence of illness (according to the so-called psychosomatic premise), but illness also affects and changes the family context. When people become sick, their families are usually concerned; treatment will involve them at an intimate level.

The doctor-patient relationship, then, is always a point of contact between the patient's family system and the physician's medical system. Even when most of the contact takes place only between patient and physician, family members are always waiting in the wings.

It is by now incontestable that family life affects the health and illness of its members. Many clinicians have commented on the links between family stress, such as the loss of a parent or a mate, and the onset or exacerbation of illness (Grolnick, 1976; Huygen, 1982; Huygen & Smits, 1983; Kellner, 1963; Klein, Dean, & Bogdanoff, 1968; Kraus & Lilienfield, 1959; Parkes, 1972). Psychosomatic medicine has advanced well beyond its beginnings (Alexander, 1932; Dunbar, 1954), and has moved to consider links between the endocrine (Selye, 1956) and the immunological (Locke, 1982) systems.

In addition, the stance that the family is the "basic unit of medical care" (Schmidt, 1978) has drawn widespread support within family medicine, and an entire literature devoted to its elaboration has been emerging.

Although other social units may involve patients in any number of ways—the school, the workplace, the church, the ethnic community, the neighborhood, the generation—none of them usually involves them so totally as does the family. More than any other system, the family serves to define, condition, promote, qualify, affirm, treat, mitigate, and otherwise create the meaning of illness in our lives. Anyone concerned with contextual medicine (Worby, 1980) must look actively at the family and seek its involvement in the patient's presenting problem.

In a way it is amazing that medicine has gone for years *without* delving more into the patient's social context. As Watzlawick, Beavin, and Jackson commented (1967), "In modern biology it would be unthinkable to study even the most primitive organism in artificial isolation from its environment" (p. 258). And yet this is what has been going on for decades. The patient is embedded in the family as a tree in the earth and cannot be understood apart from it.

Theoretical Views

Parsons' Analysis

Lawrence Henderson's 1935 essay, "Physician and Patient as a Social System," was one of the first to analyze the doctor-patient relationship from a social viewpoint. Henderson, remembered by many physicians for his role in developing the Henderson-Hasselback equation, originally was a biochemist who turned toward sociology. He taught a course in concrete sociology at Harvard, where one of his students was Talcott Parsons.

Whereas Henderson focused on the internal workings of the doctor-patient relationship, Parsons (1951) delved into the social roles of patient and practitioner.

Parsons' writings form the basis of today's analysis of the doctor-patient relationship. He saw the relationship as a necessary feature of society, patterned and regulated to be useful. According to Parsons, the relationship rests on a basic mutuality of needs and outlook: Physicians are trained in their area of expertise; patients come to them seeking help. The relationship is inherently unequal because patients are dependent, all the more so as illness often brings about a state of helplessness and regression. Patients are thus compelled to take on the sick role, which places them in a well-defined social position.

According to Parsons, this role has four characteristics:

1) Patients cannot be held responsible for their incapacity.
2) Their illness is a legitimate excuse from their usual social obligations.
3) To merit these excuses, patients must want to get well.
4) Toward this end, they must seek competent medical advice and cooperate with their physicians.

Reviewing this, Eliot Freidson (1970) has commented—a bit more wryly than Parsons—that "medicine creates the social possibilities for acting sick" (p. 206).

The practitioner's role in the Parsonian model is a functionally specialized, full-time activity, attained by special training that has imparted a minimum standard of professional competence. Practitioners must also adopt an attitude of affective neutrality toward their patients, which means approaching patients objectively and not letting subjective feelings interfere with professional judgment. Affective neutrality is the physicians' main safeguard against using patients for their own interests—sexually, financially, politically, and so on. It is the patients' guarantee, too, and thus is a cornerstone of the professional relationship.

Two other cardinal dimensions of the professional attitude, according to Parsons, are its universality and functional specificity. The former means that physicians treat *all* their patients in the same way, without bias or judgment; the second means that they limit their professional activity to what they have been trained to do.

All this implies a fundamental unity of interest between patient and practitioner, whose relationship is thus neat, mutual, and complementary.

Many sociologists have challenged Parsons' view. Freidson, for example, influenced by the social constructivist school of sociology, exposed the potential for conflict in the encounter. According to him, medicine is "engaged in the construction of illness as a social state which a human being may assume" (1970, p. 205). Medicine's monopoly includes "the right to create illness as an official social role." The patient's sense of being ill is not legitimized until the physician makes his or her diagnosis. In this lies the seed of conflict, for patients and physicians come from different worlds, each bringing different values, needs, hierarchies, and agendas with them:

> Diagnosis and treatment are not biological acts common to mice, monkeys, and men, but (are) social acts peculiar to men. Illness as such may be biological disease, but the idea of illness is not, and neither is the way human beings respond to it. Thus biological deviance or disease is defined socially and is surrounded by social acts that condition it. (Freidson, 1970, p. 205)

This understanding led Freidson to explore the *context* of illness, the meanings attributed to physical illness by patient and physician, and the motivations physicians often attribute to patients' behavior. He also criticized Parsons' neglect of chronic or permanent illness.

In examining the "professional construction of illness," Freidson highlighted the physicians' class and self-interest. Mainly in private practice, most physicians may be regarded as moral entrepreneurs, trafficking in illness as a social commodity. This leads them at times to overdiagnose or overtreat.

The strength of Freidson's analysis is his exploration of the practitioner's everyday world. Differences between doctors and patients are grounded in their stations in life, their self-interests. The medical encounter means different things to them. As Elihu Gerson (1976) noted, medicine is the physician's way of making a living, and for the patient a "grossly uncomfortable, often painful, often embarrassing, frequently terrorizing experience" (p. 220). Such a wide divergence adds tension to the encounter.

Sometimes, for example, the patient may want a prescription or a note to his employer, but the physician may not want to give it. In this case the supposed mutuality of the relationship crumbles as the two parties scuffle for control.

The physician's stance of affective neutrality is most possible when patient and physician share class and cultural backgrounds. The further apart they are, the greater the chance that their agendas will differ.

While Parsons (1951) presented the physician as benevolent and kindly, trying to help patients cope with their distress, Waitzkin and Stoeckle (1976) identified the physician as an instrument of social control. According to the latter, the physician transmits society's prevalent cultural and moral values and represents the dominant class in any society.

Others (Illich, 1976; Mishler et al., 1981; Szasz, 1974) described the physician's role in isolating groups of social deviants from the rest of society. This process has been described for the contagiously ill (Foucault, 1965), the morally degenerate or hopelessly insane (Szasz, 1974), and so on. These authors pointed out the problems that come up when illness is used to label people. Consider the following as medical "illnesses": homosexuality, menopause, pregnancy, alcoholism, frigidity, impotence, child abuse, adolescent stress reaction, senility, or school phobia.

This is where the Parsonian model falters, I believe, and a model that helps to understand conflict becomes more helpful.

Balint's Contribution

Michael Balint (1957) was a British psychoanalyst who worked for years with groups of general practitioners and studied the doctor-patient relationship intensively.

Balint began by analyzing the doctor-patient encounter. A diagnosis is negotiated by the two parties:

> The patient in his still "unorganized" state (makes) various "offers" of illness to his doctor, and the doctor (responds) to these offers by rejecting some of them and finally accepting one. An important aspect of the doctor's response is the process of elimination by appropriate physical examinations resulting in the establishment of a ranking order

> both of illnesses and of patients. Under the impact of the doctor's response a kind of "agreement" is more often than not reached between him and his patient, and the illness thus enters upon its "organized" phase. (p. 107)

Feeling bad and wondering why this is so, the patient seeks advice from the physician. Patients may have their own ideas of what is wrong. They may talk about certain symptoms rather than others in an effort to feel out the physician's responsiveness to their distress. They may have their own agenda, which determines how they will maneuver. In any case, they present a set of complaints that, in Balint's terminology, are offers: invitations to a working diagnosis. The physician may accept or reject these offers. At this stage the illness is not yet decided upon; there is no diagnosis. The doctor and patient may proceed in any number of directions. There is something to be said for keeping this phase of the illness "open" as long as possible, especially if the physician senses a complicated picture of the patient's distress.

The patient offers a series of symptoms, requests, and suggestions. At some point, the physician actively pursues one of these, and, depending on the patient's response, the illness may crystallize. At this point the illness is negotiated. Treatment, however, may have begun much earlier.

Example 2

Philip G, a 32-year-old accountant, came to the physician complaining of horrible burning in his stomach. He was afraid of an ulcer, "like my father had." He had been in good health all his life but had recently been under extreme stress at work, and he was starting to argue with his wife. At the first meeting with the physician, his history was taken and a complete physical examination done. Because the patient was so worried about an ulcer, an upper gastrointestinal tract examination series was ordered and the patient given mild antispasmodic medication. "It could be an ulcer, of course," the physician said, "but it could just as well be a couple of other things, including the effects of stress on your stomach. We'll see."

The second session a week later found Philip feeling better. The radiologic results were normal, as were routine blood tests. The physician discussed the patient's work and family situations and explained in greater detail how stress can upset one's stomach. Medication was continued.

By the third visit, two weeks later, the patient's symptoms had dwindled markedly. "I'm able to figure out when it's going to start," he said. The antispasmodic medication was continued for three months, then tapered off.

Physician and patient agreed on the diagnosis of a stress-related stomach condition.

Balint (1957) also described the physicians' usual bias against considering emotional factors (he calls them neurotic symptoms) in illness. Most physicians are likely to emphasize physical illness because they feel more comfortable with it. As in the example above, their feeling may also be linked to the patient's feeling that a physical problem is present. One consequence of this bias, however, is that the patient may become even more fixed in believing that the problem is mainly physical.

Balint's concerns for the deeper levels of the patient's problems led him to propose long sessions in which the physician explores the context of the patient's complaints, hoping thereby to get a better grasp of the meaning of the patient's complaints. One long session may actually prevent many fruitless visits for psychosomatic complaints and help patients deal more constructively with the conflicts that create emotional stress.

Example 3

Sally H, a young divorced woman, came to the physician complaining of aches in her legs and thighs. She felt her veins were "popping out." Sometimes her legs throbbed and felt hot. A friend had told her she might have phlebitis; as her mother had been ill for years with that condition, she was distraught.

Physical examination had totally negative results. Her veins did not bulge. The physician noted her to be anxious and somewhat seductive.

Because of her insistence that she had phlebitis, the physician ordered a venogram and a vascular surgery consultation. The former was negative. The vascular surgeon, also commenting on the patient's anxiety, recommended referring her to an orthopedic surgeon.

By the third visit, the patient complained of being anxious "because nobody can find out what's wrong." She had decided to visit a chiropractor. Although she denied stress in her life, further discussion revealed that she was trying to cope with job-related, financial, and personal issues all at once.

The physician offered her a long session in hopes of getting to understand better how her complaints might be related to her life. The hour was spent discussing Sally's family life—her unhappy marriage, raising her son, her disputes with her parents, and her efforts in recent months to become independent. At the end of the session, the physician prescribed a simple anti-inflammatory medication and asked her to return in a week. She accepted the formulation that the swelling in her legs might be caused by a minor muscle pull.

The next week, her symptoms were better. Although the exact cause of her problem could not be determined, patient and physician agreed that the illness was minor, that it would probably improve, and that stress would make it worse. The illness was becoming defined by negotiation.

Example 4

Balint discussed at length the physician's *response* to the patient, exploring what factors in the physician's background promoted the response. This awareness may become a therapeutic tool, as Browne and Freeling (1976), two British general practitioners influenced by Balint's work, describe in this example:

> CF was a precocious 16-year-old girl, attractive and sexually exciting to the doctor. She complained of loss of appetite, headaches, and insomnia—with a bright smile and a flash of thighs. The doctor believed that his recognition of her sexuality was important but felt handicapped by the professional dangers involved in saying this to her. In any case, he felt embarrassed. He gave her a tonic and asked about her boyfriends.
>
> CF told him vivaciously about the intricacies of her involvement with three young men, complaining that the one she liked best seemed to like her a lot, but he never spent much time with her. The doctor, feeling able to use this opening to project his own feelings, said, "Perhaps he finds you so attractive that he doesn't know what to do about it?" CF replied, "You mean he's frightened he wouldn't be able to control himself? I feel like that at times. It frightens me so much when I am attracted to boys because I want to make love with them, and then I can't eat or sleep. (p. 17)

The Carmichaels' Relational Model

In the United States, Balint's work influenced many of the founders of family medicine. Stephens (1974) spoke publicly of his debt to Balint's interest in the doctor-patient relationship with an analysis of his own.

Carmichael and Carmichael (1981) refer to three models of the doctor-patient relationship: clinical, adversarial and relational. The clinical model has a mainly biomedical orientation. The physician acts as the expert: "Management of disease is goal oriented and springs from a technological base in which success is measured in terms of the result or outcome. The relationship between the doctor and the patient is that of provider and recipient" (p. 126).

The adversarial model refers to occasions when the patient seeks something only a physician is "socially sanctioned to provide," such as a certificate of disability. Often, as we have seen, this places the physician in an adversarial relationship to the patient.

In the relational model, which the Carmichaels advocate, physicians and patients are co-participants in a process that is "not concerned with cure or control of disease, but rather with the attention, support, and comfort the patient receives" (p. 128). This model involves the development of affinity between patient and physician, a sense of intimacy, reciprocity, and continuity.

The Carmichaels may have idealized the relational model, which they believe comprises 80% of family practice. In the course of several years, a physician-patient relationship may well include aspects of all three models, and the intimacy that has developed may be accompanied by some profound conflicts as well. In essence, the relational model rests on the tacit sharing of cultural and class outlook. The greater the difference between patient and physician, the greater will be the tendency for the adversarial or clinical model to develop.

Patients may force a move from one model to another. A patient may, for example, be treated one day for a boil on the back (clinical model), come in next month complaining of depression over loss of a job (relational model), and the week afterward ask for a welfare paper and transportation voucher (adversarial model).

The Carmichaels (1981) prefer viewing the physician and patient as partners, and they value the intimacy that develops between the partners over time. Suggesting that the "family" in family medicine refers more to process than to entity, Carmichael (1976) posited this kind of rapport as the unique feature of family practice.

Byrnes and Long's Views of Style

Following R.F. Bales (1950), who fit interactive behavior into 12 categories, Byrnes and Long (1976) studied transcripts of doctors talking to patients. They described six stages of the physician's usual activity: establishing a relationship with the patient, discovering the reason for the patient's attendance, conducting a verbal or physical examination or both, considering the situation, detailing treatment or further investigation, and terminating.

After analyzing the tapes of many consultations, they concluded that styles of interaction differ among physicians. More than they realize, however, physicians adopt the same style with different patients, a style that characterizes their usual behavior. The styles may be arrayed according to how much time the physician spends in each of the above-noted phases.

The main differences between physicians' styles emerge along a spectrum of doctor-centered versus patient-centered interaction. The first refers to encounters dominated by the physician's need to find out information and dispense treatment; the latter are encounters marked by the physician's desire to listen to the patient's complaints and questions and to understand the symptoms in context.

Byrnes and Long identified four styles: silence, listening, and reflecting; clarifying and interpreting; analyzing and probing; gathering information. They asserted that physicians spend most of their time in one particular style, although they may at times move to adjacent styles. The first two styles are more characteristic of the patient-centered interaction, and the latter two, of the doctor-centered one.

The tendency to see either patient or physician in the center of the encounter spills over into the different kinds of prescriptions physicians make. Some physicians, preempting the decision-making capacity for themselves, announce a decision or try to "sell" it to the patient. At the other end of the spectrum are physicians who involve the patient actively in the decision, or who permit patients to make their own decisions.

Byrnes and Long prefer the patient-centered style. But when they tried to teach that style to physicians who followed another one, they found it difficult to change the physicians' habits.

It is not clear, however, that a patient-centered style is best for all patients. Some older, more tradition-oriented people prefer the familiar physician-centered behavior from their physician. It might even be, as Roger Bibace (personal communication, 1982) pointed out, that some types of people feel more at ease with one style or another, depending on their age, class, cultural group, and personality. The physicians' task may be to learn elements of the different styles to treat patients better. Failing this, physicians usually will find themselves with a panel of patients whom their style fits instinctively.

The Authoritarian and Mutual Models

Two kinds of doctor-patient relationships are described in the literature: the authoritarian or hierarchical model, in which doctors are the experts and patients the supplicants, and a more mutual model, in which physicians seek to use their knowledge for the patient's good, but both are involved in the process. Both kinds of relationships are useful.

The authoritarian model recapitulates the parent-child relationship. Its strength is the social and professional position of the physician, which permits the physician to help the patient better. Its weakness is the abuse of that authority by the physician.

This model has been criticized recently as if it were somehow chauvinist and denigrating. True, the traditional doctor-patient model has been associated with subordination of patients. But it is also true that the physician can get nursing care, can open doors of social bureaucracies, and can often act as an ombudsman for patients who have no resources of their own. Such influence, which stems from the physician's social authority, should not be dismissed lightly by those admitted to hospitals where they know no one and where staffing is inadequate. The physician, like it or not, may be the patient's advocate in a confusing world. Paternalism has two sides: It oppresses when abused, but it serves when used well.

In the mutual model, the physician and patient may be more equal, but that does not erase the fact that the physician has abilities the patient lacks.

What is the physicians' responsibility in this mutual relationship? Physicians, like everyone else, always put forth certain views and values, but how consciously do they promote these? Do physicians exhort patients to stop smoking? Do they try to get alcoholics to stop drinking, fat people to lose weight, hypertensive patients to reduce their salt intake? In this sense, physicians are evangelists trying to convert patients. Do they practice what they preach? Perhaps. But they always advocate, even in the most "mutual" relationship. To do otherwise abandons their duty: How can patients make decisions alone? Physicians must present facts and give an opinion so that patients may make an informed choice.

Physicians handle this by combining caring intervention and caring observation—the participant-observer position. It must matter to the physician whether or not the patient lives or dies, has pain or gains relief, is tormented or at peace. But it must somehow not be the physician's task to accomplish all this for the patient. Only the patient can take the medicine. Only the patient can lose weight, exercise, stop browbeating his wife and children.

In other words, the question of choosing between the two models of patient-practitioner interaction is a false issue. Both have their place.

Physicians, Patients, and Families

The Physician as Participant and Observer

Physicians who participate in their patients' affective life derive a significant reward from it. They become family members, like an uncle or close cousin, and may enjoy the graduations, the grandchildren, scholastic honors, promotions, new homes, and so on. Part of the reward comes also from knowing that one's caring involvement with others is appreciated.

Yet physicians must be able to manage relationships that are caring but limited. The caring comes from the physician's genuine concern and esteem for the patient, the limits from the relationship's professional character.

The Interaction of Family Members

In family practice, roles often become interchangeable. The mother may come in this week because she has a sore throat, but the next week she brings in her son who also has a cold. The father may give his wife a ride to the physician's office for her Pap smear but, a few minutes later, he may come to the physician to ask questions about his sexual performance.

The critical fact in family medicine is that the family is *the frame of reference for the physician's thinking*. One member's illness affects the others physically and emotionally in different ways. A family member may be a patient one day, a caretaker the next, a mourner a week later. A person may be simultaneously a mother, wife, daughter, sister, teacher, patient, and an active member of the church; at any given moment, she may be juggling her different roles so as to give priority to the one that seems most pressing or most important.

Nor is the family monolithic, for it is a source of great diversity. Family members share religious, class, and cultural backgrounds, but their personalities are different, their experiences vary, and conflicts abound—who loves whom the most, who takes sides against whom, who sacrifices the most, who is "nice," who is "nasty," and so on.

As family theorists know well, other family members must be kept in mind when one member comes to the helping professional as the patient. Often the presenting patient is not the only patient, as when the family is in turmoil over an alcoholic member and several different family members are involved in the problem. The physician who "takes sides" may unwittingly promote and preserve a family problem. Doherty and Baird (1983) caution the practitioner against this tendency, particularly when the patient is female and the physician male, and the absent husband is labeled the bad guy.

Example 5

Billy K's mother brought him to the doctor. "His stomach always bothers him," she said. Billy, age nine, was missing school because of persistent, severe stomach pains. Evaluation showed that the pains were indeed functional (a sign of tension), and that the main problem in the family was conflict between Billy's parents, aided by a family tendency to "fall ill" under stress. Billy's symptoms not only fit a family pattern, but they also deflected focus from the marital disputes, at the same time bringing the couple together as concerned parents.

Sometimes there is great pressure on the physician to take sides, particularly on the issue of "secrets." Sometimes a patient's relative will phone, just before the patient's appointment, telling the physician, "I just wanted you to know. He's drinking again." Or another patient will say, "You know Charlie. He hasn't been taking his medicine. Just thought you'd want to know."

In a sense, this goes with the view that the physician is the boss, the expert. Patients are only providing the doctor with information; they don't want to become involved. Some advice has to be taken in this spirit.

At other times, though, "secret" information is a sign that the family cannot cope on its own with the problem. Children are afraid, for example, to confront the father about his drinking for fear he will explode at them. Only the physician, they feel, has the authority to do this. But the astute physician realizes that he or she cannot accomplish this task alone. Much current treatment for problems of substance abuse involves mobilizing the family and breaking through the secrets.

Example 6

Repeated phone calls about Harry L's "smoking again" came from his family. Yet visit after visit, Harry, who had almost died in an intensive care unit from respiratory problems related to his heavy smoking, denied smoking more than "one or two." The physician realized she was being "triangulated"—put into a position between Harry and the family members—because the latter could not deal directly with him. To the next person who called, the physician announced, "I'm sorry. I cannot treat your father's smoking unless all of you are willing to come in and confront him with me." A family session was arranged and the dirty linen aired. Faced now with a solid front of family members and physician, Harry admitted his secret smoking. Treatment took on a new meaning, as the wife and children expressed their fears about his illness and told him about their feelings while he was ill. The secret could not have been handled otherwise.

Intimacy and Distance

The doctor-patient relationship is one of the oldest intimate relationships in history. Patients entrust the physician with their most guarded secrets. In return, the physician pledges professional expertise and concern.

The physician is forbidden virtually no area of probing. Family secrets, sexual fears and experiences, fantasies, deepest feelings, all are accessible. In addition, patients allow the physician to examine them physically, granting them intimate access denied even to wives or husbands. Doctor, patient, and the patient's family share some of life's most intense moments: the death of a loved one, a child's illness, the birth of a baby, the discovery of a dreaded disease.

Much medical practice, of course, is fairly routine: the monthly blood pressure check, diabetic monitoring, well-baby visits. Here the regularity and steadiness of contact gradually build up a sense of trust, reliability, and affection. Many sick or lonely patients enjoy the social contact of a visit to the doctor. And physicians enjoy the social and physical contact with their patients: the routines of the physical examination, touching and being touched, chatting about the family, experiencing a growing familiarity. The encounter can be a time for mutual affirmation, often accomplished by simple nods and smiles, the touch of hands, and mutual concern.

Like any other human relationship, the relationship between physicians and the families they treat may encompass all sorts of feelings. Sometimes they may be angry with each other, sometimes appreciative. They may esteem each other deeply or they may feel used and misunderstood. Patients often *want* their physician to like them and, thinking they can read the physician's signals, they may try to comply with the physician's wishes. Thus some patients try to be obedient, whereas others try to be sexy, witty, or humorous.

Over the course of time, many patients will grow fond of their doctors. They often sympathize with the doctors' fatigue and busy schedule. They inquire about their children, and are pleased when they read an article about them in the local paper. As contact builds over time, the doctor and patient grow to know each other fairly well. Some patients seem to treasure this quality of the relationship even more than the medical advice that flows through it.

Example 7

One of the first patients I cared for when I took over another physician's practice was Marie M, a 66-year-old widow who had many medical problems and woes. She immediately took on the role of my staunchest supporter among the regulars and urged me each week to remain in the practice. "We need you," she kept saying. "You're not going to leave us, are you?"

When I made the decision to remain, she swelled with pride. "See, what did I tell you? I knew you would do well if you stayed on. Tell the truth, aren't you happy you stayed? Wasn't I right? And wasn't I one of your very first supporters?" Today she continues to ask about "the wife and children, especially the little girl," and often brings in small gifts.

Not only elderly patients create familylike ties to the physician. Many other patients become interested in the physician's spouse and children, vacations, car, and hobbies. As the primary-care physician grows to know the patient, showing concern for him or her, it is natural for the patient to reciprocate.

Interest in the role of the patient's family may extend to the physician's family, too. And well it might: From recent studies of the role of the physician's own family (Crouch, 1983), it is clear that physicians' attitudes and expectations are linked in many ways to their own families—the cultural and class ties, the racial and religious identities, the financial needs and strains. Physicians who want to explore a systemic view of patients and their families will have to be prepared to turn that same view inward, exploring their own responses and their own family structure and dynamics.

Many times the physicans' responses to their patients and to patients' relatives will be troubling to them. Physicians feel angry, afraid, disgusted, enticed. Such responses are important for them to recognize, for they are often clues to what is going on with the patient, the physician, and between both.

Untoward feelings may alert physicians to being dealt with dishonestly. The queasy feeling that one gets, for example, when one is being conned for drugs is an excellent guide to diagnosing the problem. So is the frustration one experiences when dealing with patients who feel frustrated themselves and cannot focus on their problems.

Uncomfortable feelings may alert physicians to situations in which they are being manipulative. Overt sexual feelings may, for example, direct physicians to examine their own motivations. Similarly, exasperation or irritation may result from the different agendas for action the patient and physician may have. The physician may feel disobeyed and therefore angry.

The physician's feelings may alert him or her to feelings the patient is hiding. Some patients seem to get the doctor to feel what they feel. The genuinely depressed patient may bring tears to the physician's eyes. The angry patient may not express his or her anger but create contentiousness in the physician. The confused patient often has a confused physician, just as the anxious patient usually makes the physician jumpy and tense.

The foregoing does not contradict the notion of appreciating behavior in its context. Context includes not only the here and now but also images and patterns from the past that we have brought with us into the present.

Patients and physicians respond to one another in many ways. They may reenact past patterns and relationships. Patients may respond to the physician as a kindly parent whom they remember fondly, as a cruel parent they have always despised, as a kid brother or older sister, as a cute, bright grandchild. The younger male physician acts in some ways as a son to the older female patient, as a younger brother to a patient his own age who also has a younger brother, and as a parent or uncle to an adolescent patient.

Physician and patient may respond to each other in terms of fantasy: relationships they have always wished they could have or dreaded they might have. Thus the patient may treat the doctor as an idealized parental figure or as a demonic manipulative "evil scientist" prepared to do harm.

They may also respond to each other in the here and now: patient being angry with doctor for being late and charging too much, doctor being angry with patient for not taking the medicine, or each appreciating each other's honesty and integrity. These reactions are grounded in the here and now, in social roles, and in the particular kinds of people they are.

Summary

The relationship between patient, family, and physician is a dynamic, changing process. Its context determines its significance; its interactional patterns shape its meanings. It relies on many interlinked factors for its strength and effectiveness and is a blend of mutual and contradictory interests. Only a pluralistic and dialectic approach can do justice to its richness and complexity.

REFERENCES

Alexander, F. (1932). *Psychoanalytic medicine*. New York: Norton.

Bales, R.F. (1950). *Interaction process analysis*. Cambridge, MA: Addison-Wesley.

Balint, M. (1957). *The doctor, his patient and the illness*. New York: International Universities Press.

Bibace, R., & Walsh, M.E. (Eds.). (1982). Children's conceptions of health, illness, and bodily functions. In *New Directions for Child Development, 14*, 31-48. San Francisco: Jossey-Bass.

Browne, K., & Freeling, P. (1976). *The doctor-patient relationship*. Edinburgh: Churchill-Livingston.

Byrnes, P.S., & Long, B.E.L. (1976). *Doctors talking to patients*. London: Her Majesty's Stationery Office.

Carmichael, L.P. (1976). The family in medicine, process or entity? *Journal of Family Practice, 3*, 562-563.

Carmichael, L.P., & Carmichael, J.S. (1981). The relational model in family practice. *Marriage and Family Review, 4*, 123-133.

Crouch, M. (1983). Working with one's own family. Paper presented to Society of Teachers of Family Medicine, Kansas City.

Doherty, W., & Baird, M. (1983). *Family therapy and family medicine*. New York: Guilford.

Dunbar, H.F. (1954). *Emotions and bodily changes: A survey of literature on psychosomatic interrelationships*. New York: Columbia University Press.

Foucault, M. (1965). *Madness and civilization: A history of insanity in the age of reason*. New York: Random House.

Freidson, E. (1970). *Profession of medicine*. New York: Harper & Row.

Gerson, E.M. (1976). The social character of illness: Deviance or politics? *Social Science & Medicine, 10*, 219-224.

Glenn, M. (1984). *On diagnosis*. New York: Brunner/Mazel.

Grolnick, L. (1976). A family perspective of psychosomatic factors in illness. *Family Process, 11*, 457-486.

Henderson, L.J. (1935). Physician and patient as a social system. *New England Journal of Medicine, 212*, 819-823.

Huygen, F.J.A. (1982). *Family medicine: The medical life history of families*. New York: Brunner/Mazel.

Huygen, F.J.A., & Smits, A.J.A. (1983). Family therapy, family somatics, and family medicine. *Family Systems Medicine, 1*, 23-32.

Illich, I. (1976). *Medical nemesis: The expropriation of health*.New York: Pantheon.

Kellner, R. (1963). *Family ill health: An investigation in general practice*. New York: Thomas.

Klein, R., Dean, A., & Bogdanoff, M. (1968). The impact of illness upon the spouse. *Journal of Chronic Diseases, 20*, 241.

Kraus, A.S., & Lilienfield, A.M. (1959). Some epidemiological aspects of the high mortality rate in the young widowed group. *Journal of Chronic Diseases, 10*, 207.

Locke, S.E. (1982). Stress, adaptation, and immunity. *General Hospital Psychiatry, 4*, 49-58.

Mishler, E., Amarasingham, L.R., Hauser, S.T., Liem, R., Osherson, S.D., & Waxler, N.E. (1981). *Social contexts of health, illness, and patient care*. Cambridge, MA: Harvard University Press.

Parkes, C.M. (1972). *Bereavement: Studies of grief in adult life*. New York: International Universities Press.

Parsons, T. (1951). *The social system*. New York: Free Press.

Schmidt, D.D. (1978). The family as the unit of medical care. *Journal of Family Practice, 7*, 303-313.

Selye, H. (1956). *The stress of life*. New York: McGraw-Hill.

Stephens, G.G. (1974). The clinician as historian. *International Journal of Balint Groups*. Special Ed. Proceedings of Second International Congress of the Balint Society, Brussels.

Stoeckle, J.D., & Barsky, A.J. (1980). Attributions: Uses of social science knowledge in the "doctoring" of primary care. In L. Eisenberd & A. Kleinman (Eds.), *The relevance of social science for medicine*. Boston: Reidel.

Szasz, T. (1974). *The myth of mental illness*. New York: Harper.

Waitzkin, H., & Stoeckle, J.D. (1976). Information control and the micropolitics of health care: Summary of an ongoing research project. *Social Science & Medicine, 10*, 263-276.

Watzlawick, P., Beavin, J., & Jackson, D.D. (1967). *Pragmatics of human communication*. New York: Norton.

Worby, C. (1980). The family in the undergraduate medical school curriculum. Keynote address, Society of Teachers of Family Medicine Spring Conference, Kansas City, February 12, 1980.

Zola, I.K. (1966). Culture and symptoms: An analysis of patients' presenting complaints. *American Social Review, 31*, 615-630.

8

THE SINGLE ADULT

LISA C. BAKER, Ph.D. and CHRISTIAN N. RAMSEY, Jr., M.D.

The increasing variety and complexity of modern American culture are particularly descriptive of single adults. Singles are people who are divorced, widowed, or have never married; they may be parents or living with their own parents; they may be young or very old, heterosexual or homosexual, financially independent or dependent on others; they may live alone, with their children, with their family of origin, or with a roommate of the same or opposite sex; they may be committed to a single lifestyle or they may be marking time until they marry. In other words, the only thing common to all single adults is the fact that they are not legally married. The purpose of this chapter is to alert the physician to some contextual issues relevant to single people, and to suggest ways to facilitate the doctor-patient relationship when the patient is a single adult.

As is true for any patient, a physician treating a single person should take into account the whole ecology of the illness and the treatment, including the special developmental and systems issues of singleness. Developmental theory deals with the change of an organism over time; systems theory emphasizes the ecology of those changes in interaction with the environment. In creating a favorable context for disease treatment, the web of systems in which the doctor-patient relationship occurs must include attention to the relational, occupational, and temporal contexts of the person's illness. Family systems medicine has much to offer in illuminating the needs of the single adult. And because systems theory is rooted in the general notion of context, it draws attention to other systems beyond the family in which the person lives and works.

The Changing Context of Singleness

The family doctor's treatment of a single adult in the 1980s warrants some rethinking of stereotypes. The role of single adults in our culture continues to evolve in directions that unsettle ideas about the timing and meaning of family relationships. According to projections by the Joint Center for Urban Studies of MIT and Harvard University (Masnick & Bane, 1980), the number of single adults will rise more than any other population category in the United States during the next 10 years. The number of singles aged 14 or over increased nearly 70% in the 1960s and 1970s (Figure 1). Cargan and Melko (1982) showed that the population rise and the post-World War II baby boom account for about two-thirds of the increase in singles, which means that the remaining one-third of the increase must be the result of changes in social mores or other factors. One influential factor is the divorce rate, which more than doubled between 1965 and 1980, along with the interval between divorce and remarriage (Stein, 1981).

There has been a growing trend toward living alone or with nonrelatives among the never-married, the divorced, and the widowed. Between 1960 and 1975, the number of never-married adults in their twenties who headed their own households more than doubled, and most of these individuals lived alone. In 1980, an estimated 1.1 million unmarried couples were living together, more than twice as many as in 1970. Among divorced and widowed women, in particular, the number who head their own households has increased sizeably (Masnick & Bane, 1980; Stein, 1981).

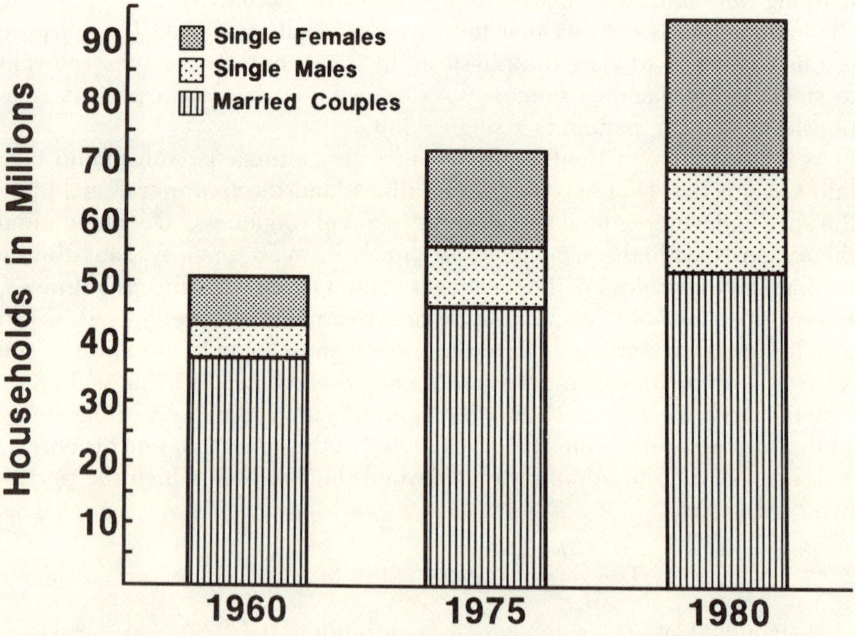

Figure 1. (From G. Masnick & M.J. Bane, 1980. Reprinted with permission.)

These facts imply that important shifts have taken place in American culture and economic structures that have created a new social climate, altering the function of and motivations for marriage and the meaning of singleness. It is no longer essential that a person live in a family unit in order to survive. An increase in options and lifespan has led to later marriages, not marrying at all, or a series of marriages interrupted by divorce or death. People now bring varied individual life experiences to their relationships (Masnick & Bane, 1980; Stein, 1981). More marriages begin with one or both partners being sexually experienced, having had several long-term relationships, and/or having maintained a household with a person of the opposite sex.

The trend toward later marriages and both partners working has made both singleness and marriage more complicated for many people. More men and women participate in joint social activities independent of marriage (Gordon, 1978). Historically, contact has gradually become less supervised and more frequent, with development of couple and group dating. Now the direction seems to be toward even more informal activity, and the rise in cohabitation among unmarried adults indicates a shift in the attitudes of the singles and the society in which they live. Marriage is no longer taken for granted as the expected and preferred lifestyle for everyone to whom it is available. For single adults who have established careers, homes, and investments, the decision to marry or remarry has been likened to the question of merging two corporations. Even for many people without extensive assets, remaining single is a preferred way of life.

Woven into these changes in family life are shifts in sex-role behavior that have had profound economic and social effects. Women and men are redefining new opportunities for women outside and for men inside the home. With more economic freedom, women become less dependent on a marriage partner for financial support. This shake-up of traditional marriage roles has called into question some basic reasons for marriage and the conduct of marital relationships. Many people find that single life offers different avenues to similar goals of companionship, productivity, and personal fulfillment, with the additional factor of increased personal freedom and flexibility.

In both popular and scholarly writings about single adults, one is struck by the disparaging, or at least ambiguous image associated with being unmarried. For the single adult, the process of making lifestyle choices may be as significant as the choices themselves, since there is little to guide them other than vague and mostly negative stereotypes. The physician can help to break the pattern of cultural negativism about singleness by allowing the patient the freedom to offer information that may or may not fit a culturally prescribed pattern.

Two stereotypes are especially common, that of the "swinging single," and of the person who is unmarried because of never being able to break away from parents. Though neither stereotype has been substantiated by data, the fact remains that the single adult must carve out a lifestyle without the benefit of a positive public image. Contradictory or negative messages come from the larger cultural system whose rules regulate and are regulated by single people's behavior. In the area of sexual behavior, for example, the message is that whatever singles do is unacceptable by traditional standards, whether that means repressing sexuality, masturbating, or engaging in nonmarital sexual activity. Although these norms are changing, single adults must still make sometimes difficult decisions about the extent and context of their sexual activity, about birth control, and about their response to the traditional dictum of "no sex outside of marriage." Sometimes single people will consult their physician about these concerns, though it may not be initially apparent that such help is being sought.

L.J. was a 24-year-old, never-married librarian from a family with strong religious beliefs and practices. To the physician who took care of her family she complained of urinary frequency. Her history, physical examination, and urinalysis results were all within normal limits. A subsequent urine culture revealed no abnormality. Pelvic examination showed that she had no hymen, and the exam was normal.

At a follow-up visit a week later, the patient complained of low back discomfort. The family physician, asking about the patient's lifestyle, sensed that the patient was using her symptoms as a "ticket" for discussion. Questions about her sexual practices revealed that the patient was sexually active and afraid of becoming pregnant. The physician was able to provide appropriate information and a method of contraception for the patient even though this was not the reason she had given for her two visits.

In our cultural system the single person is both envied and pitied, which is as much a comment on our society's ambivalence toward marriage as toward singleness. One might theorize that negative attitudes and stereotypes concerning singles are labels projected in a reciprocal way by married people *and* by singles who are uneasy about the freedom that singleness represents (H. F. Stein, personal communication, 1983). Our society has made much of the aloneness and/or loneliness that is a partner to that freedom, and many singles have reacted either by confirming the stereotype or by vehemently denying it. Either response creates a systemic pattern that family therapists would label "more of the same." To the extent that single people accept *or* rebel against the system's rules ("family myths") that devalue their life situation, they perpetuate the current patterns. Perhaps singles are given so many double messages that, unless they achieve some healthy degree of differentiation, they will be subject to the same symptomatic behavior of a family member who is continually placed in double binds by the family system.

In a content analysis of the popular literature about singleness, Cargan and Melko (1982) conclude that things may be improving: "[Singles] can [now] discuss more mundane problems, such as whether to buy a house or a condominium, without first having to argue that they are not sexually inhibited, or insist on how happy they are, or explain how it is that they happen to be single at all" (p. 65).

THE BASIC TASK: BALANCING THE NEED FOR DIFFERENTIATION AND THE NEED FOR SUPPORT

In gathering information from a single person, the physician should attend to at least three different contexts of an illness: the patient's relationships, the patient's work environment, and the timing of the patient's medical concern. The underlying task of single adults is to establish ways of relating to the systems of which they are a part that will afford the support, identity, and connectedness as well as the autonomy and flexibility they need. This task will manifest itself in attitudes toward marriage, expressions of intimacy, means of building a network of support, and feelings about aloneness. The single person, though not in a marital system, is nevertheless a part of numerous other interlocking systems.

The Patient's Relationships

One of the most common oversights of the physician is to ignore the family system of a single adult. Even when living alone, the single person may be very much a part of several family or quasi-family systems. The relationships of a single adult may involve friends, colleagues, romantic relationships, family members, and others.

The relationship with the family of origin continues to unfold and present new issues as the adult child relates to parents and siblings. One family physician noted that a 21-year-old black man had to be hospitalized for a crisis in his sickle cell disease every time he started to move out of the family home to attend vocational school. The basic task of balancing differentiation and closeness surfaces again and again through the life cycle, and it may bring special problems or unique support for the adult who is not married. If parents and siblings do a good job of letting go, the task will be easier for the single person, and vice versa (Haley, 1980).

Differentiation may be inappropriately slow or fast: Family members may collaborate to keep change from occurring, or they may dispense with a gradual process and "kick" the child out of the house. The successful or unsuccessful resolution of individual and group issues will interact with the broader family task of parent-child differentiation (Carter & McGoldrick, 1980). For example, if the parents have compensated for an empty or conflictual relationship by focusing their energies on the children, both parents and children may keep the adult child overinvolved in the family. The process may be more difficult when the first or last child is leaving, or when another sibling is left in the family spotlight.

Another important variable in the transition from family of origin to autonomous adulthood is the life situation to which the single adult moves. If the person is able to provide for the necessities of life and organize her or his resources to meet most needs previously met by family, the transition will be smoother. A recent case in our clinic involved a single parent who had returned to live with her mother after she had been unable to make it on her own in another state. As the young mother began to bring her baby to the clinic because of a variety of minor medical complaints, the physician learned about the woman's home situation. As the visits began to center more on the woman's need to talk to someone about her family stress, the physician realized the visits were the mother's excuse to come in. Taking this woman's family system into account led to a broader understanding of the medical complaints. If the physician's data gathering had been more restricted and had dealt only with somatic complaints, the patient probably would have continued to present more symptoms or she would have given up and turned elsewhere until she found someone who would listen to her.

The same differentiation must occur whether a person marries or chooses to remain single, but the process is aided for the married couple by the concrete reality of another family system. Unfortunately, singleness is often viewed as a stage at which a person is still not accorded full adult status, whereas marriage serves as a rite of passage that guarantees that a person is no longer a child. Families vary in the extent to which they view marriage as the essential prerequisite of adulthood. As the single adult gets older and moves in and out of other systems, the family may let age instead of marriage become the marker of independence. Many families have an especially difficult time seeing single women as independent adults, because women traditionally have been viewed as needing the protection and support of a family system or, more accurately, of a man. This belief is still evidenced in the traditional marriage ceremony in which the woman is transferred from one family system to another by being "given away" by her father to her husband.

The realignment of family relationships has to do with both the quality and quantity of contacts. The amount of contact with parents and siblings is one aspect of differentiation; for some people the emotional leave-taking occurs without actual physical separation. But a person can be geographically distant from the original home and still be deeply enmeshed in the family system.

G.P., a 39-year-old single woman, had not lived in her mother's home for many years, yet her life was overwhelmingly bound up with her family of origin. During a visit to her home, her family physician learned that her family's boundaries were diffuse and its organization chaotic. In addition to her own six children, she was the constant caretaker of brothers, sisters, and extended family members who drifted in and out, staying for maybe a day or maybe a year. As a result of this new information, the physician began to think of the patient's clinic visits as an attempt to define some boundaries in her life, as she came alone complaining of high blood pressure and tension headaches whenever she seemed to have lost all sense of having a life of her own. The physician realized that the mere act of seeing the woman by herself offered her a rare chance to be alone in an orderly environment where she was taken seriously as an individual.

While checking her blood pressure or doing other necessary examinations, the physician listened to the patient talk about her family and encouraged her to set appropriate boundaries in practical, concrete ways. Whenever G.P. had a plan or related an incident in which she had effectively set limits, the physician encouraged her and mentioned to her the setbacks she might expect. He tried to help her think of specific ideas, like attending church or going for walks, that would provide her with time alone or with people other than family members. By his continuing care of the patient, the physician was able to model a relationship with clear boundaries that provided security and consistency. He began seeing the patient for brief monthly "checkups," even if she had no specific physical complaint. The routine assured her that he was available to her, but that the amount of help she could expect from him was defined.

The task for the family is to develop boundaries between members that allow for individual differences without forfeiting the essential identity and loyalty of the group (Minuchin, 1974). The single adult may express continuity and discontinuity with the family of origin in concrete ways such as personal tastes, attitudes toward material possessions, decisions about employment, and sexual behavior. The family's reaction will depend on its history of dealing with the issues and its style of relating to independence in general. Another influence is the degree to which decisions are congruent or incongruent with the person's past behavior and values as perceived by the family.

Finances often serve as a metaphor for the family's progress in working through developmental issues. Parents may continue to contribute to the support of an adult child, particularly if extended education is involved. Though the givers and the recipient may have different ideas about the meaning attached to financial support, some sense of obligation is often implied or felt. At the other extreme are families who cannot provide monetary support or who deliberately withhold it. In these situations, the young adults may have the burden of independence without the means to provide adequately for their own needs.

Family systems to which the single adult belongs may extend beyond the family of origin. A divorced person may still be emotionally married, e.g., the 40-year-old patient who still has dinner with his ex-wife and children three or four times a week. Former in-laws may also be important. The extended family system may continue to be a source of blame or support for the divorced person, and the former relatives may still function actively in kinship roles for children.

The family physician should assume that the single person is involved in one or more significant systems of relationships that will influence the person's illness and subsequent treatment. Consider this case: A 24-year-old single woman came to the Family Practice Clinic with complaints of vaginal itching and burning. Discussion revealed that her real concern was that she might be pregnant and that her partner might not agree to an abortion, an alternative she preferred. As the conversation turned to contraception, the family practice resident sensed her ambivalence about the use of birth control devices. The woman felt caught between her own desire not to become pregnant and her companion's wish to have a child with her. Her response was to avoid the issue of contraception and to present to the doctor with vaginitis, which she saw as an "official" excuse not to have sexual relations. The doctor introduced the topic of contraception and talked with the patient about her mixed feelings. She decided to be fitted for a diaphragm and to talk to her partner about their conflict.

Other social systems evolve at work and in other settings, in some cases approximating the intensity or structure of family relationships. Building a foundation of emotional support is a major task for single adults. Strategies may include joining organizations (e.g., religious, athletic, political groups), developing recreational hobbies and interests, and pursuing intense emotional relationships with other people, one of whom may eventually become the marriage partner. Many churches promote the image of their fellowship as a "family" for single people. A person's living situation may also resemble a family environment. Particularly in the case of cohabitation of young single adults, living together is often a substitute for or a prelude to marriage.

The Work Environment

The meaning of work is a salient factor to consider in the treatment of a single person. People in a lower socioeconomic position may have as their goal the acquisition of the basic necessities of life, so that employment is primarily a means to that end. Middle-class people may aspire to jobs or careers with intrinsic meaning as well as financial profit. All adults must come to grips with what is necessary and satisfying in their lives, and productivity is often a part of this evaluation. A crisis or increased anxiety at work may exacerbate a physical condition such as hypertension or ulcerative colitis.

The physician needs to note the combination of unusual work-related stress and family problems. The hard-driving, divorced executive who is at high risk of a heart attack presents a case in which occupational context might interact with singleness to create a particularly vulnerable situation in which intimate support is lacking. Colleagues may fill some roles otherwise played by family members. For a middle-aged, never-married schoolteacher, for example, the discovery of her terminal cancer may cause feelings of loss like those she would feel about family members because her pupils may have become her surrogate children (Stein & Fox, in press).

The Timing of the Complaint

It is always important to note the timing of an illness, that is: Why now? Why do people have symptoms or needs at a particular time? What prompts them to seek medical care when they do? The physician needs to seek clues to the meaning of the illness within a larger constellation of events in the same way he or she takes a medical history and asks about contexts of symptoms to discover biomedical patterns.

A family-practice resident, examining a 36-year-old single woman who complained of back pain and headaches, discovered that the woman's welfare payments had stopped when she began clerical job training two weeks earlier. The woman's children had been enrolled in a daycare center for the first time. In short, the occupational change disturbed the entire system of relationships and institutions with which this family was involved. The resident talked with the patient about the multiple changes in her life, suggesting that her symptoms might be her body's way of mirroring stress. She assured her that her feelings and physical reactions were normal for a person undergoing so many major changes at once. She reminded her that there is a difference between coping poorly and coping well with a difficult situation; she told the patient that she seemed to be coping very well. The woman responded to the physician's support and encouragement, and, at last report, the patient's headaches and back pain had abated.

The sense of timing that defines the life situations a person is leaving, currently facing, and moving toward are all important to note. The physician may treat a complaint of insomnia differently if he or she knows from a conversation or a note in the chart that the patient is recovering from a divorce or the death of a spouse. Knowledge of the patient's past patterns of handling problems or stress may influence the doctor's treatment approach. In the present, a single person may be dealing with parenthood, aging parents, plans to marry, economic hardship, a physical handicap, or substance abuse. Whatever the life situation, the physician needs to assess the meaning of the medical concern in the context of the single person's present set of systems. Illness behavior may have significant meaning in more than one family system, particularly if the person is still involved with the family of origin. The future is the other timing consideration that may become important in treatment. Is a person transient or stable, secure or insecure in income and employment, increasing or decreasing responsibilities toward family of origin, moving toward marriage or continued singleness?

The Divorced Single Person

The following data illustrate the high risk of medical problems among divorced persons:

- Bachrach (1973) found that admission rates to private psychiatric hospitals of divorced and separated men were 1,904.9 per 100,000 compared to 271.8 per 100,000 for married and 927.4 per 100,000 for never-married men.
- McMurray (1970) demonstrated that the motor vehicular accident rate of persons undergoing divorce doubled during six months before and six months after the divorce.
- A study by the National Center for Health Statistics (1976), involving 88,000 households, revealed that divorced and separated persons had the highest number of visits to physicians per year and the highest yearly incidence of acute medical illnesses when compared to widowed, married, and never-married people.

Other studies have shown linkages between marital separation/divorce and deaths from suicide/homicide (Kitagawa & Hauser, 1973) and specific illnesses including tuberculosis, cirrhosis of the liver, and cancer of the lung (National Center for Health Statistics, 1976).

The physician who provides continuous care will inevitably note some marked changes in the health patterns of some patients who are becoming single again through divorce. As the family physician may be the health care provider for other family members as well, he or she should be alert for somatic difficulties in them also, as the change in the marriage reverberates throughout the family system.

The Process of Becoming Single Again Through Divorce

The physician who understands typical patterns and issues associated with divorce will do a better job in meeting the needs of patients who are making that transition and adjusting to a new life. Although the transition to divorce can be conceptualized in many different ways, the people involved perceive it as a decision, made by someone, for some reason, over some period of time, and surrounded by some circumstances.

Divorce is a complicated and bewildering occurrence that leaves both the person experiencing it and those looking on with questions about how and why it happens. The decision to divorce is based on messages from the wider cultural system whose rules about marriage have changed as expectations have moved from survival needs to companionship as the priority. These changes have been accompanied by a growing tolerance for divorce, as is evident in the trend toward more liberal divorce laws. The rising divorce rate masks the fact that desertions and unofficial separation often substituted for legal divorce in the past. Though popular opinion interprets the rise in divorce as a sign of the disintegration of the family, most family scholars disagree, believing that present-day Americans are expecting more from marriage and are less willing to settle for an unfulfilling family life (Cherlin, 1981; Crosby, 1980).

Because divorce is a process, not an event, the family physician may encounter a patient at any phase, from the early time of pressure and dissatisfaction to the time when adjustment has been made. For most people the legal divorce does not signal the end of all that is involved in becoming single again.

One of our patients complained of migraine headaches that had begun about the time he and his wife had separated. The headaches had continued to bother him until well after the divorce was granted. When he came to the clinic, the physician noted that the patient was still wearing his wedding ring, a concrete indication of what the physician then learned by asking questions—the marriage, though legally over, was still very much intact. It was helpful to the patient to understand that his mixed desires to return to his wife and to end the relationship entirely were part of a process that would probably continue until the relationship was emotionally over. The family physician knew that there are normal vacillations in a system that is evolving into a "bi-nuclear family" (Ahrons, 1980), that is, two families resulting from a divorce who are tied together by shared children. The physician understood also that people often do not think past the legal divorce, envisioning that one event as the solution to their problems; typically, new problems will emerge.

By normalizing the patient's experience, the physician helped the man to label vague feelings and to anticipate future issues that might surface as the divorce process continued:

> Almost everyone who goes through a divorce has second thoughts about it afterwards. That's normal, and it doesn't mean that you have made a mistake in getting out of the marriage. It *does* mean that there were some good things about the situation as well as the bad things that made you want to leave. No decision is 100% certain. Most of us have to be content with 60-40, 70-30, or even 51-49 decisions. Often the aftermath means some regrets or at least some doubts, and it seems that you're feeling those things now, right? It's a healthy sign that you're willing to deal with these issues in an honest way. You can expect this process to continue for a good while; it takes a long time to get out of the habit of being with someone, even it it's been a bad situation. From what you've said, I suspect that your friends, children, and parents will have some trouble adjusting to the new arrangement, and that may not always be pleasant. It sounds like your wife still has some unfinished business to work through, too, and she is expressing that by keeping you away from the children. If she would be willing to come in, I might be able to help you set up some ground rules so that everyone at least knows what to expect.

Although the ex-wife and children did not come in for a whole-family interview, the physician was able to intervene in the family system by helping the patient to adjust to the divorce.

The period of adjustment to divorce is usually understood in terms of a reaction to loss, using a stage theory such as the stages of grief as the chief descriptive model (Salts, 1979). For the family physician who may be seeing patients in the earlier stages of the transition to divorce, understanding the decision-making process is equally if not more important.

People go into relationships with certain expectations about the rewards and costs (Thibaut & Kelley, 1959), and these expectations become rules of the relationship system (Minuchin, 1974). In the language of social psychology, people get divorced when the costs of being married outweigh the benefits (Levinger, 1976). One of us (Baker, 1981) studied husbands and wives who had recently filed for divorce. We found that the breakdown of the marriage itself seems to be the focus of divorcing people, and alternative attractions and barriers act mainly as intervening variables that influence the timing and circumstances of the decision. The vast majority of our research participants reported that they did not reject the institution of marriage, but they rejected their particular marriage partner.

A person can choose how to assimilate change that alters the attractions of a relationship, picking alternatives to maintaining it or barriers to getting out. He or she may avoid the disturbances, which is a typical reaction for a period of time. The person may deny that any problem exists or deliberately decide that the change is not important enough to justify any other adjustments. Another option is to change the rules to fit the new behavior, or to change the behavior to fit the old rules. A husband may, for example, have expected his wife not to have an affair. When he discovers that she is involved with someone, he can try to get her to change her behavior to fit that idea, or he may alter his own expectations. The latter change may also cause him to change his own behavior, which may mean retaliating with an extramarital relationship of his own. Finally, an individual may decide, based on an assessment of costs and rewards, that neither the original expectations nor the new behavior is amenable to change, in which case divorce becomes the path to take. At some point, one partner reaches an "emotional point of no return" (Federico, 1979). The responses may be accomplished by several different strategies: Couples may accommodate, provoke each other, retaliate, or negotiate.

A couple is likely to go through this cycle several times, following various paths each time, before the two finally experience legal divorce. The emotional divorce takes longer.

Baker's (1981) data show that most people felt that their marriages were good at the beginning; when the relationship started to erode, about two years went by before they first thought of divorce as an option. Deciding to divorce is a complex, subtle negotiating process in which the role of leaver, decision maker, and initiator is shared. Rarely in a marriage does one person clearly see either himself or herself *or* the spouse as the one who first mentioned divorce and followed up by making the decision, leaving, and filing. Marriage partners do perceive one of the two as doing each of these things (though often they do not agree on which one it is), but the process is not made up of simple, unilateral decisions.

As the transition to divorce takes place, people go through a cognitive process of developing an account of what is happening. This continues well into the adjustment period and fills a primary need with which friends and professional care providers become involved. Much divorce counseling is aimed at helping spouses reach closure about what has happened in their marriage.

Partly in the role of listener, the physician can provide much needed support as the divorcing person tries to make sense of it all. Baker (1981) found that parents often file for divorce before talking to their children about it. The physician may be able to remind the parent that it is best to be direct in explaining the situation to the children, at the same time reassuring them that they have not caused the problems. Parents may have the best intentions in not talking to their children, or they may fail to tell them because they are not ready to admit the seriousness of the problem. Regardless of the reason, children are quick to sense tension and are likely to be confused and anxious from the double messages they get. Conversely, the uncertainty and tension may cause some parents to confide inappropriately in their children, talking to the children about the divorce before discussing it with their spouses.

Discrepancies in Divorce

If the physician sees both partners, he or she may hear two vastly different views about the marriage. Baker's (1981) study showed that the couples agreed only on who filed for divorce. She found discrepancies in the accounts of people who perceived themselves as the leavers of the marriage and those who saw themselves left, and between men's and women's experience of divorce. In general it is a harder, slower process for men than for women; the same is true for those who are left as opposed to the ones who actively leave the marriage (Brown, 1976; Crosby, Gage, & Raymond, 1980; Kressel, Jaffee, Tuchman, Watson, & Deutsch, 1980). Though every role has its unique pain, these differences should make the family physician particularly alert to the needs of men who are left by their wives, in that they can be expected to have a higher risk of illness and injury.

The following case illustrates one family physician's experience with a couple going through the transition to divorce. The patient was a 24-year-old woman who had one child. Three months postpartum, she began to have a persistent, mid-abdominal pain that would sometimes prevent her from eating. The pain was accompanied by vomiting and occasionally by severe diarrhea. An exhaustive evaluation failed to identify an organic cause and the patient did not respond to medical treatment. Meanwhile, she brought in her son several times because of multiple minor problems which could not be diagnosed specifically. During one visit, when the physician began to ask questions about her marriage, the patient broke into tears and reported great unhappiness. In a subsequent interview with the husband and wife, they said that there was little caring and no physical relationship between them. They refused to be referred for further counseling and stopped coming to the clinic. A year later the husband came in for evaluation of hypertension that had recently become a problem. He said that his wife had taken the child and left the state; the physician heard him express feelings similar to those his wife had had a year before. A few months later the physician again saw the couple together in his office when they brought their son for a medical checkup. They had decided to divorce, and she had moved back to the state so that the husband could see the child. In this case the physician's attention to the divorce process was a key factor in the medical treatment of every family member.

The Physician's Role

The physician may choose different levels of involvement in dealing with the individual, the couple, or the family on issues concerning divorce. But as family systems theorists are fond of saying, "One cannot *not* communicate." Whatever the physician does, he or she is communicating something. In the doctor-patient-family system, even if the physician decides never to discuss the divorce process, he or she is giving a message.

One choice would be simply to identify the divorcing person as at high risk of medical illness and psychological strain and to practice preventive medicine by checking up on the patient more frequently and trying to ward off illness by encouraging good nutrition, stress management, and other healthy habits. The next step would be to provide a listening ear when and if the patient needs to talk about marital problems. If the patient seems to want more time or direction in discussing divorce issues, the physician may choose to refer the patient to another professional for counseling. If the physician decides to spend time counseling the patient, he or she then has the option of asking other family members to participate in the discussions. The most active and complex role for the physician would be to counsel the entire family. Different physicians will find themselves more or less comfortable with one of these alternatives depending on their own skills and the needs of their patients.

There are several reasons a physician might choose to see the couple or family together:

- to see firsthand what the family is like instead of hearing individual family members' accounts of what goes on in the family;
- to communicate that the physician is not siding with only one family mem-

ber but is supportive of each person, even if they choose not to remain together;

- to help the couple or family come to some agreement about their future interactions, especially those concerning children;
- to determine whether or not the situation calls for a counseling referral.

One important question is whether or not one or both partners have passed the "emotional point of no return" mentioned earlier. In that case, the orientation should shift to issues of differentiation and adjustment instead of reconciliation.

Since divorce is a process that encompasses the entire family, there are issues that must be dealt with by the individuals involved (including children), the couple, and the family system as a whole (Table 1). The doctor may do a "review of systems" to learn which areas are causing problems. Perhaps members of the marital subsystem are making the transition in a fairly healthy way, but those in the parent-child subsystem or the whole family system are having problems. Divorce issues have to do with shifting boundaries that delineate who is in and who is out of the family. These changing rules extend to the social community and to the extended family, who begin to act differently as the marriage partners break the "couple front." Families will normally oscillate between stages as they develop new arrangements and expectations. The problem to watch for is when a family stabilizes at that transition, being unable to move back to the former stage or to let go and move ahead (Breunlin, 1982). Because of the practice of continuous care, the family physician is in an excellent position to watch for this problem.

Summary

The physician should be aware of the wide range of situations in which single adults live and of the implications of these factors to the provision of health care. The meaning and experience of being single are changing as demography, economics, and social mores continue to shift. There are not only more singles, but there is more diversity among them than ever before. The fundamental issues of singleness will be different for the never-married, the divorced, and the widowed person. Out of the balance of opportunities, resources, and values will grow a personal style in which a person organizes life without the benefit of a clear map of societal expectations. Whatever social networks surround the person, be they work-related, family-related, or otherwise, the family physician can use her or his understanding of illness as a process that involves all of these contexts. In many cases the family

Table 1
Issues in the Transition to Divorce: A Review of Systems

Family	*Couple*	*Individual*
Transformation to binuclear family system	Escalating conflict	*Spouses*
Change in extended family relationships	Clarifying issues	Emotional autonomy
Shifting boundaries—living arrangements, emotional bonds, rules	Deciding to divorce	Developing an "account" of the divorce
Redistribution of resources—time, money, space, energy, possessions	Disengagement	Resolving negative feelings
	Relationship to community—breaking "couple front"	Helping children deal with changes
	Negotiating changes—resources, rules	Accommodating lifestyle changes
	Closure on marriage	Establishing network of support as single person
	Establishing new parenting roles	*Children*
		Developing an "account" of the divorce
		Resolving negative feelings
		Accommodating lifestyle changes
		Accepting shift in parent-child relationship

physician has the advantage of seeing patients over time, so that she or he can modify an approach to fit the patient's changing needs.

The notion of disease as a biopsychosocial process is the heart of family medicine. This basic view shares with family systems theory the emphasis on context, and in no case is that view more important than in the life and health care needs of the single adult.

REFERENCES

Ahrons, C. (1980). Divorce: A crisis of family transition and change. *Family Relations, 29*, 533-540.

Bachrach, L.L. (1973). *Marital status of discharges from psychiatric inpatient units of general hospitals, United States 1970-1971: I. Analysis by age, color, and sex* [Statistical Note 82: National Institute of Mental Health]. Washington, D.C.: U.S. Government Printing Office.

Baker, L.C. (1981). *The transition to divorce: Discrepancies between husbands and wives*. Unpublished doctoral dissertation, Purdue University, West Lafayette, IN.

Bernard, J. (1982). *The future of marriage* (2nd ed.) New Haven: Yale University Press.

Breunlin, D. (1982, October). The clinical implications of the family life cycle. Workshop presented at annual meeting of the American Association of Marriage and Family Therapists, Dallas, Texas.

Brown, E. (1976). A model of the divorce process. *Conciliation Courts Review, 1*, 1-10.

Cargan, L., & Melko, M. (1982). *Singles: Myths and realities*. Beverly Hills: Sage Publications.

Carter, E.A., & McGoldrick, M. (1980). *The family life cycle*. New York: Gardner Press.

Cherlin, A. (1981). *Marriage, divorce, and remarriage*. Cambridge, MA: Harvard University Press.

Crosby, J.F. (1980). A critique of divorce statistics and their interpretation. *Family Relations, 29*, 51-58.

Crosby, J.F., Gage, B.A., & Raymond, M.C. (1980, October). *The grief resolution process in divorce*. Paper presented at annual meeting of the National Council on Family Relations, Portland, OR.

Federico, J. (1979). The marital termination period of the divorce adjustment process. *Journal of Divorce, 3*, 93-106.

Gordon, M. (1978). *The American family: Past, present, and future*. New York: Random House.

Haley, J. (1980). *Leaving home*. New York: McGraw-Hill.

Kitagawa, E.M., & Hauser, P.M. (1973). *Differential mortality in the United States: A study in socioeconomic epidemiology*. Cambridge, MA: Harvard University Press.

Kressel, K., Jaffee, N., Tuchman, B., Watson, C., & Deutsch, M. (1980). A typology of divorcing couples: Implications for mediation and the divorce process. *Family Process, 19*, 101-116.

Levinger, G. (1976). A social psychological perspective on marital dissolution. *Journal of Social Issues, 32*, 21-47.

Masnick, G., & Bane, M.J. (1980). *The nation's families: 1960-1990*. Cambridge, MA: Joint Center for Urban Studies.

McMurray, L. (1970). Emotional stress and driving performance: The effect of divorce. *Behavioral Research in Highway Safety, 1*, 100-114.

Minuchin, S. (1974). *Families and family therapy*. Cambridge, MA: Harvard University Press.

National Center for Health Statistics (1976). *Differentials in health characteristics by marital status: United States, 1971-1972*. Vital and health statistics. Series 10:104. Washington, DC: U.S. Government Printing Office.

Salts, C.J. (1979). Divorce process: Integration of theory. *Journal of Divorce, 2*, 233-240.

Stein, P. (Ed.). (1981). *Single life*. New York: St Martin's Press.

Stein, H.F. & Fox, D.P. (in press). Work as family: Occupational relationships and social transference. In H.F. Stein & M. Apprey (Eds.), *Context and dynamics in clinical knowledge*. Charlottesville: University Press of Virginia.

Thibaut, J.W., & Kelley, H.H. (1959). *The social psychology of groups*. New York: Wiley.

9

EVALUATING AND COUNSELING ADOLESCENTS

SERGIO HENAO, M.D.

My purpose here is to address some general issues a family physician may think about when dealing with families who have adolescent children. Specific clinical problems are discussed in other chapters of this book.

The Biological Context

In evaluating an adolescent, the physician's first priority is to assess the patient's physical health. This is amply covered in medical textbooks; there is, however, an aspect of the biological basis of behavior that deserves special consideration here. Terms like personality traits, constitution, or temperament have been used to describe this. Thomas and Chess (1984), who conducted the most comprehensive studies of these traits from early infancy to adult life, chose "temperament" to indicate a set of behavioral characteristics that are present at birth and represent the constitutional substratum for the development of individual behavior. This behavior is "the result of a continuously evolving interaction between a child with his individual characteristics (temperament) and significant features of his intrafamilial and extrafamilial environment" (Chess & Thomas, 1977, p. 219). They developed nine categories to describe temperament and to analyze the evolution of this temperament from infancy into adulthood: activity level, rhythmicity (regularity), approach or withdrawal, adaptability, threshold of responsiveness, intensity of reaction, quality of mood, distractability, and attention span. Based on these temperamental characteristics they classified children as "easy," "difficult," and "slow-to-warm-up." Parental attitudes and behavior under normal circumstances do not seem decisive in the development of these characteristics during the first year of life.

The expression of the child's temperament will, however, be determined and shaped by interaction with familial and environmental factors. At a particular time in the child's development the child's behavior will be determined by the fit between these various forces. No single set of temperamental characteristics is predictive of psychopathology even for the temperamentally "difficult child." The eventual outcome in terms of normal or abnormal functioning is determined by the interaction of temperamental, familial, and social influences.

These concepts have important implications for counseling parents and their adolescents. If, within the normal range of variations, a child exhibits a high level of motor activity, a short attention span, a low threshold of responsiveness, and tendency toward intense reactions as part of his or her temperament, the probabilities of that child's developing behavioral disturbances may well depend on the parents' level of tolerance and comfort with these characteristics. Impatient, anxious parents may respond negatively to this child, which may exacerbate the problem. A particularly stressful period in a family's life cycle also may disrupt the parents' ability to deal with this child and lead to the eruption of behavioral problems even though the parents were previously well adjusted to the child's temperament.

Such a situation is illustrated by the case of a 14-year-old boy who was brought to my office because of his undisciplined behavior at home and at school. His father had died six months before in a fishing accident. The child had been difficult to discipline before the father's death, but had not been a behavioral problem because of his father's firm and loving attitude. The mother, devastated by the loss of her husband, was so incapable of managing her son that she sent him to a military school.

Thomas and Chess (1984) stressed the importance of what they call "unpredictable events or changes in life situations" as well as "unpredictable changes in the individual" in determining a child's eventual behavior and the outcome of a particular situation. In illustrating this, they described the case of a child whose behavioral problems had developed during her preschool years (p. 7).

The child had a difficult temperament, to which her father responded with rigid demands for quick, positive adaptation, and hostile criticism and punishment when the girl could not meet his expectations. The mother, who was intimidated by both her husband and daughter, was vacillating and anxious with the child. As the girl's symptoms worsened, she entered psychotherapy but achieved only modest improvement. At age nine, the girl blossomed with musical and dramatic talent, which brought her favorable attention and praise from teachers and other parents. This talent also rated high in her parents' hierarchy of desirable attributes. Her father began to see his daughter's intense, explosive personality not as a sign of a "rotten kid," his previous label, but as evidence of a budding artist. As he began to make allowances for the child's "artistic temperament," the mother was able to relax and relate positively to her daughter. The girl was allowed to adapt at her own pace, and by adolescence all evidence of her neurotic symptoms and functioning had disappeared. Early adult follow-up at age 22 showed that she had continued to function well.

Assessment of an adolescent's temperamental characteristics is essential in counseling adolescents who have behavioral problems, as well as their parents. It is also evident that the complexity of interaction between temperament, family, and social characteristics as well as unforeseen events at any level—individual, familial, or social—make predictions hazardous indeed.

The Family Context

Traditionally, growing up and moving out of the family has been considered a major developmental task of adolescents and, until recently, developmental theorists paid little attention to developmental stages after adolescence. This has changed, however, with the research on adult development (Gould, 1972; Levinson, 1977), which was heralded by Erikson's eight ages of man (1950). These studies showed that a human being's psychological evolution does not stop in adolescence but continues throughout life, and they provided evidence "that the adult period is a time of active and systematic change" (Gould, 1972, p. 531). The child going through adolescence, with all its physical and developmental changes, is intimately engaged with adults, primarily his or her parents, who are themselves experiencing developmental changes, probably those of their own mid-life transition.

The psychological functioning of family members depends in many respects on their own and others' psychological developmental stage. This may seem so obvious that one should not mention it. Yet the professional psychiatric literature has been so dominated by an individual-oriented theory of development that the multifactorial and systemic view has received scant attention.

Hartmann (1958), for example, preferred the study of ego development and function in what he called the "average expectable environment." One can hardly imagine what this might be. Discussing adolescent rebellion, Marohn (1980) wrote: "I am not so concerned with those familial, social, environmental, cultural, or political factors which sustain, stimulate or provoke adolescent rebellious behavior. Rather, I am interested in the psychic and psychological configurations which resonate with and precipitate states of mind readily expressed in overt rebellion" (p. 175). As this kind of emphasis is presented as a personal intellectual preference, which puts it beyond argument, one might not realize that, given the impossibility of isolating human beings from their social context, this is a theoretically untenable proposition.

The interdependence of individual behavior and its social context was brilliantly illustrated in the neurobiological research of Jose Delgado (1969), who used remote radio stimulation of the members of a monkey colony. These studies had the advantage of preserving the natural social structure of monkey colonies as opposed to previous experiments performed with isolated individual monkeys. These colonies usually have a clearly defined leader who determines feeding, mating, and other activities. Radio stimulation of the leading monkey's brain produced increased aggressivity and attacks against other competing males of the colony but not toward a favorite female partner. Depending on the stimulated monkey's social rank, aggressive attacks were modified; a low-ranking monkey whose rage center was stimulated might show no aggressive response. In Delgado's view, the expression of behavior depends on social setting. He concluded that: "We cannot be free from parents, teachers, and society, because they are the extracerebral sources of our minds" (p. 243).

Clearly, the behavior of adolescents must be evaluated in the social context of the family, especially the parents', because individual psychological development does not take place inevitably and independently of that social context. A rigid, tyrannical father or a depressed, alcoholic mother may play a crucial role in what otherwise may be perceived as adolescent turmoil or adolescent pathology. These problems may not become evident if the physician evaluates the adolescent without simultaneously assessing the family context. The adolescent's rebelliousness may be a reaction to the parents' rigidity and vice versa.

Family research has shown also that optimum level of family functioning may not be necessary for the development of healthy, normal children. Parents may have significant psychopathological problems and still manage to perform adequately as parents (Masterson, 1967a). Westley and Epstein (1969) reported similar findings.

Lewis, Beavers, Gossett, and Phillips (1976) found that children from families they termed "competent but pained" developed and functioned normally. Difficulties in the parents' relationship led to relatively benign mother-son and father-daughter alliances that did not become a source of conflict. The longitudinal studies of Thomas and Chess (1976) also showed that, even in families that had long-lasting conflicts and illness, some of the children improved or even recovered. Thomas and Chess believe that what differentiated the adolescents who did improve from the ones who did not was the adolescents' ability to shift interests and emotional commitments to extrafamilial activities or people.

Family Triangles

The study of families has led to the observation of family alliances and coalitions which are "familiar" to many of us in very personal ways. A common observation about these coalitions is that they often involve three persons in a family, two taking sides against the third, and are therefore called "triangles" by family theoreticians.

Bowen (1966) wrote:

> The basic building block of any emotional system is the triangle. In calm periods, two members of the triangle have a comfortable emotional alliance, and the third, in the unfavored outsider position, moves either toward winning the favor of one of the others or toward rejection, which may be planned as winning favor. In tension situations, the outsider is in the favored position and both of the emotionally overinvolved ones will predictably make efforts to involve the third in the conflict. When tension increases, it will involve increasing outside members, the emotional circuits running on a series of emotional triangles. (p. 356)

This type of triangulation is normally present in human relations, but when it becomes rigid and repetitive it may lead to psychological and behavioral problems, especially if children are involved. Usually in these cases one parent, the mother, is overinvolved with the adolescent, while the father is peripheral and often criticized by the mother and child. The parents may have a conflictual relationship which causes one of them gradually to develop a coalition with the child across generational boundaries.

This situation is illustrated by a 17-year-old girl who was brought to my office because she was anxious, shy, and socially isolated. The father spent a great deal of time away from the family. He often complained that his wife was a poor mother who did not know how to help their daughter. The mother resented her husband's lack of support, but instead of settling this issue with her husband she became increasingly enmeshed with the daughter in an effort to become a better mother. She did this while experiencing a mixture of strong feelings of anger, guilt, and insecurity, all of which made her mothering more difficult and inadequate. The daughter, on the other hand, grew more insecure and dependent, which in turn precipitated more angry tirades from the father, and so on.

Sometimes in an unstable coalition each parent may try to win the child to his or her side, while the child will be afraid of choosing sides lest his or her behavior be interpreted as supporting one parent against the other. This is often seen in younger children and in child custody cases. As the child grows older a more stable and rigid coalition may develop.

Another form of triangulation is the classic process of scapegoating in which both parents are united in their attacks ("the child is bad") or exaggerated concerns ("the child is mad"). The parents' alliance may also serve the function of protecting the marriage and distracting from any marital conflict the parents may be unwilling to face. Often the coalitions involve three generations—as, for example, when grandparents, who consider their divorced daughter immature and inadequate as a mother, become overinvolved in the care of their grandchildren. Because of the increased existence of single-parent households, it is then important for the physician to investigate all, not only nuclear, family involvements. The raising of adolescent children is particularly difficult for single, working mothers when grandparents become too involved. The involvement of grandparents in the care of children in single-parent families is not necessarily pathological; it may be necessary for family survival, as is very commonly seen in poor black families.

As I have said, conflict between parents does not necessarily mean that the children will function abnormally. As Bowen (1966) observed:

> The fact that there are some families with intense marital conflict and no impairment of children is evidence that marital conflict does not, within itself, cause problems in children. The fact that serious impairment of children can develop in calm harmonious marriages is further evidence that the impairment of children can occur without conflict. (p. 361)

On the basis of his experience with families, Bowen believes that marital conflict and immaturity is manifested in three basic ways: overt marital disharmony and conflict; physical, psychological, or social dysfunction in one spouse; involvement of children through some of the mechanisms already discussed.

One may find one or all of these in a family, and the preponderance of one or the others may change depending on the family's life cycle or on unexpected events. Adolescence, with its major tasks of transformation of the child into an independent adult, is often a junction at which a child becomes involved in the chronic marital conflicts of his or her parents. Adolescent behavior becomes then the arena for marital battles.

The family physician will do well to remember that descriptions of triangulations and coalitions are artificial concepts and that each family needs to be evaluated on its own merits and in its own context. These concepts are maps, perhaps convenient ones, but a map is not the territory. It is not helpful, therefore, to point out these dynamics to the family because the labels will either anger them if they do not want to acknowledge their problems, or discourage them even more if they already know them. Families in which an adolescent is involved in a chronic conflictual relationship are better referred to professional therapists.

The Cultural Context

The adolescent's cultural context is the only other one I will discuss here. What might be considered mature behavior for a nonreligious Protestant adolescent girl in a large city might be thought abnormal and immoral for her Catholic counterpart living in a small town.

The psychiatric literature is filled with controversies on this issue with statements ranging from the extreme biological and individual orientation—Berman's (1970) pronouncement that "the basic dynamics of adolescent psychology are the same for all mankind"—to Prelinger's (1974) view that adolescence is a culturally created stage of life. Perhaps such a diversity of opinions arises from indiscriminate and unsophisticated use of terms such as puberty and adolescence. Puberty is the biological phenomenon of sexual maturation, while adolescence is its psychosocial correlate. Puberty is universal; adolescence is individually and culturally variable (Gadpaille, 1977).

Adolescent Turmoil as a Cultural Myth

Not only the general public but many health professionals believe that adolescence is a time of great conflict and turmoil. People jokingly commiserate with parents of adolescent children. This cultural tenet may in turn perpetuate an attitude toward adolescent children that will bring about the dreaded behavior. If one believes, for instance, that adolescents are rebellious, one may ask them to do something in a loud and demanding voice. This behavior, in turn, is most likely to stimulate a rebellious and defiant attitude in the adolescent. In other words, the danger of this belief is that it may easily become a self-fulfilling prophecy. To a great degree the belief in the inevitability of adolescent crises and turmoil comes from the professional literature. In her classic paper on adolescence, Anna Freud (1958) stated categorically that "there is, first, the ever recurrent question whether the adolescent upheaval is welcome and beneficial as such, whether it is necessary and, more than that, inevitable. On this point, psychoanalytic opinion is decisive and unanimous" (p. 267). And further: "The adolescent manifestations come close to symptom formation of the psychotic or dissocial order and merge almost imperceptibly into borderline states, initial, frustrated or fully-fledged forms of almost all the mental illnesses" (p. 267).

Anna Freud's paper had a profound influence on psychiatric theory and many other authors postulated similar views (Blos, 1962, 1967; Erikson, 1956) based for the most part on clinical experience. Recently, however, the collection of data from a small number of patients has shifted to studies based on normative data from large sample populations. This research shows a much less tumultuous adolescence than what had originally been portrayed in classic psychoanalytic writing, raising questions about the validity of sweeping generalizations about the inevitability of the adolescent turmoil syndrome.

Douvan and Adelson (1966), who studied a large number of high school students, concluded that these adolescents generally trusted their parents, derived much of their self-esteem from parental approval, and shared a core of common values with them. Rebellion was chiefly evident in disagreements about such things as music and dress. The teenagers showed little evidence of inner turmoil or ego disruption.

Having studied an older population of well-adjusted college freshmen, Grinker (1962) reported that they had impressive ego strength, supportive interpersonal relationships, and a healthy sense of self-esteem. There was no indication of severe inner turmoil or identity crises.

The Offers and their colleagues (Offer, Marcus, & Offer, 1970; Offer & Offer, 1969; Offer, Sabshin & Marcus, 1965), in the most comprehensive and persuasive studies of normal adolescent development to date, reported rebellion in early adolescence was present but not impressively so. They interviewed 73 boys in two high schools six times over a seven-year period. The children's and parents' chronic disagreements were related to such issues as household chores, dress, and curfew. There was no evidence of delinquency or emotional upheaval. The adolescents did not present serious changes in affect although they reported temporary periods of anxiety, depression, guilt, and shame. Only 7% of the group experienced significant emotional problems.

Clearly these data do not support the idea that normal adolescence is a period of severe inner turmoil, significant behavioral problems, or significantly conflictual relations with adults. The longitudinal studies of Thomas and Chess (1976) also showed that not all adolescents go through a period of major turmoil even when they are developing and coping on a healthy level. Furthermore, as Thomas and Chess pointed out, "The evidence from this group of adolescents indicates no a priori conclusion can be drawn as to the significance of the presence or absence of adolescent turmoil in any specific youngster. Each case has to be evaluated individually and in the perspective of the overall behavior and functioning" (p. 542).

Perpetuating the belief that adolescents must negotiate a period of inner turmoil and chaos has led to two other erroneous beliefs. One is that, since all adolescents must experience this upheaval, the ones that don't must be abnormal in some way. Here again, Anna Freud (1958) believed that the absence of this turmoil is

> a sign to be taken seriously. These are children who have built up excessive defenses against their drive activities and are now crippled by the results, which act as barriers against the normal maturational processes of phase development. They are, perhaps more than any others, in need of therapeutic help to remove the inner restrictions and clear the path for normal development, however "upsetting" the latter may prove to be. (p. 265)

It is then logical that, if adolescent turmoil is part of normal development, adolescents will "grow out of it." Research evidence already presented, as well as research by Masterson (1967a, 1967b, 1968), Masterson and Washburne (1966), Weiner and Delgado (1976) and Rutter, Graham, Chadwick, and Yale (1976), showed this to be an unfortunate view. These studies indicated that adolescent symptoms persist and become more differentiated over time, that psychiatric diagnosis may be difficult in adolescence, but that normal adolescent stress is clearly different from psychiatric disturbance. An excellent review of research on the validity of the concept of adolescent turmoil as a normal developmental stage may be found in Blotcky and Looney (1980).

Oldham (1978) summarized the main findings of these studies:

- Adolescents normally maintain psychic equilibrium as they struggle with developmental tasks.
- Adolescent development is usually associated with successful social and family adjustment which persists into early adulthood.
- Adolescent "turmoil" is normatively manifested by mild forms of depression and anxiety and minor disagreements with authority figures.
- Symptoms other than mild depression and anxiety often indicate psychiatric illness and may warrant professional attention.

- Adolescent symptom patterns tend to persist and become more differentiated over time.
- Adolescent "turmoil" is distinguishable from psychiatric illness but may intensify coexisting disorders.
- Difficulties in differential diagnosis during adolescence have more to do with obscurities inherent in psychiatric diagnoses themselves than with the presence or absence of "turmoil." (pp. 273-274)

Counseling by the Family Physician

A few of the adolescents seen by a family physician may need referral to a child psychiatrist or other mental health professional. This is particularly important in cases of severe psychopathology such as psychosis, drug abuse, or anorexia nervosa. These problems are discussed in subsequent chapters.

The great majority of adolescent patients do not need special referral. An alert and sensitive physician may be able to help many of these children and their families as well as prevent the development of more serious problems.

The term *counseling* has been used widely to indicate short-term, educational, and supportive guidance, as opposed to more intense, longer term child or family psychotherapy. In my view, in practice both terms overlap a great deal but the distinction is still a useful one. Thomas and Chess (1984) have successfully used what they call "parental guidance" with the children in their longitudinal research, which now covers more than 20 years. In their sample of 133 subjects followed from infancy to early adulthood they found that, with few exceptions, the patients treated with the parental-guidance approach recovered and were functioning well in adolescence and early adult life.

The basic emphasis of this treatment approach is on changing the parents' behaviors and attitudes towards their children. Before this can be done, however, one must give the parents support and understanding; if not done, parents will take the physician's suggestions as criticisms and will tend to react defensively, even though they may recognize the validity of the physician's comments. This is particularly true when parents need to be more consistent in disciplining their children. Once parents feel supported and understood, they will be more willing to explore alternative ways of behaving. The physician should present his or her suggestions as possible alternatives to be explored rather than the only appropriate solution to obvious problems the parents have created. Often the difficulties parents present are related to a poor fit between the child's temperament and a parent's attitudes. A child who is naturally timid, for example, may have a father who wants him or her to be outgoing and extroverted. In these cases, a simple explanation of this interaction may contribute to the parents' willingness to explore new behaviors. Sometimes the counseling may be directed at changing adverse environmental influences such as inappropriate school placement.

This approach does not attempt to change the parents' personalities or what may be conflicts in the marital relationship. Even when marital conflict is evident, it is better to concentrate on the children's problems as presented by the parents, at least at first, because the apparent marital conflict may be secondary to tensions generated by trying to cope with the children's problems. When relationships with the children are discussed first but there is indeed a longstanding marital conflict, the parents may spontaneously request help for this. At that point the physician may decide to refer them for marital therapy.

The emphasis of this approach is on changing the parents or at least on counseling primarily the parents. It is important to remember, however, that as the adolescent grows older he or she may need to be seen individually to be able to describe problems and concerns freely. A family systems orientation does not preclude sessions with individual family members; on the contrary, in many cases, particularly with adolescents, this may be necessary. I use the term *counseling* here, independent of emphasis on parent or child or both, and with the assumption that the family physician will maintain a family systems perspective no matter who is the counseled person.

The following are some additional considerations in planning family counseling.

Time

Family physicians need to realize that this kind of work requires time and effort. Family counseling may be very rewarding, but it may also be very frustrating if physicians are ambivalent about the time and money it may cost them. Most cases may be handled in a few sessions, but sometimes complicated situations will consume much time and energy. If physicians are undecided about this or a family begins to consume too much time, they should be referred to a mental health professional.

The Patient Is Always Right

Physicians should not argue with the patient—it takes a great deal of skill to turn an argument into a productive exchange. This does not mean avoiding firmness when necessary, but instead of arguing physicians should accept the family's wishes and point of view about their problems and their plans for changing them. If, for instance, the physician suggests that parents monitor their adolescent son's school performance more closely, and they refuse to do it, it may be better to drop the suggestion and wait to see if they become more receptive to the idea after a while. Sometimes the family physician may be able to use indirect or paradoxical methods (see Chapter 5 on the strategic approach), but for the most part these methods require time and special skills.

Listening and Clarifying

These are valuable, time-honored techniques but they are predicated on the assumption that the family doctor has time to sit down, listen carefully, and ask clarifying questions. Listening is not a passive activity. It requires concentrated effort and focused attention.

Using Common Sense

As someone has said that common sense is the least common of all senses, I may be excused for bringing up its importance. Even if a commonsense approach turns out not to work, it deserves a good try. Many people, at least in psychotherapy, believe that common sense has often been tried by the patient or family and therefore it is useless to try it again. In my opinion, common sense does not exist in the abstract and what may appear as common sense to the physician may have never occurred to the family. Common sense is affected by education, experience, and cultural beliefs. What looks like common sense to one person may look different to another.

One of my patients, for example, was a mother who believed that letting her anxious 12-year-old son sleep with her when he had insomnia made sense. When I explained to her why it made sense to stop it, she did so.

The Physician's Personality

This, perhaps the most crucial element in the physician's professional success, is particularly decisive in dealing with patients' psychological problems. If the physician is anxious or depressed, or optimistic and hopeful, all of this will be reflected in his or her work. Not that the physician has to be a model of mental health, but the quality of counseling is closely related to the quality of the physician's mental health. The physician who is anxious and irritable with his or her own children will find it difficult to persuade anxious, irritable parents to be calm and understanding with their children.

An old Sufi story illustrates this issue. Mulla Nasrudin, the legendary sage of Sufi stories, was visited by a mother who was worried about her son's excessive eating of sugar. She wanted him to tell her son to reduce sugar consumption, and she hoped that Nasrudin's authority might impress the youngster. Nasrudin asked her to bring her son in one week. When the two came, he asked them to return in two weeks. When Nasrudin finally saw them, he simply told the child to stop eating so much sugar. Surprised, the woman later asked him privately why it had taken him so long to talk to the child. Nasrudin responded that, before admonishing the child, he wanted to be sure he could stop eating so much sugar himself.

Investigating the Attempted Solutions

This issue has been covered extensively in Chapter 5, but it is so crucial that it deserves to be mentioned again. Clinical experience has shown that, when problems become repetitive and seem insoluble, careful analysis of the solutions will usually show that some single solution has been tried again and again despite the fact that the attempted solution never solved the problem. This leads to a vicious cycle not much different from the situation of a car stuck in the sand and the driver's insistence on solving the problem by pushing on the gas pedal. The result: wheel-spinning.

An example of this is the case of the mother I have mentioned. The child could not sleep, so the mother lay down with him to help him go to sleep. Subsequently, the child would become nervous if mother did not lie down with him, so mother did, and so on. The investigation of these attempted solutions will provide information to the physician about what not to do and will provide an opportunity to explore other possible solutions.

Clearly the main issue for adolescents and their families is the successful negotiation of their separation and the further development of the child into a mature and independent adult. This requires the child to become mature enough to leave and also the parents to be mature enough to let go.

This issue has been beautifully put by Kahlil Gibran in the *Prophet* (1923).

Your children are not your children.
They are the sons and daughters of Life's longing for itself.
They come through you but not from you,
And though they are with you yet they belong not to you.
You may give them your love but not your thoughts,
For they have their own thoughts.
You may house their bodies but not their souls,
For their souls dwell in the house of tomorrow, which you cannot visit,
not even in your dreams.
You may strive to be like them, but seek not to make them like you.
For life goes not backward nor tarries with yesterday.

REFERENCES

Berman, S. (1970). Alienation: An essential process of the psychology of adolescence. *Journal of the American Academy of Child Psychiatry, 9*, 233-250.

Blos, P. (1962). *On adolescence*. New York: Free Press.

Blos, P. (1967). The second individuation process of adolescence. *Psychoanalytic Study of the Child, 22*, 162-186.

Blotcky, M.J., & Looney, J.G. (1980). *Adolescent Psychiatry, 8*, 184-199.

Bowen, M., (1966). The use of family theory in clinical practice. *Comprehensive Psychiatry*, 7(5), 345-374.

Chess, S., & Thomas, A. (1977). Temperamental individuality from childhood to adolescence. *Journal of the American Academy of Child Psychiatry, 16*(2), 218-226.

Delgado, J.M.R. (1969). Physical control of the mind. *Toward a psychocivilized society*. New York: Harper & Row.

Douvan, E., & Adelson, J. (1966). *The adolescent experience*. New York: Wiley.

Erikson, E.H. (1950). *Childhood and society*. New York: Norton.

Erikson, E.H. (1956). The problem of ego identity. *Journal of the American Psychoanalytic Association, 4*, 56-121.

Freud, A. (1958). Adolescence. *Psychoanalytic Study of the Child, 13*, 255-278.

Gadpaille, W.J. (1977). Adolescence: Developmental phase or cultural artifact. *Adolescent Psychiatry, 5*, 143-150.

Gibran, K. (1923). *The prophet*. New York: Alfred A. Knopf.

Gould, R.L. (1972). The phases of adult life: A study in developmental psychology. *American Journal of Psychiatry, 129*, 521-531.

Grinker, R.R., Sr. (1962). Mentally healthy young males (homoclites). *Archives of General Psychiatry, 6*, 405-453.

Hartmann, H. (1958). *Journal of the American Psychoanalytic Association, Monograph Series No. 1 Ego psychology and the problem of adaptation*. (D. Rappaport, Trans.). New York: International Universities Press. (Original work published 1939).

Levinson, D.J. (1977). The mid-life transition: A period in adult psychological development. *Psychiatry, 40*, 99-112.

Lewis, J.M., Beavers, W.R., Gossett, J.T., & Phillips, V.A. (1976). *No single thread: Psychological health in family systems*. New York: Brunner/Mazel.

Marohn, R.C. (1980). Adolescent rebellion and the task of separation. *Adolescent Psychiatry, 8*, 173-183.

Masterson, J. (1967a). *The psychiatric dilemma of adolescence*. Boston: Little, Brown.

Masterson, J. (1967b). The symptomatic adolescent five years later: He didn't grow out of it. *American Journal of Pyschiatry, 123*, 1338-1345.

Masterson, J. (1968). The psychiatric significance of adolescent turmoil. *American Journal of Psychiatry, 124*, 1549-1554.

Masterson, J., & Washburne, A. (1966). The symptomatic adolescent: Psychiatric illness or adolescent turmoil. *American Journal of Psychiatry, 122*, 1240-1247.

Mead, M. (1928). *Coming of age in Samoa*. New York: Morrow.

Offer, D., Marcus, D., & Offer, J.L. (1970). A longitudinal study of normal adolescent boys. *American Journal of Psychiatry, 126*, 917-924.

Offer, D., & Offer, J.L. (1969). Growing up: A follow-up study of normal adolescents. *Seminars in Psychiatry, 1*, 45-56.

Offer, D., Sabshin, M., & Marcus, D. (1965). Clinical evaluation of normal adolescents. *American Journal of Psychiatry, 121*, 864-872.

Oldham, D.G. (1978). Adolescent turmoil: A myth revisited. *Adolescent Psychiatry, 7*, 267-279.

Prelinger, E. (1974). Crises of identity. In M.D. Hays (Ed.), *The identity crises*. New York, National Project Center for Film and the Humanities.

Rutter, M., Graham, P., Chadwick, O., & Yale, W. (1976). Adolescent turmoil: Fact or fiction. *Journal of Child Psychology and Psychiatry and Allied Disciplines, 17*, 35-56.

Thomas, A., & Chess, S. (1976). Evolution of behavior disorders into adolescence. *American Journal of Psychiatry, 133*(5), 539-542.

Thomas, A., & Chess, S. (1984). Genesis and evolution of behavioral disorders: From infancy to early adult life. *American Journal of Psychiatry, 141*, 1-9.

Weiner, I., & Delgado, A. (1976). Psychopathology in adolescence. *Archives of General Psychiatry, 33*, 187-193.

Westley, W.E., & Epstein, N.B. (1969). *The silent majority*. San Francisco: Jossey-Bass.

10

FAMILY DIMENSIONS OF HEALTH CARE FOR THE AGED

ERNEST FRUGÉ, Ph.D. and GEORGE NIEDEREHE, Ph.D.

Over the coming years, most primary-care physicians will be treating increasing numbers of elderly patients whose medical problems are embedded in unique psychological, social, and economic contexts. We believe that understanding these special conditions will enhance the delivery of effective health care to elderly patients. We shall review aspects of family systems that should be considered when assessing and treating aged patients: the current status of the elderly person in the American family; the primary-care physician's role in treating elderly patients and their families; and family dynamics that may influence elderly patients' diagnoses and treatment.

The Family Context of the Elderly Population

Family Structure

In recent years, the proportion of older people in our society has risen dramatically, primarily because of the declining birth rate and a general increase in longevity. In 1900, only 3 million persons (4% of the U.S. population) were 65 years old or older. In 1980, the elderly accounted for 11% of the population, and it is predicted that by 1990 this age group will number 29 million (Soldo, 1980).

The group generally identified as "old people" encompasses two generations, people from 65 to more than 100 years old. About 40% of this group is older than 75 and 8% is older than 85. Women outnumber men in the

Work on this chapter was partially supported by NIMH Research Grant #MH 35400 to the second author, "Family Dynamics and the Care of Aged with Dementia."

over-65 age group (14.3 to 9.8 million), the preponderance of women increasing with the age of the sample. Among those older than 85, women outnumber men two to one (Shanas & Sussman, 1981). It is this group of "old-old" people (older than 75) who are most likely to be frail or to have serious health problems, and to depend on their families for social and material support. They are also the most rapidly growing segment of the elderly population.

The radical shift in the proportion of senior people in our society is reflected in a changing family structure. As with all changes, there are accompanying challenges, opportunities, and drawbacks. A longer life span, and smaller families whose children are closely spaced, have allowed more people to share the second half of their lives in intact family constellations (spouse, adult children, and grandchildren) and deepened the potential range and richness of family relationships. Yet, at the very time that middle-aged adults are freed from child rearing, they are increasingly likely to face new responsibilities for a frail elderly parent. For the frail elderly, a smaller family means fewer children who can help and, for the children, it means fewer brothers and sisters who can share the burden of caring for disabled parents.

Myths and Facts about Aging in American Families

Perhaps as a result of the tension that arises from rapid changes in society, myths and stereotypes about what it means to grow old in American families are plentiful: for example, that the family life of the aged is bleaker today than it used to be. A related stereotype holds that the aged in our society live in isolation, rejected by and alienated from their own families because family ties and values have broken down. These views are often born of the myths of bygone golden days in which the elderly supposedly spent blissful lives, in the bosom of their close-knit, extended families who were bound together by love and a shared sense of respect and obligation. Modern historians provide considerable evidence that three-generation families living together were actually rare, and that economic necessity, as much as familial love and concern, was the root of family solidarity in the past.

The stereotypical view of aging generally is a negative one, and it is often linked with discrimination against the elderly. "Ageist" views are so pervasive in our society that health care professionals are apt to be as unenlightened as others. Many physicians have negative attitudes about the medical and social conditions they associate with elderly patients (Geiger, 1978; Gorlin & Zucker, 1983; Klein, Najman, Kohrman, & Munro, 1982; Spence, Feigenbaum, Fitzgerald, & Roth, 1968). A recent large study of physicians in Michigan showed that 59% of general practitioners do not visit elderly patients in nursing homes, and nearly 20% said they simply do not like old people (Mitchell, 1982). It is thus very important for professionals to carefully examine the assumptions they spontaneously carry into their contacts with the aged and their families, and to replace informally acquired biases with accurate information about the family context of aging.

Some interrelated misconceptions that portray the family life of the elderly in negativistic terms deserve to be examined. Our objective is to present a realistic view of most elderly people as neither alienated from their families nor entirely dependent on younger generations for meaning and vitality.

Misconception #1: Most older people live alone, apart from their families. Families do, in fact, provide the most common living arrangement for older people regardless of age, gender, or race. Usually, the "family" consists of an elderly married couple, but there are striking gender differences in marital status. Women over 65 are only half as likely to be married and three times as likely to be widowed as men, reflecting the tendency for men to have shorter life spans and to marry younger women. Over the next decades, there will be more older women without spouses.

Most older people like to balance autonomy and privacy in their personal lives, while maintaining contact with their younger-generation family members. Although most live a relatively short distance from at least one close relative, most older people prefer to live independently. In a survey of widows, for example, Lopata (1973) found they preferred not to live with offspring. The widows' reasons were clear—they wanted to be boss in their own kitchens, and they did not want to change lifestyles or contend with rowdy grandchildren. But this does not mean that older people are cut off from their families.

Misconception #2: Most older people have infrequent contact with offspring because of the geographic mobility of families and a general weakening of family ties. Although few aging parents live with their offspring, contemporary families maintain a high degree of interaction between the generations. According to a 1962 survey by Shanas, Townsend, Wedderburn, et al. (1968), only one in 10 elderly citizens had not seen one of his or her children in the preceding 30 days. A 1974 sampling in Los Angeles found that 56% of older Mexican Americans, 40% of the white, and 33% of the black elders had seen one of their children the day before (Bengtson & Treas, 1980). The preferred pattern of frequent interaction while maintaining separate households has been called "intimacy at a distance" (Rosenmayr, 1968).

Misconception #3: Most families have a "generation gap" that involves serious strains between generations. On the contrary, a wider generation gap tends to be seen when one compares age groups in general across the culture than between generations in a given family. Most family members, especially the older ones, think of their relationships as warm (Bengtson, 1971). Although the elderly tend to disengage from formal and peer group relationships that do not satisfy them, they clearly maintain immediate family ties and a sense of emotional solidarity with kin (Brown, 1974).

This sunny view of emotional solidarity between family generations needs to be balanced, however. In terms of consensus on values, developmental concerns and interests obviously change across the life span. As Cohler (1983) suggested, while younger adults in their child-rearing years are primarily interested in creating interdependent relationships, older adults are typically more concerned with autonomy and fulfilling personal desires that may have been set aside in order to support others. Thus, even though family relationships remain important, they are not older persons' only concern. Family relations may even be a source of stress if they are burdensome or otherwise less than ideal or interfere with the developmental urge toward greater personal autonomy (e.g., having to support an incompetent adult child or having to take up primary responsibility for the parenting of grandchildren) (Cohler, 1983). Likewise, the decrease of autonomy that usually accompanies aging at some point and the attendant need for material and even physical assistance from adult children may be expected to lower the elderly parent's morale (Seelbach, 1977; Seelbach & Sauer, 1977).

Misconception #4: Old people are primarily recipients in intergenerational exchanges, receiving more than they give. There is a general tendency for family members to turn to kin for aid, rather than to either friends or outside agencies (Sussman, 1965). Hill, Foote, and colleagues (1970) found this to be true of all three generations in a crisis. Surprisingly, the older person is frequently the donor in family exchanges. Shanas et al. (1968) reported that not only did three-fifths of elderly Americans receive help from children, but more than half reported they gave help. Other observers have suggested that more aid flows from the older to younger generations than the other way around. Societal provision for the elderly and historical shifts that have made education the basis of financial security have largely eliminated economic reasons for the imposed togetherness of families. Yet, the elderly in particular, and society in general, continue to believe that the younger generation has significant responsibilities toward its elders. More older women tend to expect their adult children to fulfill these responsibilities than do elderly men (Seelbach, 1977; Seelbach & Sauer, 1977). Adult children typically go to great lengths to live up to these expectations (Shanas, 1960; Simos, 1973).

Misconception #5: Many elderly people must be maintained in public institutions because their families abandon them when they become seriously ill. Many observers agree that constraints on family resources will naturally follow the shrinking of family size, and that in the future "aspects of housing, recreation, health care, and income maintenance now provided by younger generations to their elderly parents and grandparents will need to be provided by society at large" (Shanas & Hauser, 1974, p. 91). Yet it is a mistake to believe that society is becoming responsible for supporting old people because families no longer care for their elderly members. The increased demand for societally supported services for the aged is a direct reflection of the rising numbers of the aged, and not of diminished family support. In fact, rather than "dumping" their ill elderly relatives into public institutions, most family members go to great lengths to maintain the relative in a natural family setting. A national survey in 1975 found 95% of all elderly living in the community and not in institutions (Bengtson & Treas, 1980). It is older people without kin who are most likely to be institutionalized. Furthermore, the family decision to institutionalize an elderly relative usually occurs only after all other family resources and alternatives have been exhausted, and often after the physical ability of other family members to maintain the dependent elder outside the institution has for some reason broken down (Lowenthal, 1964).

The available evidence uniformly dispels negative stereotypes about the lack of solidarity in the family life of older people. Most older people are not isolated; family relationships are warm; the older person is frequently the donor in family exchanges; and norms of filial loyalty endure. The average elderly American prefers to be as autonomous as possible, electing a variety of social involvements to produce a meaningful and vital existence. Nevertheless, the family provides the most dependable, significant, and enduring interpersonal relations. The significance of family ties is apt to become most apparent at times of illness or other personal need, when the increasing dependence of the older person typically calls for the heightened involvement of other family members.

Elderly Patients and Health Care: Family Aspects

Illness and Symptom Reporting

The elderly patient may encounter a variety of difficulties in obtaining appropriate, comprehensive, and cost-effective health care. Some of these difficulties are related to negative stereotypes about the way aging affects health and the use of health care services.

Misconception #6: Aging is virtually synonymous with illness. A common belief in our culture is that old age is always associated with illness and loss of independence. Indeed, the occurrence of disease and disability rises sharply with age, but these two dimensions must be clearly differentiated; illness in old age does not invariably mean loss of independence or even a restricted lifestyle. Although 80% of the elderly report at least one chronic health condition, only about 4% of people over 75 are bedridden at home and about the same number are bedridden in institutions (Levy & Glantz, 1981). Most elderly people are ambulatory, mentally alert, and self-sufficient.

Still, the stereotype about aging and illness bespeaks a certain truth: Because of the greater prevalence of illness, old people are relatively heavy users of health care. Most primary-care physicians can expect to see a large proportion of elderly patients among their clientele. According to figures cited in several sources (Libow & Sherman, 1981; Wetle, 1982), although persons over 65 comprise only 11% of the population, they account for 29% of total personal health care expenditures ($41.3 billion of $142.6 billion). The elderly are the leading consumers of pharmaceuticals, purchasing 25% of all prescription drugs and a larger percentage of nonprescription drugs. They account for 40% of acute hospital bed days and 95% of bed days in long-term care. Their length of voluntary hospitalization during acute illnesses is 32% longer than that of middle-aged individuals (11.6 days compared to 8.8 days). Nursing home care cost 10 billion dollars in 1976 and 21.6 billion dollars in 1980. The clustering of diseases also increases with age.

These numbers primarily reflect the fact that disease occurs disproportionately during the later years of life, a reality that must be faced. The danger with stereotypic thinking that equates aging with disease and disability, however, is that it blurs the tremendous variations among older persons in terms of their health status and potential for successful treatment. Despite the increased risk of illness, many older persons stay healthy to advanced ages or can be treated successfully. The negative, "ageist" bias that is shared by so many elderly people, their families, and health care professionals (Butler & Lewis, 1973) may lead to inaccurate reporting of illness, misdiagnosis, complications in treatment, or, even worse, may become a self-fulfilling prophecy because of failure to treat the treatable.

Misconception #7: Most elderly patients are hypochondriacal. The evidence suggests the opposite—much "suffering in silence." Brody, Kleban, and Moles (1983) sampled 132 old people to identify their day-to-day mental and physical symptoms and what was done about them. Those surveyed had an average of six diagnosed chronic health problems, yet on a day-to-day basis, they reported virtually no symptoms of diagnosed or undiagnosed disorders to health care professionals. The patients and families tried to treat the symptoms themselves.

Some elderly persons *are* hypochondriacal complainers, just as others tend toward minimizing or denying their physical problems. Most elderly people, however, rate their own health accurately, in comparison to physicians' ratings and other behavioral indicators (Heyman & Jeffers, 1963; Maddox & Douglas, 1973). Underestimation of one's health in later life is abnormal and has been associated with a history of clinical depression and poor social adjustment (Maddox, 1962; Shanas et al., 1968). According to Costa (1985), excessive somatic complaining at any age is linked with neuroticism, and the research evidence indicates that neither neuroticism nor complaining increases as a function of normal aging.

Actually, older people (at least the current generation) may seem to emphasize somatic factors when they experience a general absence of well-being because they are not likely to identify and acknowledge psychological, emotional, and interpersonal factors that may be contributing to their situation. They often present their difficulties as somatic, perhaps because of the perception that with age physical ailments are more significant, the cultural acceptability of physical problems in old age, insensitivity to psychological notions, inability to articulate emotions, or distrust of the mental health profession. Clearly, frank depression and milder feelings of demoralization or dysphoria are quite prevalent among the older population, but relatively few of these cases come to the attention of mental health professionals. The vast majority of elderly persons with such problems remain untreated, self-treated, or see primary-care physicians (Blazer & Williams, 1980; Regier, Goldberg, & Taube, 1978; Sparacino & Ronchi, 1982).

The Health Care System and the Aged

The physician's response to these types of situations will be influenced by his or her perceptions of elderly patients and of the role of their families in their health care. The response will also, of course, be guided by the organization of the health care system in which the physician and patient are operating. Two aspects of the current health care system have particular relevance for elderly patients.

Difficulty #1: Our health care system is fragmented and passive. The elderly are at a disadvantage because health care systems generally must be activated by the patient or patient advocates, and require mobility, familiarity with insurance rules, and adequate income and social support (Libow, 1981). This delays the early detection of disease and early intervention when a favorable outcome is most likely (Wetle, 1982). Libow (1981) suggested that a simply organized system of health care for the elderly could be achieved by integrating health care components that already exist in many communities.

When older patients present relatively trivial somatic complaints that may represent feelings of depression or other nonphysiological problems, the physician must determine how the underlying problems are to be recognized and dealt with. The patient's malaise is often linked to family issues and relationships. Other family members may collude in somatizing a psychological problem, and encouraging or demanding somatic treatment, rather than having to acknowledge and take responsibility for broader family issues. Physicians may unwittingly collude in this process by prescribing medications, when educating or counseling the family would be more appropriate. They may do this, even though they recognize the nonphysiological factors, because the latter seem too complicated to deal with, the amount of time required is more than they prefer to spend on a case, or the family presses the physician to avoid nonphysical problems.

To respond effectively to these clinical realities, the physician may have to establish linkages with other kinds of professionals and services. Because of their unique place in the social and medical structure, primary-care physicians can link the patient and family to both medical and nonmedical community resources, and they may find increasing numbers of elderly patients and families seeking their help to gain this access. The physician's role with the elderly is complex—assessing the patient in his or her family context, helping the patient navigate through the health care system to ensure coordinated service delivery, and linking the patient and family to nonmedical community services for economic and social support. Social services may include groups that offer companionship and recreation, as well as self-help groups for families caring for more severely disabled elderly members. Experienced geriatricians strongly recommend a multidisciplinary team approach to the elderly patient and family. Such an approach improves the scope of technical expertise, generates alternative treatment strategies, prevents therapeutic nihilism, and generally enhances the patient's health and morale (Libow, 1981).

Difficulty #2: Medications are likely to be misused. The use and misuse of medications is a clear example of how fragmentation of medical services interacts with the health behaviors of elderly people and their family members and exacerbates serious gaps in health care. More than 85% of elderly patients take drugs, prescribed by a physician or self-prescribed, of which 25% may well be ineffective or unneeded (Lamy, 1979). Despite a general paucity of knowledge about pharmacokinetics in the elderly, we know that elderly people are more vulnerable to negative side effects than younger people, and that most drug interactions are unpredictable and potentially harmful. Old people also tend to be treated in many different clinical settings, typically without informing their primary-care professionals. It is common to find elderly outpatients taking eight to 10 different prescriptions or more.

Polypharmacy may become self-perpetuating as more medicines are added to control what are actually side effects of other medicines. Family members sometimes participate unintentionally in the misuse of drugs by increasing or decreasing dosages without medical advice in an effort to increase effect, reduce the threat of dependence, or decrease side effects. A recent report concluded that 20% of the patients entering the geriatric service of a large hospital showed evidence of disorders directly attributable to the effects of prescription drugs (Levy & Glantz, 1981).

To complicate matters, elderly people often use over-the-counter (OTC) medications without informing a primary-care provider. In the Brody et al. (1983) study mentioned earlier, about 70% of drugs taken in response to chest pain were either OTC or could not be identified by the patients. The chest pains had previously been diagnosed by a physician, and medication had been prescribed. Polypharmacy should thus be a primary consideration in evaluating the elderly patient, and families should be asked routinely to bring in the entire collection of medicines in the older person's home. Considerable family education about the proper use of medications is often needed, as are efforts to coordinate treatment plans with other medical specialists involved in the patient's total care.

A Family Perspective in Assessing Elderly Patients

Accurate diagnosis and treatment of elderly patients require familiarity with parameters of "normal" biological, psychological, and social functioning of aging individuals. Gerontology is a relatively new area of specialization, and many assessment procedures have not been validated for elderly populations. There are many useful reviews of geriatric medicine (e.g., Besdine, 1980; Libow, 1981; Rowe & Besdine, 1981), and of aging and mental health issues (Birren & Sloane, 1980; Busse & Pfeiffer, 1977; Butler & Lewis, 1973; Gaitz, 1978; Zarit, 1980). Several authors have recommended comprehensive assessment procedures for elderly patients (Cohen, 1977; Libow, 1981; Tager, 1980). Comprehensive schedules such as the Older Americans Resources and Services (OARS) Multidimensional Functional Assessment

Questionnaire (Pfeiffer, 1975) tap various areas of the patient's functional capacities and life situation.

The crucial liaison between the elderly patient and the physician is typically a member of the patient's family. Therefore, baseline information about the family system of elderly patients should include a picture of who is in the family, where they live, their health and social status (e.g., marital status, occupation, and any major problems), predictable patterns of reaction to illness or other stressors, and the quality of family relationships. The physician usually collects this general information gradually as he or she cares for various family members over the years. To get a good family history of new patients, a more detailed inquiry is necessary. A genogram, a schematic representation of the family, may be useful (Walsh, 1980). The genogram can be expanded to include significant nonfamily social relationships (e.g., visiting nurses, church groups, other health professionals).

To assess the general quality of family relationships, the physician should ask how often the elderly patient has contact with various family members, what usually takes place (e.g., phone or letter contacts, assistance with chores or money matters), and how emotionally close they are. As these relationships are described, the physician should note the quality of attachment in the relationships (e.g., positive versus negative), what is exchanged (e.g., financial or emotional support), and how problems are managed (e.g., covert manipulation versus open debate or conflict). These descriptions will give the physician a sense of the elderly patient's place in the family. Asking the same questions of different family members helps to produce a more complete, and often more balanced, view. Meeting with family members as a group offers an incomparable opportunity to observe patterns that the family may or may not report in individual interviews.

Assessing the emotional attachment of family members is of particular importance for understanding how the family is reacting to an ill elderly member. Remnet (1979) suggests attending to these questions:

- Is the family in a current state of crisis because of the failing capacities of one of its members?
- Are other stresses impinging on the system?
- Has the family system changed over the years to meet the needs of its members?
- Is change acknowledged and accepted?

In relation to the older person:

- Who is assuming responsibility for what?
- Is the responsibility realistic?

- Have all family members been involved in the plan?
- Have the expectations of each family member been explored and defined?
- Is the current plan considered permanent or temporary? (p. 209)

With all of this information, the primary-care physician is able to form hypotheses about family dynamics that may be interfering with the health and care of the elderly patient—how, for example, efforts to protect the elderly patient's feelings may have led to delay in diagnosis or noncompliance with medical regimens. In this volume, Weakland and Fisch outline a useful method of detecting how the very action family members take to manage difficulties may actually maintain or worsen problems. Herr and Weakland (1979) elaborated this approach in an excellent book on counseling elderly people and their families.

Just as the standard review of medical history and current health status contributes important information about the patient's social adaptation, domains of assessment usually considered "psychological" contribute much to understanding the patient's family adaptation. Health-related habits (for example, nutrition and exercise) and health knowledge and attitudes (perhaps fear of hospitals) may reflect family patterns rather than the patient's idiosyncratic characteristics. A comprehensive assessment should include a review of the older patient's past functioning and current behavior in the home and family. Establishing the patient's objective level of intellectual and physical abilities in tasks required for daily living is particularly important when treating elderly patients who have obvious or suspected disabilities. This baseline of capabilities also allows the physician to examine whether physical, psychological, and/or social factors may be contributing to lower levels of functioning than the patient is capable of, or what has been termed "excess disability." Fleisher (1979) reviewed a series of objective measures that may be useful to practitioners in assessing mental status (Alpaugh & Haney, 1978); self-care skills and abilities for daily living (Lawton, 1971); and morale and life satisfaction (Lawton, 1971; Nydegger, 1976).

Problems associated with aging routinely present challenges in differential diagnosis. In the next section we give several case examples, focusing on family dynamics that can influence the presenting problem and on the potential for family-based interventions.

Common Clinical Problems of the Elderly and Their Families

Psychosocial Transitions in the Life Cycle—Retirement

Mr. B. brought his 16-year-old daughter, Lucy, to a physician because she complained of recurrent headaches, mild nausea, and lethargy. The symptoms usually occurred in the morning, and Lucy had missed a great deal of school. Physical examination revealed no detectable reason for the complaints. Taking the family history, the physician learned that Lucy was the second of two children from Mr. B.'s third and current marriage. He was 67 years old, had worked around the world as an engineer, and described himself as a consultant currently between jobs, although he had not worked for three years and his company had retired him. Lucy's mother was Taiwanese and 20 years younger than her husband. After the birth of their first child, Mr. B. relocated his family to the United States. He insisted that the children be reared here, but he preferred to work overseas, because of the higher income. Until he retired, he had visited his family only a few times a year during brief vacations.

When interviewed with his wife and their two children, Mr. B. was reluctant to talk about anything other than Lucy's problem. He now labeled his daughter's behavior as faking and part of her "rebellion." Interrupting, Mrs. B. said that her husband's previous marriages had ended because he was too domineering and that the three children from these marriages despised him. Since his retirement, she said she and her husband often fought. Mr. B. began to accuse his wife of undermining his authority with the children. Lucy joined in, saying she would never leave her mother alone with her father because they often got into physical fights, and her mother needed protection. Bob, Lucy's older brother, was a high school dropout. Mr. B. said he was pushing Bob through a welding course in trade school. Bob maintained he had no opinions about the family's state of affairs. He was quiet throughout the interview, occasionally chuckling when the argument between other family members reached peak levels.

Predictable events occur as individuals grow older that constitute major transitions in social role and functioning. These major transitions include the passage from parent roles as the youngest child matures into adulthood, retirement from a paid work role, personal incapacitation through illness, and loss of a spouse and other family members through death. The family described here was struggling with at least two major transitions of aging, Mr. B.'s retirement from his work roles and the couple's passage from parental roles, which corresponds to the adolescent's transition into adulthood.

Retirement entails a voluntary or involuntary termination of significant relationships that give individuals a sense of worth and identity. Family members usually draw on their mutual love and experience to support one another through such times of stressful change. In some cases, however, the unique dynamics of a family exacerbate the stress typically associated with transitions, and individual members may become ill. In this case the transition was especially difficult in that the family members had inflexible patterns of organizing their activities. Mr. B. was accustomed to directing the work of many people on large projects and could not accept his forced retirement. Mrs. B. was accustomed to a substantial income, to infrequent visits from a husband much older than herself, and to an almost exclusive relationship with the children. The couple had not had much opportunity to work as a team and had developed a rigid, predictable pattern of managing conflict. Everyone in the family, including Mr. B., agreed he had always been a complete dictator while at home on vacations. Mrs. B. had always followed his orders begrudgingly, and when he returned to work she returned to her own life, seeking personal satisfaction in her relationship with her children. Now she had to contend with a severe drop in income, her husband's constant presence, the prospect of her children's growing up and out of the family, and being left alone with a belligerent, domineering husband. As Mr. B. tried to cope with his damaged self-esteem by escalating his domineering behavior, Mrs. B. undercut his authority and clung more tightly to her children, stating that she only wanted to protect them and herself from her husband's harsh ways.

This case illustrates that problematic situations in a family are frequently maintained and exacerbated by the simple repetition of ineffective coping strategies—the attempted solutions become a problem (Herr & Weakland, 1979). Mr. B. was trying to help his family and marriage with a hard-nosed management approach that he had found successful in the business world. He acknowledged that, since his retirement, his history of prolonged absences from the family made him feel that he had to ensure a positive and meaningful relationship with his children, but there was a desperate quality in his unrelenting, domineering style. Mrs. B., in turn, intensified her alliance with the children against her husband, which fueled the children's rebellion against their father and reduced the chances for the couple's collaboration.

Family members usually retire from work a long time after they have raised their children. In this family, however, since Bob and Lucy were born relatively late in Mr. B.'s life, the stress of Mr. B.'s forced retirement overlapped with Lucy's adolescence. To mature, the adolescent must, in a sense, "retire" from childhood and, for parents, adolescence involves another sort of "retirement." As with retirement from work, the "retirement" from parenthood may bring a new sense of freedom and identity and/or a profound sense of loss in purpose or meaning. In a systemic way within families, life cycle transitions for one person generally mean complementary transitions and adjustments for other family members.

Usually, if there are difficulties with a transition of aging (such as retirement), the symptoms will be manifested by the elderly family member—but not always. In this case Lucy was the identified patient. Lucy's physical symptoms can be seen as a somatic index of the family's strain in adjusting to several major social transitions associated with aging, as well as in coping with Lucy's own developmental issues.

An underlying issue is that family members tend to be threatened by the separations and losses implicit in all major transitions (Boszormenyi-Nagy, 1972). Family members may try to avoid the grief of these losses by projecting unwanted feelings onto other family members and by clinging to old solutions that have become ineffective. Rather than dealing directly with issues stemming from his retirement, Mr. B. could be seen as projecting his doubts about his own competence onto his son and pushing him to succeed.

A primary-care physician is often in a position to counsel people about major upcoming transitions before they occur by inquiring routinely, for example, about the retirement plans of middle-aged patients. Once the primary-care physician diagnoses a problem as resulting from a family's difficulty in coping with transitional issues, she or he may elect to counsel the family or refer them to a mental health professional who has expertise in family therapy.

We suggest that the physician first try to moderate frank discussion with family members about the major transitions they are coping with. Often communication has been blocked. The open exchange of thoughts and feelings in the presence of a trusted physician will often allow the family to develop innovative coping responses. If factual information does not seem to make a difference, if suggestions are solicited but never adequately followed, or if family conflict is so rampant as to preclude any cooperative efforts, then interventions that attempt to modify the redundant, maladaptive patterns of family relationships are indicated. In cases like the B. family conflicts may be so extreme as to preclude cooperation with any professional.

Depression

After seeing a TV special about Alzheimer's disease, Mrs. Y. called her physician with questions about her father, Mr. G. She believed her father, then 70, needed a checkup. He was new in town and as yet had no personal physician. Mrs. Y. said that her father was having difficulty with his memory and asked repetitious questions. She knew he was taking at least two medications for arthritis and high blood pressure. The physician asked her to invite her father to make an appointment.

During the examination Mr. G. was generally cooperative but reserved. He was not sure why his daughter had arranged the appointment. Things were generally fine, he said, and he had no complaints to speak of. When pressed a bit with more specific questions, he mentioned his arthritis, high blood pressure, and cataracts that prevented him from driving. He admitted to becoming somewhat more absentminded over the past few years, feeling slowed down and often having restless sleep. He attributed this to "growing old." He reported that recurrent sinus infections often ruined his appetite.

On physical examination, the only abnormal finding was a very mildly elevated blood pressure. On the mental status exam, Mr. G. was well oriented but he made some errors in recalling brief stories. While copying designs he also complained that his arthritis limited his dexterity. He spoke in short sentences and grew somewhat more brusque with the physician during the neurological exam.

Mr. G. had worked for the railroads for 29 years, 18 years of which were in management. He had retired five years previously, had been divorced for eight years, and enjoyed a bit of yardwork and watching TV. Since his move to the city five months before, his main social contact had been his daughter. Mrs. Y. had asked her father to make the first appointment in order to "meet" a local physician who might be involved in his future care. When briefly interviewed, Mrs. Y. added concerns about her father she had not discussed with him and did not want him to know she had mentioned. Mrs. Y said her father seemed to be afraid to do things by himself. Her eyes teared as she talked about calling him during the day only to hear his listless voice. Tears continued to well up as she recounted her husband's criticisms about the time she was spending with her father. Mrs. Y. was a 52-year-old housewife. Her two daughters were grown, married, and living in distant cities. A year before she had suggested that her father move to be near her after his poor vision had caused him to have an auto accident and he was compelled to quit driving.

Depression is a complex biopsychosocial phenomenon, involving diverse symptomatic aspects and etiological factors that are poorly understood. Symptomatically, it may encompass not only depressed mood, but other components such as self-criticism, complaints of symptomatic distress, reduced activity level, sleep disturbance, and disturbed vegetative functioning. Epidemiologically, the incidence of depression is highest in middle age, and only slightly lower in old age because recurrence and incomplete remission rates rise with age (Silverman, 1968). Depression is the most common psychological disturbance of the elderly (Epstein, 1976). The frequency of diagnosable clinical depressions is probably no greater among the aged than among other age groups, but states of mild depression, dysphoria, apathy, or demoralization that fail to meet standard clinical criteria for psychiatric disorder are common among the elderly (Blau & Berezin, 1975; Blazer & Williams, 1980).

Although there is no evidence for the traditional category of "involutional melancholia" as a distinct subtype, the patterns of depressive symptomatology tend to be different in elderly compared to younger populations. Self-deprecation is less common; paranoid symptoms, when present, are less ominous; somatic complaints and hypochondriacal features and complaints about memory loss are among the most salient features of depressive syndromes in late life (Kahn, Zarit, Hilbert, & Niederehe, 1975; Pfeiffer & Busse, 1973; Zung, 1980). For more information on symptomatology, the reader is referred to general readings on depressive syndromes in the elderly (Blazer, 1982; Post, 1976; Stenback, 1980; Zung, 1980).

Depression and physical illness certainly should not be considered mutually exclusive, and they are frequently associated in the aged. Since depression may be a by-product of physical illness, physical causes for somatic symptoms, such as sleep difficulties, should be identified and treated, or ruled out (Salzman & Shader, 1979; Verwoerdt & Dovenmuehle, 1964). On the other hand, depression may contribute to and magnify the impairments brought on by ill health. Alleviation of depression can enhance the overall functioning of the patient even if the physical aspects of the illness are untreatable. As mentioned earlier, the vast majority of depressed aged patients are treated only by primary-care physicians, and not by mental health personnel. Beck and Beck (1972) offer a rapid screening procedure for use in family practice to help in identifying depressed patients.

The differential diagnosis of organic from depressive disorders in the aged is generally considered one of the most difficult in psychiatry (Butler & Lewis, 1973). Various observers have described a pattern termed "pseudodementia" or "pseudosenility," in which symptoms resemble an organic brain syndrome, but seem to be an atypical form of depression responsive to antidepressant treatments (Libow, 1973; Wells, 1979). The label is less descriptive of the symptoms than of the tendency of clinicians mistakenly to diagnose senile dementia while ignoring the affective symptoms (Kiloh, 1973).

In our case example, serious organic causes (including medication effects) were ruled out as bases for Mr. G.'s mild symptoms of memory loss, sleep disturbance, poor appetite, and virus infections. He disliked cooking and ate balanced meals only when dining with his daughter. The pattern of his symptoms, as well as his tense and somewhat defensive style, fit the picture of depression.

While there is ample evidence for the utility of pharmaceutical interventions with many depressed patients (Zung, 1980), the role of the family in the development and maintenance of depression tends to receive less attention. Many researchers, however, have identified social or interpersonal stressors as the primary precipitants of depressive episodes. The precursor events tend to involve other persons exiting from, or entering into, the patient's social field in ways that involve some blow to the patient's self-esteem (Leff, Roatch, & Bunney, 1970; Paykel, Myers, Dienelt, Klerman, Lindenthal, & Pepper, 1969).

Mr. G. certainly had had to deal with several significant losses including a divorce, retirement, failing eyesight and, more recently, the move away from his home community. Although at first very reticent to talk about his feelings, he seemed more relaxed during the second interview. He said he had been happier in his hometown but "gave up" driving and had not been able to see his old friends as often. His friends had similar problems with transportation. He had begun to feel blue and had accepted with some relief the invitation to move closer to his daughter. Mr. G.'s voice took on a noticeable emotional edge when he spoke of "giving up" driving. His relatively frail physical condition and Mrs. Y.'s desire to help him had led to his becoming detached from a meaningful set of nonfamily relationships. Also, his loss of mobility, while he was still relatively capable in other ways, was a continuing source of self-criticism.

From a family systems perspective, depression is not an individual phenomenon, and "every depressive needs a partner" (Rubinstein & Timmons, 1978, p. 16). Depressive symptoms are maintained by covert unresolved conflict between family members around feelings of deprivation, resentment, and a struggle for power to determine who is to be taken care of. Frequently, a third party is recruited to maintain a dyadic balance.

As Mrs. Y. gave her view of the family relationships it became clear that, as an only child, she had been the third party, stuck between her mother and father. She said she had always loved and respected her father, but she described him as strict and as having traveled a great deal on business. She was uncertain about why her parents had divorced. She thought that her mother, who initiated the divorce, had wanted more affection from Mr. G. Apparently her mother had longed for, then despaired of, obtaining the father's support and affection. As a child, Mrs. Y. had felt closer to her mother and had wished, along with her mother, for the father's attention. Mrs. Y.'s increased involvement in her father's life at this time was part of a continuing attempt to reach out to him, albeit with mixed emotions. She had also experienced some of her mother's anger toward him. Not only was her husband complaining about the time she was spending with her father, but Mrs. Y. was beginning to feel apprehensive about her own decision to have her father move near her. She had felt sorry for him, but now it seemed that the harder she tried to help, the more he seemed to be turning inside himself, doing less and becoming bitter. Mrs. Y. felt uncomfortable talking about it to her mother, and had been having less phone contact with her recently.

A predictable pattern of social response is associated with the behavior of depressed persons (Coyne, 1976a; Gallagher & Frankel, 1980). Family members and significant others may begin by offering the depressed person assurance and support, but the depressed person's behavior continues and others start to see it as a plea for prolonged support. As this goes on, the significant other becomes frustrated, expressing anger or withdrawing from the patient, and leaving the patient convinced of his or her own worthlessness. Depressed persons play an active role in producing such negative reactions in others (Coyne, 1976b; Lewinsohn & Lee, 1980). Depressive persons' interactions are characterized by repetitious cycles with characteristic verbal (e.g., demands, reassurance) and nonverbal (e.g., eye contact, voice tone) components for each participant. Mrs. Y. and her father interacted awkwardly and actually spoke very little to each other. The uncomfortable shifts in power and responsibility that occur when an adult child begins to care for an elderly parent's basic needs were obvious in this situation.

The most straightforward suggestion to increase this father's and daughter's morale was to counsel them both on ways to increase the father's social network of friends and activities. This was designed to provide entertainment and a new sense of community to the old man, and to reduce some of the strain on the daughter. With Mrs. Y., it was also helpful to discuss the history of her role between her parents. She began to wait longer between calls and mailed her father information on schedules of public transportation. As a result of these interventions, Mr. G. became involved with a very active church, Mrs. Y. relaxed, and the expression of complaints was reduced.

Special steps may be required in the case of elderly patients who are frankly hypochondriacal, which can be seen as a functional equivalent of depression. Treatment recommendations are discussed by Busse and Pfeiffer (1977), and they may include such steps as placebo medications and regular but brief office appointments.

Cognitive Impairment

Over a period of years, Mrs. R. developed memory problems. She first had trouble remembering activities that had been planned, and developed the habit of repeatedly asking questions of her husband to keep herself on track. These symptoms progressed rather rapidly to the point that she was having trouble remembering her husband's name and finally began to confuse him with her first husband. Though Mr. and Mrs. R. had been married

44 years, at one point she wanted to have a marriage ceremony to make sure they were really married. Although Mrs. R. still tried to participate in conversations, when she talked beyond simply agreeing or disagreeing, her speech became highly abstract, ranging from more or less philosophical statements to ramblings about how people should be protected from one thing or another.

Mr. R. was a large, even-tempered man who brought his wife to appointments by public transportation. Though several extensive workups had all produced the diagnosis of Alzheimer's disease, and though her loss of functions had stabilized over the past year, Mr. R. remained anxious for information about his wife's condition. At first, his only complaint was that she often woke him in the middle of the night for no apparent reason. During the second interview, he admitted with great regret and apprehension to having nearly "killed" his wife accidentally by overmedicating her. He was worried also about how soon she might become nonambulatory and incontinent. He had a work-related back injury and feared that he would no longer be able to care for her if she had to be lifted. The couple survived on his social security payments. Mrs. R. had never worked and was ineligible for benefits. The couple had five children, two of whom lived in town and helped the father by "watching mother" at times.

Intellectual impairment in older patients is encountered fairly often by the medical practitioner. The kind of cognitive changes Mrs. R. showed were clearcut and extensive. Marked intellectual decline in an older patient, even when it is considerably less severe than in the case example, is *not* part of the normal aging process, and should never be written off by the physician as "just aging." Whereas some mild cognitive changes routinely accompany the aging process, these changes are rarely of a magnitude to interfere with the individual's ability to perform daily living tasks autonomously.

A large proportion of older persons have less formal education than do younger patients. Physicians must simplify their language to communicate with these patients effectively. Differences in vocabulary plus the cognitive changes of normal aging are apt to increase the amount of time the physician needs to spend with the older patient. Failure to allot more time to communicating with older patients may result in the incomplete reception or understanding of the information the physician is trying to convey, followed often by the patient's failure to carry out treatment recommendations properly.

Rather than representing normal aging, intellectual decline in the aged that interferes with daily functioning is often a sign of physical illness. This is true especially when the changes are marked and obvious, regardless of whether they have developed rapidly or slowly. Dementing brain diseases account for much of the severe intellectual decline seen in late life, but other common health problems also may have a dramatic effect on the older patient's alertness and cognition. These problems include cardiovascular disease, malnutrition and vitamin deficiency, metabolic disturbances, and the effects of overmedication or drug interactions. Intellectual decline is associated in general with reduced life expectancy. It should alert the physician's concern and spur an aggressive diagnostic effort to uncover causes for the intellectual impairment.

"Dementia" is a behavioral pattern characterized by a general decline of intellectual and psychomotor abilities, but it also involves changes in personal habits, interpersonal behavior, and affective expression. The term is correct only when there is concomitant evidence that the patient's behavioral changes are irreversible and stem from brain pathology. Only 4% to 6% of the total elderly population has the moderate to severe cognitive impairment that suggests a dementing brain disease, but the prevalence rate may rise to 20% or more after age 80 (Kay, 1972). The traditional clinical features of dementia, such as impairment of memory, orientation, judgment, comprehension, and lability or shallowness of affect, are familiar to most practitioners (Busse, 1973). The patient may have hallucinations, especially at night when general environmental stimulation is reduced, and express paranoid ideation and delusions. Behavioral disturbances include restlessness, sleeplessness, wandering, incontinence, aggressiveness, and agitation.

Except for brain biopsy or autopsy, no tests can positively identify dementing diseases. Dementia is thus "a diagnosis of last resort" (National Institute on Aging Task Force, 1980) properly arrived at only by a process of exclusion, after ruling out all more identifiable and treatable factors. Recent research suggests that the majority of late-life dementias are caused primarily by Alzheimer-type degeneration; cerebral arteriosclerosis is much less common than has been believed. The reader is referred elsewhere for reviews on the basic clinical features of dementia and its treatment and differential diagnosis (Karasu & Katzman, 1976; Libow, 1973; Pearce & Miller, 1973; Wang & Busse, 1971; Wells, 1978, 1979).

In contrast to the dementing diseases, other medical conditions may produce *acute* conditions, in which the cognitive decline is *reversible*. Common behavioral manifestations of an acute condition, today officially designated as "delirium," are fluctuating levels of awareness, hallucinations, disorientation, anxiety, and impaired attention, concentration, and retention. With appropriate identification and treatment of the factors that cause the dysfunction (e.g., congestive heart failure, nutritional deficiencies, infectious processes, metabolic imbalances, temporary toxic conditions), there is a high recovery rate; however, there is also a substantial risk of death in these cases. It is quite common for persons with these conditions to show exacerbated cognitive dysfunction because of changes in their health and environment and the accompanying stress. Some family issues in dealing with patients who have acute brain dysfunctions are discussed by Rynearson (1977).

Like depression, syndromes of cognitive impairment should be seen as complex biopsychosocial phenomena in which personality and the social environment play major roles (Kahn, 1971). There may be little that can be done about cerebral damage and neuronal loss, but psychosocial factors (as well as reversible medical problems) are often more amenable to treatment, which may lead to substantial improvements in the patient's level of functioning (Wang & Busse, 1971).

The nature of the family system is a major factor in how much the inherent stressfulness of the situation will be moderated or exacerbated, both for the affected older person and the caregiving family members. As we have said, families do not abandon their elderly members when dementia or other disabilities develop. Rather, as exemplified by Mr. R., spouses, adult children, and other relatives play an active role in caring for the disabled elderly, both at home and in linking them to the health care system.

Family members typically go to great lengths to fulfill their sense of loyalty and responsibility to the impaired relative. Much evidence suggests that, in providing this care, they may themselves be at high risk for incurring social isolation or disruption of work roles, for developing emotional and physical problems, or for encountering family conflicts or other problems (Sainsbury & Grad de Alarcon, 1970). In one recent study, 87% of caregivers to the demented aged cited chronic fatigue, anger, or depression as a problem, and they often had difficulty differentiating among these feelings (Rabins, Mace, & Lucas, 1982).

An elderly patient's cognitive impairments create the need for greater collaboration between the physician and the family in the patient's care. Since the prognosis for demented patients is one of variable but general decline, physicians often think there is little they can offer the family once the diagnosis has been made. The physician can help, however, by giving the family information about the illness, helping the family to solve problems encountered in caregiving, supporting the primary caregivers emotionally, and assisting with difficult decisions such as placing the patient in a nursing home. Discussions of the issues involved in these family situations and ways of helping the family cope with them can be found in various sources (Niederehe & Frugé, 1984; Ware & Carper, 1982; Zarit & Zarit, 1982). The physician can also help to lower family stress, in part by the judicious prescription of medications that help to control such difficult patient symptoms as belligerence and nocturnal restlessness.

For patients in severe cognitive decline (dementia), the caregivers have major needs that physicians should be aware of. The family members typically need to receive information about the nature and prognosis of the patient's disorder, engage in problem solving about coping with the patient's behavioral problems, and develop strategies for maximizing the patient's level of functioning. They may also need permission to attend to their own needs and connections to supportive social and health services (Zarit, 1979).

Families often do not receive sufficient information about dementia. On the other hand, they are often stunned by the diagnosis and have difficulty taking in detailed information at first. Over time, they will have many questions and worries about the illness. Families thus need to hear simple explanations. The information may need to be repeated patiently several times as the families gradually accept the reality of the situation and encounter new problems. Several informative books are available, specifically for families caring for a demented family member (Mace & Rabins, 1981; McDowell, 1980; Powell & Courtice, 1983; Reisberg, 1981). Practitioners in urban areas might also refer families to local chapters of the Alzheimer's Disease and Related Disorders Association, a self-help group for families dealing with the problems and strains presented by relatives who have dementia.

Family members are understandably interested in prognosis and possible cures. It is difficult to dissuade people from quack cures without destroying hope. Instead of telling families that the illness usually involves a progressive decline, the physician should emphasize how each person's illness follows a different course that is hard to predict, but mention that no cures have been substantiated by research (Zarit, 1980).

In offering emotional support to caregivers of demented patients, the physician should recognize and accept that the family may be experiencing anticipatory grief over the loss of a loved one (Herr & Weakland, 1979). The loss of communicative ability and personality in the loved one is often experienced as a partial death. Other behavioral changes may also leave family members emotionally traumatized. Some elderly paranoid patients are, for example, much more hostile to close family members than they are to strangers. Such radical change in the behavior of a loved one is extremely painful to caring family members. They may also feel guilty when they are provoked to frustration and anger. The professional can help the family to reduce the guilt and express the grief that is a natural response to the situation. Confusion about how to interpret the patient's actions is another source of emotional stress. Clarifying the diagnosis and discussing how the disease typically affects behavior helps the family to decide which behaviors of the patient result from disease-related deficiencies and which deserve to be seen as intentionally motivated.

Family meetings can be very helpful in problem solving. Whole-family meetings permit the professional to collect family history, detail problem areas and family coping strategies, and directly observe the patient-family interaction. It is important to determine what specific behaviors are most problematic for the caregivers, how the caregivers explain the cause of the problem, how they deal with the situation, and the outcome of their strategies both for the patient and themselves. A careful analysis of these components can lead to clear hypotheses about what works, what does not work, and which changes may improve outcomes.

Caregiver and patient distress can be reduced by simply offering information that changes the caregivers' view of the situation and that, in turn, changes their activity with the patient. Mr. R., for example, thought that his wife's memory problems were the result of laziness and that disciplined practice could alleviate them. According to Weston, Reeves, and Zarit (1980), however, home-based memory training efforts may have little effect on demented patients but may depress caregivers by highlighting the severity and irreversibility of their relative's deficits. Helping Mr. R. to understand and accept Mrs. R.'s objective limitations changed his expectations and well-intentioned efforts to help, and reduced the frustration experienced by both. On the other hand, some caregivers block the competencies of patients by expecting too little of them. Too much well-intentioned assistance can promote apathy and despair in the patient. Family members should be encouraged to allow the patient maximum self-sufficiency, to supplement the patient's material resources judiciously, and to offer just enough concrete assistance to compensate for the elderly person's objective limitations.

Often, when there is no spouse, one of the adult children is designated by the family to carry the main burdens of caregiving. In this situation the health care professional may seek to distribute responsibilities by involving more of the family system in the patient's care. Sometimes the selected caregiver is the least loved of the children, who is motivated to seek parental favor, expiate guilt, or block the other siblings from involvement (Cath, 1972). In this situation the whole family, particularly the caregiver, may resist the professional's effort to distribute responsibility. Not infrequently, family crises resulting from parental ill health reawaken old conflicts and sibling rivalries. Assessing the history of family relationships will provide important information about the caregiver's motivation, style, and possible areas of resistance to suggestions.

Families are often advised to place their cognitively impaired relatives in nursing homes. This bias toward institutionalization is itself partly based on assuming that dementia inevitably follows the pattern of decline seen in institutionalized patients. Observations of elderly demented patients kept at home versus those institutionalized, however, suggest that patients kept in their own homes have fewer behavioral problems and maintain their competencies better (Zarit, 1980). Many problems displayed by the institutionalized elderly may result from their impaired ability to cope with a changed environment and the concomitant overuse of medications. Even brief disruptions in environment, such as hospitalization, may produce symptoms of disorientation in vulnerable older persons. Family members should be advised that such symptoms may be reversed once the home situation is reestablished. At the same time, the needs of all family members must be taken into account (Soyer, 1972). At times, nursing home placement may be indicated as the lesser evil, in light of the ill effects that home care may have on the caregiver or other family members. The professional is often a supportive and reasonable sounding board, as the family struggles with such troublesome and ethically complex decisions.

REFERENCES

Alpaugh, P., & Haney, M. (1978). *Counseling the older adult: A training manual*. Los Angeles: Andrus Gerontology Center, University of Southern California.

Beck, A.T., & Beck, R.W. (1972). Screening depressed patients in family practice: A rapid technique. *Postgraduate Medicine, 52,* 81-85.

Bengtson, V.L. (1971). Inter-age differences in perception and the generation gap. *Gerontologist, 11*(4, pt. 2), 85-90.

Bengtson, V.L., & Treas, J. (1980). The changing family context of mental health and aging. In J.E. Birren & R.B. Sloane (Eds.), *Handbook of mental health and aging* (pp. 400-428). Englewood Cliffs, NJ: Prentice-Hall.

Besdine, R.W. (1980). Geriatric medicine: An overview. *Annual Review of Gerontology and Geriatrics, 1,* 135-153.

Birren, J.E., & Sloane, R.B. (Eds.) (1980). *Handbook of mental health and aging*. Englewood Cliffs, NJ: Prentice-Hall.

Blau, D., & Berezin, M.A. (1975). Neuroses and character disorders. In J.G. Howells (Ed.), *Modern perspectives in the psychiatry of old age* (pp. 201-233). New York: Brunner/Mazel.

Blazer, D. (1982). *Depression in late life*. St. Louis: C.V. Mosby.

Blazer, D., & Williams, C.D. (1980). Epidemiology of dysphoria and depression in an elderly population. *American Journal of Psychiatry, 137,* 439-444.

Boszormenyi-Nagy, I. (1972). Loyalty implications of the transference model in psychotherapy. *Archives of General Psychiatry, 27,* 374-380.

Brody, E.M., Kleban, M.H., & Moles, E. (1983). What older people do about their mental and physical health symptoms. *Journal of the American Geriatrics Society, 31*(8), 489-497.

Brown, A.S. (1974). Satisfying relationships for the elderly and their patterns of disengagement. *Gerontologist, 14,* 258-262.

Busse, E.W. (1973). Mental disorders in later life—Organic brain syndromes. In E.W. Busse & E. Pfeiffer (Eds.), *Mental illness in later life* (pp. 91-106). Washington, DC: American Psychiatric Association.

Busse, E.W., & Pfeiffer, E. (1977). Functional psychiatric disorders in old age. In E.W. Busse

& E. Pfeiffer (Eds.), *Behavior and adaptation in laterlife* (2nd ed., pp. 158-211). Boston: Little, Brown & Co.

Butler, R.N., & Lewis, M.I. (1973). *Aging and mental health: Positive psycho-social approaches*. St. Louis: C.V. Mosby.

Cath, S.H. (1972). The geriatric patient and his family: The institutionalization of a parent—A nadir of life. *Journal of Geriatric Psychiatry, 5*, 25-46.

Cohen, G.D. (1977). Approach to the geriatric patient. *Medical Clinics of North America, 61*(4), 855-866.

Cohler, B.J. (1983). Autonomy and interdependence in the family of adulthood: A psychological perspective. *Gerontologist, 23*, 33-39.

Costa, P.T. (1985). Longitudinal stability of personality and its relation to health perceptions. In C.M. Gaitz, G. Niederehe, & N.L. Wilson (Eds.), *Aging 2000: Our health care destiny* (Vol. 2). New York: Springer-Verlag.

Coyne, J.C. (1976a). Depression and the response of others. *Journal of Abnormal Psychology, 85*, 186-193.

Coyne, J.C. (1976b). Toward an interactional description of depression. *Psychiatry, 39*, 28-40.

Epstein, L.J. (1976). Depression in the elderly. *Journal of Gerontology, 31*, 278-282.

Fleisher, D. (1979). The practitioner's role: Assessment and response. In P.K. Ragan (Ed.), *Aging parents* (pp. 175-189). Los Angeles: University of Southern California Press.

Gaitz, C.M. (1978). Aged patients, their families and physicians. In G. Usdin & C.K. Hofling (Eds.), *Aging: The process and the people* (pp. 206-239). New York: Brunner/Mazel.

Gallagher, D., & Frankel, A.S. (1980). Depression in (an) older adult(s): A moderate structuralist viewpoint. *Psychotherapy: Theory, Research, and Practice, 17*, 101-104.

Geiger, D. (1978). How future professionals view the elderly: A comparative analysis of social work, law, and medical students' perceptions. *Gerontologist, 18*, 591-594.

Gorlin, R., & Zucker, H.D. (1983). Physicians' reactions to patients. *New England Journal of Medicine, 308*, 1059-1063.

Herr, J.J., & Weakland, J.H. (1979). *Counseling elders and their families*. New York: Springer.

Heyman, D.K., & Jeffers, F.C. (1963). Effect of time lapse on consistency of self-health and medical evaluations of elderly persons. *Journal of Gerontology, 18*, 160-164.

Hill, R., Foote, N., Aldous, J., Carlson, R., & MacDonald, R. (1970). *Family development in three generations*. Cambridge, MA: Schenkman.

Kahn, R.L. (1971). Psychological aspects of aging. In I. Rossman (Ed.), *Clinical geriatrics* (pp. 107-113). Philadelphia: J.B. Lippincott.

Kahn, R.L., Zarit, S.H., Hilbert, N.M., & Niederehe, G. (1975). Memory complaints and impairment in the aged: The effect of depression and altered brain function. *Archives of General Psychiatry, 32*, 1569-1573.

Karasu, T.B., & Katzman, R. (1976). Organic brain syndrome. In L. Bellak & T.B. Karasu (Eds.), *Geriatric psychiatry* (pp. 123-140). New York: Grune & Stratton.

Kay, D.W.K. (1972). Epidemiological aspects of organic brain disease in the aged. In C.M. Gaitz (Ed.), *Aging and the brain: Advances in behavioral biology* (Vol. 3, pp. 15-27). New York: Plenum.

Kiloh, L.G. (1973). Unmasking pseudodementia. *Geriatrics, 28*, 20-25.

Klein, D., Najman, J., Kohrman, A.F., & Munro, C. (1982). Patient characteristics that elicit negative responses from family physicians. *Journal of Family Practice, 14*(5), 881-888.

Lamy, P.P. (1979). Considerations in drug therapy of the elderly. *Journal of Drug Issues, 9*(1), 27-45.

Lawton, M.P. (1971). The functional assessment of elderly people. *Journal of the American Geriatrics Society, 19*, 465-480.

Leff, M.J., Roatch, J.F., & Bunney, W.E. (1970). Environmental factors preceding the onset of severe depressions. *Psychiatry, 33*, 293-311.

Levy, M., & Glantz, K. (1981). Drug misuse among the elderly. *Journal of Drug Education, 11*, 62.

Lewinsohn, P.M., & Lee, W.M.L. (1980). Assessment of affective disorders. In D.H. Barlow (Ed.), *Behavioral assessment of adult disorders* (pp. 129-179). New York: Guilford Press.

Libow, L. S. (1973). Pseudo-senility: Acute and reversible organic brain syndromes. *Journal of the American Geriatrics Society, 21,* 112-120.

Libow, L.S. (1981). General concepts of geriatric medicine. In L.S. Libow & F.T. Sherman (Eds.), *The core of geriatric medicine: A guide for students and practitioners* (pp. 1-15). St. Louis: C.V. Mosby.

Libow, L.S., & Sherman, F.T. (Eds.). (1981). *The core of geriatric medicine: A guide for students and practitioners*. St. Louis: C.V. Mosby.

Lopata, H.Z. (1973). *Widowhood in an American city*. Cambridge, MA: Schenkman.

Lowenthal, M.F. (1964). *Lives in distress: The paths of the elderly to the psychiatric ward*. New York: Basic Books.

Mace, N.L., & Rabins, P.V. (1981). *The 36-hour day: A family guide to caring for persons with Alzheimer's disease, related dementing illness, and memory loss in later life*. Baltimore: Johns Hopkins University Press.

Maddox, G.L. (1962). Some correlates of differences in self-assessment of health status among the elderly. *Journal of Gerontology, 17,* 180-185.

Maddox, G.L., & Douglas, E.B. (1973). Self-assessment of health: A longitudinal study of elderly subjects. *Journal of Health and Social Behavior, 14,* 87-93.

McDowell, F.H. (Ed.). (1980). *Managing the person with intellectual loss (dementia or Alzheimer's disease) at home*. White Plains, NY: The Burke Rehabilitation Center.

Mitchell, J. (1982). *Medicare access to physician services in nursing homes*. Health Care Financing Administration Grant No. 95-P-97885/1-02, unpublished.

National Institute on Aging Task Force. (1980). Senility reconsidered. *Journal of the American Medical Association, 244,* 259-263.

Niederehe, G., & Frugé, E.D. (1984). Dementia and family dynamics: Clinical research issues. *Journal of Geriatric Psychiatry, 17*(1), 21–56.

Nydegger, C. (Ed.). (1976). *Measuring morale: A guide to effective assessment*. Washington, DC: Gerontological Society.

Paykel, E.S., Myers, J.K., Dienelt, M.N., Klerman, G.L., Lindenthal, J.J., & Pepper, M.P. (1969). Life events and depression: A controlled study. *Archives of General Psychiatry, 21,* 753-760.

Pearce, J., & Miller, E. (1973). *Clinical aspects of dementia*. London: Baillière-Tindall.

Pfeiffer, E. (Ed.). (1975). *Multidimensional functional assessment: The OARS methodology*. Durham, NC: Center for the Study of Aging and Development, Duke University.

Pfeiffer, E., & Busse, E.W. (1973). Mental disorders in later life: Affective disorders; paranoid, neurotic, and situational reactions. In E.W. Busse & E. Pfeiffer (Eds.), *Mental illness in later life* (pp. 109-144). Washington, DC: American Psychiatric Association.

Post, F. (1976). Diagnosis of depression in geriatric patients and treatment modalities appropriate for the population. In D.M. Gallant & G.M. Simpson (Eds.), *Depression: Behavioral, biochemical, diagnostic, and treatment concepts* (pp. 205-231). New York: Spectrum Publications.

Powell, L.S., & Courtice, K. (1983). *Alzheimer's disease: A guide for families*. Reading, MA: Addison-Wesley.

Rabins, P.V., Mace, N.L., & Lucas, M.J. (1982). The impact of dementia on the family. *Journal of the American Medical Association, 248*(3), 333-335.

Regier, D.A., Goldberg, I.D., & Taube, C.A. (1978). The de facto US mental health services system. *Archives of General Psychiatry, 35,* 685-693.

Reisberg, B. (1981). *A guide to Alzheimer's disease: For families, spouses and friends*. New York: Free Press.

Remnet, V.L. (1979). Alternatives in health care services. In P.K. Ragan (Ed.), *Aging parents* (pp. 206-220). Los Angeles: University of Southern California Press.

Rosenmayr, L. (1968). Family relations of the elderly. *Journal of Marriage and the Family, 30,* 672-680.

Rowe, J.W., & Besdine, R.W. (Eds.). (1981). *Health and disease in old age*. Boston: Little, Brown.

Rubinstein, D., & Timmons, J.F. (1978). Depressive dyadic and triadic relationships. *Journal of Marriage and Family Counseling, 4,* 13-23.
Rynearson, E.K. (1977). The acute brain syndrome: A family affair. *Psychiatric Annals, 7,* 11-14.
Sainsbury, P., & Grad de Alarcon, J. (1970). The psychiatrist and the geriatric patient: The effects of community care on the family of the geriatric patient. *Journal of Geriatric Psychiatry, 4,* 23-41.
Salzman, C., & Shader, R.I. (1979). Clinical evaluation of depression in the elderly. In A. Raskin & L.F. Jarvik (Eds.), *Psychiatric symptoms and cognitive loss in the elderly* (pp. 39-72). Washington, DC: Hemisphere Publishing Co.
Seelbach, W.G. (1977). Gender differences in expectations for filial responsibility. *Gerontologist, 17,* 421-425.
Seelbach, W.C., & Sauer, W.J. (1977). Filial responsibility expectations and morale among aged parents. *Gerontologist, 17,* 492-499.
Shanas, E. (1960). Family responsibility and the health of older people. *Journal of Gerontology, 15,* 408-411.
Shanas, E., & Hauser, P.M. (1974). Zero population growth and the family life of old people. *Journal of Social Issues, 30*(4), 79-92.
Shanas, E., & Sussman, M.B. (1981). The family in later life: Social structure and social policy. In R.W. Fogel, E. Hatfield, S.B. Kiesler, & E. Shanas (Eds.), *Aging: Stability and change in the family* (pp. 211-231). New York: Academic Press.
Shanas, E., Townsend, P., Wedderburn, D., Friis, H., Milhoj, P., & Stehouwer, J. (1968). *Old people in three industrial societies*. New York: Atherton Press.
Silverman, C. (1968). *The epidemiology of depression*. Baltimore: Johns Hopkins University Press.
Simos, B.G. (1973). Adult children and their aging parents. *Social Work, 18,* 78-85.
Soldo, B.J. (1980). America's elderly population in the 1980s. *Population Bulletin, 35*(4), 3–48.
Soyer, D. (1972). The geriatric patient and his family: Helping the family to live with itself. *Journal of Geriatric Psychiatry, 5,* 52-65.
Sparacino, J., & Ronchi, D. (1982). Psychotherapy for Medicare patients: Can psychologists do the job? *Psychological Reports, 50,* 1103-1115.
Spence, D.L., Feigenbaum, E.M., Fitzgerald, F., & Roth, J. (1968). Medical student attitudes toward the geriatric patient. *Journal of the American Geriatrics Society, 16*(1), 976-983.
Stenback, A. (1980). Depression and suicidal behavior in old age. In J.E. Birren & R.B. Sloane (Eds.), *Handbook of mental health and aging* (pp. 616-652). Englewood Cliffs, NJ: Prentice-Hall.
Sussman, M.S. (1965). Relationships of adult children with their parents in the United States. In E. Shanas & G. Streib (Eds.), *Social structure and the family: Generational relationships* (pp. 62-92). Englewood Cliffs, NJ: Prentice-Hall.
Tager, R.M. (1980). Physical assessment, In S.H. Zarit (Ed.), *Aging and mental disorders: Psychological approaches to assessment and treatment* (pp. 161-183). New York: Free Press.
Verwoerdt, A., & Dovenmuehle, R.H. (1964). Physical illness and depressive symptomatology. *Journal of Gerontology, 19,* 330-335.
Walsh, F. (1980). The family in later life. In E.A. Carter & M. McGoldrick (Eds.), *The family life cycle: A framework for family therapy* (pp. 197-220). New York: Gardner Press.
Wang, H.S., & Busse, E.W. (1971). Dementia in old age. In C.E. Wells (Ed.), *Dementia* (pp. 152-162). Philadelphia: F.A. Davis.
Ware, L.A., & Carper, M. (1982). Living with Alzheimer disease patients: Family stresses and coping mechanisms. *Psychotherapy: Theory, Research and Practice, 19,* 472-481.
Wells, C.E. (1978). Chronic brain disease: An overview. *American Journal of Psychiatry, 135,* 1-12.
Wells, C.E. (1979). Pseudodementia. *American Journal of Psychiatry, 136,* 895-900.
Weston, J.M., Reeves, K.E., & Zarit, S.H. (1980). Effects of training on severe memory loss.

Paper presented at the 33rd Annual Scientific Meeting of the Gerontological Society, San Diego, California.
Wetle, T. (Ed.). (1982). *Handbook of geriatric care*. East Hanover, NJ: Sandoz.
Zarit, S.H. (1979). The organic brain syndromes and family relationships. In P.K. Ragan (Ed.), *Aging parents* (pp. 237-257). Los Angeles: University of Southern California Press.
Zarit, S.H. (1980). (Ed.). *Aging and mental disorders: Psychological approaches to assessment and treatment*. New York: Free Press.
Zarit, S.H., & Zarit, J.M. (1982). Families under stress: Interventions for caregivers of senile dementia patients. *Psychotherapy: Theory, Research and Practice, 19*, 461-471.
Zung, W.W.K. (1980). Affective disorders. In E.W. Busse & D. Blazer (Eds.), *Handbook of geriatric psychiatry* (pp. 338-367). New York: Van Nostrand Reinhold.

III.
CLINICAL APPLICATION OF A FAMILY SYSTEMS APPROACH

11

THE FAMILY AND SUBSTANCE ABUSE

M. DUNCAN STANTON, Ph.D. and JUDITH LANDAU, M.D.

When a practitioner encounters a person who is abusing drugs or alcohol, several questions seem appropriate to ask. The first is: Why is this person using substances now? In other words, what events and patterns in this person's life have catalyzed or contributed to drug- or alcohol-taking at this time? Is there something distinctive about his or her life, or stage in life, that has led to substance abuse? Why is he or she appearing now, instead of six months ago, or two years hence? What is going on at present that led or contributed to the current problem?

In this chapter, we shall attempt to deal with these questions in a framework that includes the substance abuser's "significant others"—usually the family—and pay particular attention to the context of the abuse or addiction. Given certain conditions, substance abuse may be a means of adapting to changes in the family's life cycle and, contrary to popular belief, may in effect be "functional" within the family system.

First, however, it is necessary to look at the problem from a perspective that may reveal why such "undesirable" behavior might be adaptive and functional. This notion is not proffered as an "excuse" for abuse. The idea is to place it in a framework that divests it of some of the blaming it can engender, thus setting the stage for intervention and treatment. Such a perspective promotes change and improvement without placing the practitioner in a position in which he incurs defensiveness and inordinate resistance by patient and family. To this end, several important concepts that bear on drug and alcohol abuse by a family member will be explicated.

Applying a Conceptual Framework

To intervene effectively in a substance-abusing family, the practitioner needs to understand the concepts that have emerged in the family therapy field concerning family dynamics, structures, and patterns. Many of these have been presented in the earlier chapters of this book. Such formulations differ from conventional views of patients, their families, and ideas of how symptoms develop within them. Too often in the past a simplistic view of the family has predominated. Except for consideration of the early developmental years, the family has until recently been viewed as a more or less inert influence which, at worst, can bring additional stress on the symptomatic member. The family's importance in symptom *maintenance* generally went unrecognized. When the family was mentioned, discussion usually focused on, for example, mother-addict or father-addict dyads, or on the characteristics of these people as individuals. The concept of the family as a *system of people* composed of the members *and their interactions* is relatively new. In other words, individually and dyadically oriented concepts are no longer in tune with what we have learned about families during the past 25 to 30 years (Stanton, 1980b).

In families in which a young person is abusing drugs or alcohol, the prototypic pattern shows that one parent is intensely involved or enmeshed with the abuser, while the other parent is more punitive, distant, or absent (Stanton, 1979a). Usually the overinvolved, indulgent, overprotective parent is of the opposite sex of the abuser's, although this varies among cultural groups, and in some abusers' families the same-sex parent or both parents may show such enmeshment. Sometimes the overinvolvement (intergenerational coalition) may reach the point of incest, especially in families in which the drug abuser is female.

Until recently, the extent to which substance abusers are involved with their families of origin (parents, grandparents, siblings) has tended to be overlooked. To be sure, it has not necessarily been obvious that, for example, addicts in their late twenties and early thirties would still be involved with their parents. Their age, submersion in the drug subculture, frequent changes of residence, possible military service, and other characteristics all seemed to imply that they were cut off, or at least distanced, from one or both parents. Thus they were predominantly viewed as "drifters" or "loners" with few or no primary ties.

Emerging research challenges this notion. In reviews of 17 studies and reports in which patterns of parent-addict contact were examined, the first author (Stanton, 1980a, 1980b; Stanton, Todd, Heard, et al., 1978; Stanton, Todd, & Associates, 1982) found increasing evidence that, despite their frequent protestations of independence and their efforts to protect their parents, the majority of addicts maintain close family ties. Even if they do not reside with their parents, they may live nearby, and the frequency of contact is high. The general findings are that two-thirds of U.S. male addicts under age 35 (most being in their middle and late twenties) either live with their parents or see their mothers daily, while 80 to 90% see one or both parents weekly. Perzel and Lamon (1979) indicated that 42 to 48% of polydrug abusers live with their parents, compared to 21% of patients with other psychiatric diagnoses and 7% of a group of comparable "normals." Further, this phenomenon does not seem to be limited to North America, as 80% of the addicts in Italy and Thailand, 67% of those in Puerto Rico, and 62% of the addicts in England have been reported to be living with their parents. These multiple findings document the loose boundaries (enmeshment) that seem to exist between most addicts and their parents or parent surrogates, and they hint at the possible importance of the family of origin in the addiction process.

It is easy for the physician to be caught in the myth that the addict is either "enmeshed" or "cut off" (out of touch) from his or her family, and that these are unrelated family patterns. It is common, however, for the addict to be at times close, at other times distant, from the family. Even if one pattern predominates, a multiperson behavioral cycle is involved. The cycle may include siblings and other relatives who maintain indirect communication between the addict and his or her parents. The apparent closeness and distance are merely polar extremes of an unresolved conflict in the transition that occurs during the family life-cycle stage of "leaving home" (Landau, Griffiths, & Mason, 1982).

Triads

The concept of triads or triangles being involved in people's interpersonal problems and symptoms has been a cornerstone of family therapy. Assuming that a triad is involved in the problem is an almost invariably correct assumption. Usually the triad involves two adults and the identified patient. If the symptomatic person is a young man who abuses drugs, for example, one commonly observes that his mother lavishes affection on him because she is not getting enough time and attention from his father. Conversely, the husband may retreat because his wife undercuts him—as, for example, when he tries to discipline the son appropriately. Further, the drug-abusing son may serve a function for the parents, either as a channel for their communication or as a disrupter whose distracting behavior keeps the parents' fights from crystallizing; he may seek a "sick state" to position himself, childlike, as the focus of his parents' attentions. This kind of thinking is attuned to the whole family system and shows how all members may together become caught in a repetitive, dysfunctional pattern.

An adult may become a heavy drinker when his job and family escalate their respective demands on him to the point at which he can no longer satisfy both; the drinking serves as a withdrawal from an impossible situation and also as a way of getting both systems to relax their demands.

In some substance abusers' families of origin, one parent (often the father) is absent. In such cases, one would think that a triadic model would not apply, and that a dyadic framework, that is, one encompassing mother and son, would be more fitting. It would also seem to be more parsimonious and less complicated. Nonetheless, we have found (Stanton et al., 1978) that when the matter is pursued closely a third member generally emerges as an important participant in the interaction. Usually the triadic system takes a less obvious form, like a covert disagreement between mother and grandmother or mother and ex-husband. This is consonant with a point made emphatically by Haley (1976) that at least two adults usually are involved in an offspring's problem and that clinicians should look for a triangle consisting of an overinvolved parent-child dyad and a more peripheral parent, grandparent, or parent surrogate. Thus, in addition to the (male) addict and his mother, the triad may include mother's male friend, an estranged father, a grandparent, some other relative, or even a therapist or agency. These alternative systems seem to exhibit patterns and cycles similar to those in which both parents are present, and they often revolve around interruption by the abuser of conflicts between adult members. Achieving separation and independence is even more of an issue in single-parent families, however, since the single parent may be left alone with few interpersonal supports if the drug abuser departs.

Family Homeostasis and the Family Addiction Cycle

Families have a sense of balance and stability. When disruptions occur in this balance, built-in, "homeostatic" compensatory mechanisms take hold to return the family to stability. This regulation is manifested by a series of repetitive family behavior patterns. A particularly cogent depiction of family homeostasis emerges from observations of the families of heroin addicts. Stanton and associates (Stanton, 1980a; Stanton et al., 1978) have noted that drug-taking is often part of a cyclical process that involves three or more individuals, commonly the addict and two parental figures. These people form an intimate, interdependent, interpersonal system. At times the equilibrium of the system is disturbed, as when discord between the parents rises to the point of impending separation. When this happens, the addict becomes activated, his or her behavior changes, and he or she creates a situation that dramatically *focuses attention upon himself or herself*.

The behavior can take a number of forms. For example, he or she may lose his or her temper, come home high, commit a serious crime, or overdose on drugs. Whatever its form, however, the action allows the parents to shift focus from their marital conflict to a parental overinvolvement with the offspring. In effect, the movement is from an unstable dyadic interaction (i.e., parents alone) to a more stable triadic interaction (parents and addict). By focusing on the problems of addiction, no matter how severe or life-threatening, the parents choose a course that is apparently safer than dealing with long-standing marital tensions. Consequently, after the marital crisis has been successfully avoided, the addict shifts to a less provocative stance and begins to behave more competently.

This is a new step in the sequence. As the addict demonstrates increased competence, indicating the ability to function independently of the family—for example, by getting a job, getting married, enrolling in a drug treatment program, or detoxifying—the parents are left to deal with their still unresolved conflicts. At this point in the cycle, marital tensions increase and the threat of separation arises again. The addict then behaves in an attention-getting or self-destructive way, and the dysfunctional triadic cycle is again completed.

In this framework, then, the drug taking is part of a *family* addiction cycle. Although a particular person abuses drugs or alcohol, this should not be seen as his or her action alone. It is one bit of behavior in a temporal *sequence* of behaviors that involves several people, predominantly family members. All are part of the repetitive process. Attending to the behavior of only one member necessarily limits both one's understanding and one's therapeutic options.

The addiction cycle may vary in intensity. It may occur in subdued form in treatment sessions or during day-to-day interactions and conversations in the home. For example, a parent hinting at vacationing without the spouse may trigger a spurt of loud talking by the addict. If the stakes are increased, the cycle becomes more explosive and the actions of all participants grow more serious and more dramatic; the parents' threats of divorce, for example, might be followed by the addict's overdosing. Whatever their intensity level, such patterns are regularly observed by clinicians and researchers. Thus, when viewed from this perspective, the behavior of the addict serves an important *protective* function and helps to maintain the homeostatic balance of the family system.

In addition to the family, the addiction cycle may include other systems, such as courts, schools, hospitals, and other "helpers," as the following case example shows.

Case example. Twenty-three-year-old Jim had been addicted to opiates for seven years (Heard, 1982). He lived with his parents and two younger sisters. Recently his paternal great-aunt had moved into the home, usurping

Jim's room and serving as a source of conflict between his parents. Jim reacted to the family conflict by exploding emotionally at the other members and then admitting himself to a drug treatment hospital unit for detoxification. Several days later he discharged himself against medical advice, before he had completed detoxification, and returned home. The therapist (David Heard, Ph.D.) soon learned that this was a rather common pattern for Jim and his family. In fact, he had unsuccessfully attempted to detoxify in this way nine times in the previous five or six years: Tension would mount in the family over some issue, Jim would blow up, enter the hospital, and then abort his treatment. In each instance the hospital would admit him without conditions or without involving his family, and each time the result was the same. The pattern kept repeating itself even though hospital staff members were aware of his multiple admissions and failures. In other words, a repetitive cycle that had originally begun among family members had been expanded to include the hospital. The institution provided a convenient "steam valve" and had unwittingly become an essential element in the process. Thus the expanded therapeutic system, including hospital, physicians, and staff, was an integral part of the homeostasis. The addiction cycle involved multiple systems, rather than only the addict and his family.

The importance of observing the symptom within its wider behavioral context is apparent in this example. To be effective, the physician needs to know the conditions leading up to and surrounding a particular behavior or symptom.

Family Role Selection

Family members are assigned particular roles in their families, often before they are born. The roles depend on multiple variables like birth order, gender, energy level, and what is transpiring in the family at the birth. A child born during a period of parental bereavement will have different experiences from those of a child born at a time of joy or financial success. In extreme cases a child may be "assigned" to one parent as belonging to him or her, while the other parent may "adopt" a later child. Sometimes a parent or parents "buy" freedom from their own parents by giving away a child to the older couple to raise. The role of "black sheep" is often assigned to one member in each generation of a family, as is the role of the "responsible" or "parentified" child. Reilly (1976) noted that the naming process is important, as children are sometimes raised in the role of the person, usually a relative, after whom they are named; he observed also that substance abusers are sometimes named after relatives who have an addiction problem. To believe, then, that the environment is the same for all children in a family is to make a grave miscalculation. Family members are *not* treated identically, although less dysfunctional or less disturbed families will allow offspring more role flexibility. This point is important for drug and alcohol treatment because it concerns the issue of why all siblings do not take drugs with equal frequency, especially if all of them have equal opportunity to observe the drug-taking patterns of their parents. "Modeling" parents' behavior is only a partial explanation for drug-taking behavior.

The "Identified Patient" or "Scapegoat"

From a family viewpoint, difficulties or symptoms one member experiences are part of a total family process in which that one member is labeled as the problem. This viewpoint contrasts with the more traditional notion that blame and responsibility must be laid at the feet of either the substance abuser or the parents. To counter the natural tendency to ascribe blame, it may be helpful to view symptomatic members as sacrificial persons (Stanton, 1977). They give up their reputations and well-being in the service of their families. They may protect their families from the intrusion of outside helpers by drawing attention to themselves and their problems. Trying to cope with their troubles may be a rallying point which brings their families together; in some families it seems that no one else can unite the system and, if the substance abuser's problem disappears, the family becomes fragmented. Of course symptom bearers also perpetuate the problem, sometimes even in the face of growth or improvement in other family members; they may try to get the family to return to the old homeostatic condition.

This view of symptomatic members as sacrificial is radically new to some people, and it may be hard to believe. Perhaps one has to observe the phenomenon in order to be persuaded. One may have to see, for example, how a son avoids success and realization of his potential so as to prevent his uneducated father from appearing as the least competent family member. Perhaps one has to observe a child who is the identified patient burst out with symptoms when the parents begin to move toward divorce, thus reuniting them around helping him or her and postponing the separation. Whatever the case, this process takes place in many families and acknowledging it may help to understand why symptoms occur as they do.

Case example. Marty, age 14, was a compulsive polydrug abuser who had attemped suicide twice and had a history of running away. His drug abuse had caused his expulsion from school. In desperation his parents had him admitted to a hospital. In family therapy sessions Marty made a concerted effort to keep the therapists (the second author and Nancy Fox, Ph.D.) focused on him and his problems. Each time the therapists asked the parents anything about themselves, Marty became intrusive and vociferous, to the extent of blowing a handmade paper trumpet to detour the therapists' efforts. It became evident that the therapy should initially focus on helping the parents to unite in relation to their son.

For a number of sessions the therapy remained centered on how to deal with Marty. This restructuring move enabled the parents to work together toward mutually acceptable goals. At this stage their marriage was not addressed, as they were not ready to face the problems of their own relationship. It is generally wisest not to deal with marital issues early in such treatment (Haley, 1980), at least until success is attained both with the presenting problem and, where appropriate, with parenting issues.

Once the parents had succeeded with Marty, by controlling him in sessions and making him adhere to hospital rules, they felt safe enough to reveal that their marriage had been on the rocks for 22 years. The mother had been drinking heavily for a long time, and Marty was almost the only topic on which she and Marty's father communicated. When the issue of separation and divorce was raised in therapy, Marty's behavior became intolerable, and both parents focused on him instead of completing the discussion. Repeatedly and emphatically the therapists had to redirect the parents from their attention to Marty. Finally, as Marty realized that his parents were indeed capable of dealing directly with each other—even if this meant divorce—his unruly behavior abated. He no longer had to sacrifice himself, because his mother and father were facing the real issues in the family. By the time of Marty's discharge from the hospital five weeks after admission, his parents had separated. A follow-up six months later indicated that the parents had remained separated while sharing parenting responsibilities and that the mother had stopped drinking. Marty, who was relating well to both parents, was doing well in school, had ceased his drug abuse and running away, and was no longer showing indications of depression.

Family Life Cycle

Failure to resolve family life-cycle transitions often is a major factor in substance abuse. Among families of youthful drug abusers, problems at two particular life-cycle stages appear to be unduly common. The first of these is the beginning adolescence of the identified patient-to-be (Landeau & Stanton, 1983). The young person is going through the normal but often troublesome process of growing up, experimenting with new behaviors, becoming self-assertive, and developing close (usually heterosexual) relationships outside the family. Drug experimentation is now more a part of the process than in the past.

As Kandel, Treiman, Faust, and Single (1976) propose, there are three stages in adolescent drug use, each having different concomitants. First is the use of legal drugs, like alcohol, and this is mainly a social phenomenon. The second involves use of marijuana and is also primarily peer-influenced. The third stage, frequent or compulsive use of other illegal drugs, seems to be contingent more on the quality of the parent-adolescent relationship than on other factors. Thus, these authors conclude from their studies that more serious drug misuse is predominantly a family phenomenon. Not infrequently, the young abuser was a "favorite child" or the "easiest to raise" during his or her earlier years, but now the child is a problem. This seems to be tied, again, to the family's inability to adjust to the adolescent's growing independence and, especially, to the initial heterosexual involvement with peers, as occurs when dating begins. The young person is becoming less available and less attached to the family, who cannot tolerate the competition and threatened loss.

The second important life-cycle stage for families of youthful drug abusers is the point at which it is appropriate for the young person to leave home (Haley, 1980). Since he or she seems to be badly needed by the family, the threatened departure heralds parental panic. The family then becomes stuck in a chronic, repetitive process centered on the young member's leaving home; sometimes this happens quite overtly and goes through a number of cycles, the young person moving out of the home and then back in again. The pressure not to leave may be so powerful that the family will endure (and even encourage) terrible indignities such as lying, stealing, and public shame, rather than take a firm position in relation to this offspring. The family may also protect the young person from outside agencies, relatives, and other social systems. Rather than accept responsibility, family members may blame external systems, like peers or the neighborhood, for the drug problem. When the parents take effective action, such as evicting their addicted offspring, they often undo their actions by encouraging his or her return. They seem to be saying, "We will suffer almost anything, but please don't leave us." Thus it becomes nearly impossible for the addict to negotiate a way out of the family, and he or she will slip into greater abuse as a means of resolving the bind (Stanton, 1980a; Stanton et al., 1978; Stanton, Todd, & Associates, 1982). Again, the transition from drug use to abuse is an example of a family's conflict around a transitional stage in its life cycle (Landau, in press; Landau, Griffiths, & Mason, 1982).

For adult substance abusers who develop drinking problems, other life-cycle stages frequently are related to the onset or exacerbation of the problem. Loss of a job or retirement are common ones, i.e., the risk of alcoholism increases among the jobless. Among women who develop drinking problems in middle age, the "empty nest" syndrome is often reported to be related to the onset of their drinking (Curlee, 1969). Finally, many substance abuse problems arise after a bereavement, especially if the lost family member was "powerful" and the death unexpected (Coleman & Stanton, 1978; Stanton & Coleman, 1980).

Comparisons with Other Symptoms or Disorders

Since a number of disorders, in addition to drug abuse, show a pattern of overinvolvement by one parent and distance or absence by the other, the question arises as to how drug abusers' families differ from other dysfunctional families. Stanton and associates (1978, 1982) have tried to clarify this issue, drawing from the literature and their own studies. In brief, the cluster of distinguishing factors for addict families seems to include the following:

(a) There is a higher frequency of multigenerational chemical dependency —particularly alcohol among males—plus a propensity for other addiction-like behaviors such as gambling and watching television (such practices provide modeling for children and may also develop into family "traditions").
(b) Compared, in particular, to families of persons who have schizophrenic or psychosomatic disorders, families of addicts seem to express conflict more primitively and directly.
(c) Alliances among family members are often quite explicit (versus covert), for example, between addict and overinvolved parent, and are usually viewed as very "close" by the family.
(d) The kind of blurred communications and ambivalent mother-child patterns seen in schizophrenic families are not as common in addict families.
(e) Addicts may have a peer group or subculture to which they retreat briefly following family conflict—the illusion of independence is greater.
(f) Mothers of addicts display "symbiotic" child-rearing practices longer into the life of the child, and they show greater symbiotic needs than mothers of schizophrenic and normal persons.
(g) There is a preponderance of death themes and premature, unexpected, or untimely deaths in the family.
(h) The symptom of addiction provides an illusion of independence, of being or appearing to be simultaneously dependent and individuated at several levels, from the individual-pharmacological level to that of the drug subculture.
(i) The rate of addiction among immigrants' offspring raised in the family's new culture is higher than might be expected, suggesting the importance of acculturation and parent-child cultural disparity in addiction.

Clinical Considerations

In this section we shall give some guidelines that the primary-care physician might want to apply when dealing with a substance abuse problem.

Symptom Context

When encountering an identified substance-abusing person in a clinical situation, the practitioner should consider the questions posed at the beginning of this chapter: Why is this person appearing now? Why did he or she not show up six months ago, or two years hence? What is going on at present that has led or contributed to the current problem? One way of approaching such questions is to try to get an overall view of the problem—to see it in its context. This includes determining what interpersonal systems, particularly the family, are involved. One might ask the patient with whom he or she is living. Who raised him or her? Even if the patient is an adult, it may be advisable to ask, Where are the parents, or the people who raised him or her? How often does the patient see or talk on the phone to these people? Who are the most "powerful" people in the family? Who gets most upset when the problem occurs? The physician wants to keep an eye out for important, often influential, but "hidden" family members who may not be identified without a little probing (in one of our addiction cases, no change could take place until an uncle, who was head of the family and lived 1,000 miles away, approved the therapy). The purpose of this line of inquiry is to find out who else might be involved in the interpersonal sequence of behaviors that precede and succeed the symptomatic behavior, thus providing clues to the family or other systems in which the problem occurs. The physician might even ask specifically about the behavior of these significant others in the sequence. In our experience, however, most people do not think in terms of such sequences, and because such questions might sound like these others are being blamed, most patients need to be led gently through the questioning.

It is helpful to remember that symptoms often occur when a person is caught in an impossible situation and feels unable to escape (Haley, 1976). The physician, then, will want to know about the conflicting forces buffeting and entrapping the patient. With which systems does he or she interact? What triads or triangles (in which the patient is one element) are involved? Is there a struggle between two parents, between the requirements of job and family, between growing up and staying home, between a parent and the patient's spouse? All answers to such questions may give clues on how the symptom may provide a "way out" or serve some other function.

In the first interview, or as part of routine initial information-gathering, it is always wise to ask about issues of alcohol and drug taking—both prescribed and nonprescribed—among family members. These questions should be posed in a factual, nonemotive way, so that they are not construed as blaming. They are asked at this point because the family is usually in crisis and is more willing to reveal or admit to such practices among its members. Later on, family members tend to be more guarded and reluctant to disclose information of this sort.

In addition to identifying the people involved, the physician must determine the family life-cycle stage and the transitional point that bear on the problem. We have found the family life-cycle concept invaluable diagnostically. The clinician wants to determine who is growing up, is leaving home, has obtained or lost a job, is faced with retirement, has died, has left or is threatening to leave the family. In fact, Noone (1979), in a study of heroin and barbiturate addicts, examined the contiguity of family additions, losses, threatened losses (e.g., heart attacks, diagnoses of cancer in a family member), or retirement, to drug-related behavior by the addict. He found that in 86% of the cases at least one such event had occurred in the family at about the same time the addict was described as first developing a drug-abuse problem. Similar events occurred also in concert with most overdoses (80%), arrests (80%), and points when the addict entered treatment (67%). These data underscore the utility of viewing drug taking vis-à-vis life-cycle events, with their attendant changes in the family structure.

Families are usually unaware of any connection between the onset of problems and life-cycle/structural changes. For example, a couple was recently referred to the first author because of marital problems; the husband had also been "slacking off" at his sales job, was occasionally abusing tranquilizers, and had been drinking heavily—a dangerous pharmacological combination. The couple placed the beginning of their problems about 11 months earlier but could not explain why things had begun to deteriorate at that time. A few minutes later in the interview the first author asked each of them where their parents were. It was revealed that the husband's mother (with whom he had been very close and somewhat joined in a coalition against his wife) had died 11 months ago. Despite the obvious importance of this event, however, the couple had not associated it with their subsequent difficulties. In addition to the loss, and the husband's probably unresolved mourning, the mother's death had led to a shift in the structure of the couple's relationship. No longer allied with and dependent upon his mother's support (and possibly her pulling him away from the marriage), the husband had turned to his wife for support and closeness. Because a long-time balance had been maintained in the marriage, in which the wife had remained somewhat distant in order to offset the opposing dyad of husband and mother-in-law (and perhaps not get too close to her husband as a result of the pull from her own family), she was not prepared to embrace her husband so suddenly. She could not readily throw off the old homeostatic/structural pattern. She repelled him and their struggles intensifed, developing into a series of battles, threats to leave each other, and symptomatic behavior on the part of the husband. Through it all, the importance for their marriage of the major change/loss that had occurred had escaped them completely.

In contrast to this case, it is not uncommon for a married woman who becomes an abuser of, for example, sedatives, to be experiencing the loss of a spouse (rather than attempting to reject a husband who is trying to get closer or more dependent on her). The loss may not be total but may result from his becoming more involved in work (especially if he is an ambitious, high-achieving man), thus giving her less time, attention, and support. She might be caught between (a) the positive features of the change (e.g., higher income and social status, or recognition that his work is important because he is involved, for instance, in a helping profession), and (b) the negative aspect that her own needs are being addressed even less than before. The drug taking becomes an escape from this approach-avoidance conflict associated with familial/marital change.

While the connection between family life-cycle change and symptom onset may, in a given case, be clear to the physician, he or she should not necessarily expect the patient or family to be overly receptive to his "astute interpretation." Some people will find such insights very helpful. Others may deny any such connection. The extent of their receptiveness seems to depend greatly on how the issue is broached.

A Nonblaming Approach

It is sometimes easy for practitioners to become impatient, even irritated, with substance abusers, especially in view of the apparent self-destructiveness of their behavior. Many such patients may also be quite deceptive, which is frustrating to the professional who is trying his or her best to be helpful and to provide good treatment; the physician may feel like a defense attorney whose client will not tell the truth, severely handicapping the attorney's efforts. Nonetheless, it is rarely effective to permit oneself the emotional luxury of slipping into a lecturing or blaming stance with these patients and their families. Such a response by the practitioner is neither tactically nor theoretically sound. A negative reaction by the physician will usually turn off the client, causing further misrepresentation or withdrawal from treatment. These patients are usually tremendously defensive, and "blaming" causes them to muster massive resistance to what they see as a pejorative label.

They may respond either by arguing with the physician or by side-stepping the issue or the treatment entirely. Further, if a substance abuser can be seen as caught in a web of conflicts in his or her interpersonal system, to saddle him or her wholly with the blame is to oversimplify a complex process, possibly leading to the patient's being scapegoated by the physician. If a problem like an addictive cycle resides in a family system in which each person (including, of course, the identified patient) is a contributor, singling out one member has great limitations. By exhorting the identified patient to "grow up" or "shape up," the physician places himself or herself in direct competition with the whole system, in relation to the abuser. As the patient's system of significant others usually is more important to him than is the physician, the patient is much more likely to respond to the needs of the former than to the dictates of the latter. The patient may feel trapped and will get out of the bind in the best way he or she knows, sometimes by lying, other times by noncompliance or escape.

For the same reason, it also helps very little for example, to blame an abuser's parents, either when seeing the father or mother alone or conjointly. Drug addicts, in particular, are extremely protective of their families, whether conscious of this or not. Sensitive therapists learned long ago not to take sides with a patient against parents, because this usually leads to increased and sometimes subtle resistance by all members. Even if the abuser ostensibly agrees with the physician, the message being conveyed is that, if the parents and family are brought in for evaluation or treatment, they will be exposed to what the patient perceives as outright attack. The patient will rarely let this happen, responding instead with a litany of reasons why the parents cannot be present now or in the future. A nonblaming stance by the practitioner is more likely to elicit additional information that will be valuable in establishing a treatment plan.

The physician may find it useful to *ascribe noble intentions*, rather than blame, to the participants in the drug abuse drama (Stanton et al., 1982). This turning the resistance back on itself has been termed "positive interpretation." The strategy helps to remove defensiveness and may even lead the patient and family toward beneficial change. The practitioner might, for instance, praise a drug abuser for his or her efforts to "keep the family together" by providing "excitement" and giving the parents a job on which to work together, which helps to unite them. The physician may note how the patient "really must care" about the family to go to such lengths to accomplish this. The phrasing of the message is important; if it is stated with a negative tag attached (e.g., "You are keeping them together when they really dislike each other and can't get along"), the patient's response will again be one of opposition. The message must have no negative or judgmental feature because this could cancel out its positive aspect. The physician must be careful also not to smile or appear uncomfortable when making positive interpretations so as not to seem sarcastic and insincere.

As another example of positive interpretation, a clinician could note how helpful a sedative-abusing person's behavior is to his or her spouse. A woman might be told that, by being a problem, she makes her husband look more competent in contrast; she provides him with a concern and a kind of job in caring for her, allowing him to feel important and helpful. In other words, by endangering her own mental and physical health, she is giving her ambitious, busy husband an excuse to leave his demanding job and spend time at home. In a sense, he can devote time to his marriage with a clearer conscience about "neglecting" his work. Thus she deserves praise for her "sacrifice" and for helping her husband sort out his priorities.

This example is not meant to imply that the physician should openly condone or encourage a spouse's substance abuse. The intent is to reframe an existing situation in positive terms to avoid the automatic resistance that follows blaming. If the patient is not blamed, he or she becomes free to be more receptive to other means of coping and may even suggest alternatives (e.g., socializing more, mobilizing family and other supportive networks, becoming involved in activities) that will draw him or her out of the substance-abuse cycle.

A common reaction to positive interpretation is for the patient and family to be caught off guard, and even, initially, to be bewildered. They expected to be told to stop what they are doing and they may also have anticipated being blamed. Hearing their behaviors put in a positive light, they are less likely to counterattack or otherwise resist and may feel more amenable to opening the door to change. One reason why this approach may work is that many people with problems often *do* feel as though they are "working overtime" to help their family members. They see themselves in the same positive light as the interpretation. They feel unappreciated, and the physician who recognizes this gains considerable leverage simply by conveying understanding of their predicament. In any event, these techniques have been developed by therapists who deal with many resistant families and patients; if properly applied, the method may help to set the stage for improvement.

Interventions

In the past, rarely has a primary-care physician developed the skills for working with and attempting to change family interaction patterns. Thinking in terms of a whole family system when one has been accustomed to dealing with individual problems is difficult, and different skills are required for treating a system. What must be done, usually, is to try to change the family's interactions *within the actual session*. This can be done by restructuring (Minuchin, 1974) for both diagnostic and intervening purposes. For instance, a "distant" father and his drug-abusing son might be encouraged, while in the office, to interact around a common interest or goal, while the physician subtly supports the mother and keeps her out of the father-son conversation (perhaps by sitting next to her and talking softly to her during the father-son interchange). The ease or difficulty with which the two males talk provides diagnostic information and gives the physician clues as to whether they need to be pushed a little harder to talk amiably. The physician may want to test other hypotheses by changing family seating arrangements and seeing what happens. The extent to which the physician engages in such interventions depends on his or her interest in experimenting and on the time available. The physician should probably avoid being too passive during the process. If he or she is not fairly active, working to bring about change in the session, the family's behavior patterns will remain unaltered and the members will continue to interact much as they do outside the treatment setting (Stanton, 1979b).

At times the severity of a patient's substance-abuse problem may reach life-threatening proportions, while the family denies the problem or takes no responsibility to help. The physician must then force the family to face this harsh reality—to point out that the identified patient may commit suicide or otherwise die unless something is done soon. In our experience, such reality facing is much less likely to be effective when it is directed to the patient alone; some reasons for this have been presented earlier. Instead, the likelihood for action and change is greater if the severity of the problem is conveyed to the family (and parents) *directly*. In other words, the whole system is addressed. This removes the identified patient from center stage and may mobilize positive actions and support from the family.

The intervention is more likely to succeed, however, if the physician follows a certain sequence. If, for instance, the physician wants to raise the concern of a father who claims to have given up on his substance-abusing son, the father should first be given credit for his concern. He could be told, "You care more about your son than you are letting on, otherwise you wouldn't be here today. My bet is that you would be the first to bail him out if he got into trouble" (a not uncommon pattern in substance-abusers' families). The physician might even argue mildly with the father about this, pressing home the positive side of the father's contribution. Once this is done, chances are better that the father will concur when the practitioner follows with a statement such as: "If something isn't done quickly, your son will soon be dead. But I can't prevent this myself. I need your help. After all, you are the people who care about him and who are important to him."

This kind of approach could, of course, be taken with both parents (as a unit), a spouse, or others. When the physician believes he or she must take a strong stand (and we would recommend that such a posture be assumed only under exceptional circumstances), the statement should be prefaced with an almost equally strong dose of positive interpretation.

Referral

Naturally, most primary-care physicians do not become deeply involved in psychotherapy of families of substance abusers. But, by observing and gathering relevant information about an abuser's familial and interpersonal context, the practitioner serves both patient and family in an important way by obtaining data needed for an appropriate referral. Once the physician identifies the family members involved in the problem, and the transitional family life-cycle stage that has not been resolved, he or she can convey this information to the person to whom the family is referred. For patients referred for psychotherapy in whose cases family factors seem to be important, the physician may, of course, want to involve a practitioner who is comfortable in dealing with whole families—perhaps one who practices routinely in this way. Whatever the situation, by obtaining a clearer picture of the substance-abuse problem in its interpersonal/familial context, the primary-care physician advances his or her own commitment to sound clinical judgment and effective treatment.

REFERENCES

Coleman, S.B., & Stanton, M.D. (1978). The role of death in the addict family. *Journal of Marital and Family Therapy*, *4*, 79-91.

Curlee, J. (1969). Alcoholism and the "empty nest." *Bulletin of the Menninger Clinic*, *33*, 165-171.

Haley, J. (1976). *Problem-solving therapy*. San Francisco: Jossey-Bass.

Haley, J. (1980). *Leaving home: Therapy with disturbed young people*. New York: McGraw-Hill.

Heard, D.B. (1982). Death as a motivator: Using crisis induction to break through the denial system. In M.D. Stanton, T.C. Todd, & Associates, *The family therapy of drug abuse and addiction*. New York: Guilford.

Kandel, D.B., Treiman, D., Faust, R., & Single, E. (1976). Adolescent involvement in legal and illegal drug use: A multiple classification analysis. *Social Forces*, *54*, 438-458.

Landau, J. (in press). *The family in transition: Theory and practice*. New York: Guilford.

Landau, J., Griffiths, J., & Mason, J. (1982). The extended family in transition: Clinical implications. In F. Kaslow (Ed.), *The international book of family therapy*. New York: Brunner/Mazel.

Landau, J., & Stanton, M.D. (1983). Families with adolescent substance abusers: Therapeutic intervention. *Focus on Alcohol and Drug Issues*, *6*, 2-3, 20.

Minuchin, S. (1974). *Families and family therapy*. Cambridge, MA: Harvard University Press.

Noone, R.J. (1979, April). *Drug abuse behavior in relation to change in the family structure*.

Paper presented at the Third Pittsburgh Family Systems Symposium, Western Psychiatric Institute and Clinic, University of Pittsburgh, PA.

Perzel, J.F., & Lamon, S. (1979, August). *Enmeshment within families of polydrug abusers*. Paper presented at the National Drug Abuse Conference, New Orleans.

Reilly, D.M. (1976). Family factors in the etiology and treatment of youthful drug abuse. *Family Therapy*, 2, 149-171.

Stanton, M.D. (1977). The addict as savior: Heroin, death and the family. *Family Process, 16*, 191-197.

Stanton, M.D. (1979a). Drugs and the family: A review of the recent literature. *Marriage and Family Review*, 2, 1-10.

Stanton, M.D. (1979b). Family treatment approaches to drug abuse problems: A review. *Family Process, 18*, 251-280.

Stanton, M.D. (1980a). A family theory of drug abuse. In D. Lettieri, M. Sayers, & H. Pearson (Eds.), *Theories on drug abuse: Selected contemporary perspectives* (National Institute on Drug Abuse Research Monograph Series No. 30). Washington, DC: U.S. Government Printing Office.

Stanton, M.D. (1980b). Some overlooked aspects of the family and drug abuse. In B. Ellis (Ed.), *Drug abuse from the family perspective: Coping is a family affair* (National Institute on Drug Abuse and DHHS publication No. [ADM] 80-910). Washington, DC: U.S. Government Printing Office.

Stanton, M.D., & Coleman, S.B. (1980). The participatory aspects of indirect self-destructive behavior: The addict family as a model. In N.L. Farberow (Ed.), *The many faces of suicide*. New York: McGraw-Hill.

Stanton, M.D., Todd, T.C., Heard, D.B., Kirschner, S., Kleiman, J.I., Mowatt, D.T., Riley, P., Scott, S.M., & Van Deusen, J.M. (1978). Heroin addiction as a family phenomenon: A new conceptual model. *American Journal of Drug and Alcohol Abuse*, 5, 125-150.

Stanton, M.D., Todd, T.C., & Associates (1982). *The family therapy of drug abuse and addiction*. New York: Guilford.

12

EATING DISORDERS

JOHN SARGENT, M.D. and RONALD LIEBMAN, M.D.

Anorexia nervosa and bulimia are prototypic examples of biopsychosocial disorders (Garfinkel & Garner, 1982). Both disorders have profound physical and psychological consequences for the individual patient, and their incidence is increasing (Halmi, Falk, & Schwartz, 1981; Willi & Grossman, 1983). The patient's family is intensely involved in efforts to respond to the symptoms. The culture at large reinforces concern and effort about one's body shape, as well as the idea that one's body shape reflects one's vitality and energy and is a vehicle for social advancement. Currently there are many difficulties in our culture with eating, diet, and adaptation to body shape. Anorexia and bulimia represent specific syndromes of disturbed eating behavior and psychological adjustment that may become life-threatening and interfere seriously with individual and family function.

Eating disorders represent diagnostic and therapeutic challenges for the physician. The physician must complete physical, psychological, and familial assessments and direct the interventions necessary to support the patient's recovery and improvement in overall adaptation. The physician can also play a role in altering the cultural pursuit of thinness which reinforces disturbances in eating patterns in vulnerable individuals in vulnerable families. This chapter focuses on the individual physical and psychological features and familial features associated with anorexia and bulimia, as well as the role of the physician in the diagnosis and treatment, and highlights a model of physician-therapist collaboration in the treatment of eating disorders.

Syndrome Description

Anorexia Nervosa

Anorexia nervosa is the diagnosis applied to individuals who demonstrate a relentless pursuit of thinness and an absolute refusal to maintain minimum normal body weight (Bruch, 1973, 1978; Crisp, 1980; Garfinkel & Garner, 1982). They achieve weight loss by reducing their dietary caloric intake, especially of foods containing carbohydrates and fats. Some patients lose weight by using diet pills, laxatives, or diuretics, and by vomiting. The patient's body image is markedly disturbed. She* feels fat even when underweight and believes strongly that she needs to continue dieting to lose more weight. The term anorexia is, in fact, a misnomer because there is no loss of appetite, only the absolute control of appetite by the patient. Although the diagnosis of anorexia nervosa per se requires that no other physical and psychiatric disorder be present to account for the weight loss, the syndrome may occur in association with chronic underlying physical or psychiatric illness. Recently, there has been a significant increase of anorexia and bulimia in diabetic patients (Hillard & Hillard, 1984); and we have treated patients who have heart disease, cancer, and kidney disease and who, during treatment for those diseases, also developed anorexia nervosa.

Most criteria for the diagnosis of anorexia require patients to have lost at least 25% of their ideal body weight (Feighner, Robins, Guze, Woodruff, Winokur, & Munoz, 1972). We recommend, however, that diagnosis and treatment of anorexia occur at any point when a thin patient is below a healthy weight for her age and height, but continues to diet and believes strongly that she needs to lose more weight.

Ninety-five percent of anorectic patients are women. The onset of the disorder occurs most often in adolescence and currently one out of 200 adolescent girls develops the symptoms of anorexia (Garfinkel & Garner, 1982). Anorexia has recently been reported among older women, most frequently beginning after the birth of a child or another significant stress of adult life. No specific organic etiology has been identified for the disorder. It may and often does become chronic, with an estimated mortality of 5-10% of cases (Garfinkel & Garner, 1982).

Physical features. The primary physical features of anorexia nervosa are those associated with starvation as well as complications from specific weight loss methods the patient may be using. Anorectic patients have significant abnormalities in endocrine function associated with starvation-induced hypothalamic disturbances (Crisp, 1980; Garfinkel & Garner, 1982; Lippe, 1983; Schwab, 1981). Women are amenorrheic. The amenorrhea may precede significant weight loss and persist for a time after the patients regain

*Throughout this discussion, although anorexia and bulimia are seen in males, the feminine pronoun is used to reflect the higher frequency of these disorders in females.

normal weight. Patients generally have low body temperature, low pulse, and low blood pressure; they may have significant gastrointestinal complaints, including abdominal pain and a feeling of bloating when eating small amounts of food. At significantly low weight (weight loss of more than 30%), patients have muscle-wasting weakness and slow movements. Their hair may be markedly thinned and they may develop fine lanugo hair over the body. Patients usually complain of being cold when others are warm, but their thyroid hormone levels are generally within normal limits. At moderate amounts of weight loss (less than 25%), there are generally no other significant physical disturbances and most laboratory findings are within normal limits. Patients may have slight leukopenia with white-blood counts in the range of 4000 and increased hemoglobin, usually because of chronic dehydration. Among patients whose weight loss is achieved solely by dieting, death from cardiovascular collapse generally occurs after more than 40% weight loss. Patients may show marked changes in cognition, thinking slowly and in a constricted, rigid fashion. They may identify problems in concentrating. At levels of severe weight loss, an organic psychosis may occur in which the patient hallucinates and becomes acutely disturbed and disoriented. Patients who are using laxatives or vomiting as a means of achieving weight loss may also have markedly altered electrolytes, with vomiting resulting in hypokalemic alkalosis and laxative use leading to dehydration.

Resumption of normal dietary intake and cessation of vomiting generally lead to physical recovery and normalization of these physical signs and symptoms. Some patients, after prolonged periods of malnutrition, may have gastrointestinal complaints, malabsorption, and diarrhea upon refeeding (Russell, Freedman, Feiglin, Jeejeebhoy, Swinson & Garfinkel, 1983; Schwab, 1981). This is rare, however, and generally occurs only in patients whose dietary intake has been fewer than 500 calories a day for several months. Concern about cardiovascular difficulties upon refeeding (Brotman & Stern, 1983; Powers, 1982) has arisen because dramatic increases in caloric intake from 500 to between 3500 and 5000 calories a day over a short period resulted in cardiac failure in some patients. This was reversed when caloric intake was reduced. For patients recovering from anorexia, moderate caloric intake of 2500 to 3000 calories a day after slowly increasing it by 200 to 300 calories daily has not been associated with harmful physical effects.

Psychological and behavioral features. Patients with anorexia nervosa have characteristic psychological and behavioral disturbances. They deny other problems and say they feel fine, have no physical complaints, and only need to lose a few more pounds. Yet they demonstrate a pervasive sense of helplessness and ineffectiveness (Bruch, 1973, 1978), are markedly nonassertive, and do not make decisions easily. The anorectic person is perfectionistic and not satisfied with current or previous accomplishments. Her self-esteem is low and she may describe herself as feeling out of control except for weight loss, which gives her a sense of mastery and control. She generally does not disagree overtly and yet maintains a stance of intractability through resistance. She may be withdrawn and difficult to engage in conversation. She is usually brought to the physician's attention by someone else (most often her parents) rather than coming independently and voluntarily. Individuals with anorexia also are often highly sensitive and very closely attuned to the moods and feelings of those around them. They may be very attentive to their parents' feelings and highly concerned about their families' well-being.

Anorectic patients may have bizarre or unusual eating habits; they may eat compulsively and some refuse to eat in the company of others. They generally say they do not like others watching them eat, and they may become extremely distressed when comments are made about how or what they are eating. Anorectic persons may also exercise compulsively, in a ritualistic fashion, not for fun, but for the effect of exercise on caloric consumption and weight loss. Most patients continue to attend school or work and make strong attempts to maintain their performance. This may lead some anorectic adolescents or college students to study excessively for hours at a time. This increase in studying probably reflects concentration problems induced by weight loss and malnutrition (Garfinkel & Garner, 1982).

The patient usually is socially isolated and withdrawn from peers and peer-group activities. She may seem sullen and defiant, becoming highly emotional and exceedingly upset when frustrated, and demonstrating marked shifts in mood and significant irritability. Her relationships with others tend to be dependent, shallow, and easily disrupted. The symptoms of anorexia may appear after a significant psychosocial stress like loss of a boyfriend, divorce, or death of a parent, or after the patient has developed increased body awareness or is disappointed in her accomplishments or attractiveness. In general, individuals who develop anorexia have been unhappy and dissatisfied with themselves for some time before they begin dieting and losing weight. This sense of dissatisfaction and poor self-esteem, when coupled with increased emphasis on one's body shape as well as successful dieting, reinforces the dieting behavior. Dieting and weight loss then lead to a worsening of the patient's psychological state and growing social withdrawal, which in turn strengthen the focus on weight and dieting.

Subtypes of anorexia. There seem to be at least two distinct subtypes of anorexia nervosa (Strober, 1983). The first includes patients who achieve weight loss exclusively through caloric reduction and dietary restriction. In this group, binge eating and purging by vomiting or laxative abuse are rare. Most patients are socially withdrawn and usually in early adolescence at the onset of symptoms. These patients rarely have an impulse disorder like drug or alcohol abuse or sexual promiscuity. Their behavior style generally is obsessive with markedly overcontrolled behavior. They have few friends and few interests. These patients tend to have few physical complications associated with mild weight loss, and the current evidence is that they may respond better than those in the other subgroup to effective treatment (Halmi & Falk, 1982; Minuchin, Rosman, & Baker, 1978; Strober, 1983; Swift, 1982).

A second subtype includes patients who experience periods of starvation that alternate with binges associated with extreme efforts at purging. They may vomit or use laxatives excessively after what the patient believes to be a period of overeating. The binge may not necessarily involve an excessive amount of calories, but for the patient it may be a frightening experience of losing control, to which she then responds by attempting to get rid of the calories consumed. These patients generally develop symptoms at an older age with the peak occurring in late adolescence or early adulthood. They may engage in drug or alcohol use, or episodes of sexual promiscuity. They may have great difficulty with social relationships and love affairs. Their weight may fluctuate widely during weight loss or weight gain periods. Patients may have suicidal ideation and a history of previous suicide attempts. Generally, these patients have severe physical difficulties associated with their anorexia, including electrolyte abnormalities and dehydration following periods of purging, and they may have more physical complications associated with weight gain.

Differential diagnosis. The differential diagnosis for anorexia nervosa includes other causes of weight loss and appetite restriction. It is rare for significant organic illnesses to mimic the psychological and behavioral features of anorexia and its purposeful and relentless course. Chronic gastrointestinal disease, including Crohn's disease or ulcerative colitis, may be accompanied by reduced food intake, diarrhea, gastrointestinal bleeding, and evidence of malabsorption. Patients who have cancer may also have significant weight loss and reduced appetite, but the purposeful nature of weight loss of anorexia will be absent. Central nervous system tumors and Addison's disease have also, at times, been confused with anorexia. It is our strong impression, however, that in the appropriate age range, history and physical examination clearly differentiate anorexia from chronic illness.

Bulimia

Patients who have bulimia eat excessively and then follow those periods of overeating with episodes of purging either by vomiting, laxative abuse, or diuretic use (Boskind-White & White, 1983; Cauwels, 1983). We reserve the term bulimia for patients who are of at least normal weight at the time of diagnosis. The weights of most solely bulimic patients vary between normal and 10-15% above. Some descriptions of anorexia indicate that about one-third of patients who experience a period of weight loss may go on to periods of binging and purging as they regain and maintain normal weight (Garfinkel & Garner, 1982). Other bulimic patients may never have been significantly underweight but have recurrent episodes of overeating and purging. The frequency of binges generally varies among patients and it may vary also for any individual patient. Some patients may go days or weeks without binging or purging; others may do this daily or several times a day. The exact incidence of bulimia is unknown, although recent studies of the eating habits of female college students indicate that 10-20% engage in this behavior (Halmi, Falk, & Schwartz, 1981). Bulimia also occurs much more frequently in women (80-90% of cases). The age of onset of bulimia is generally late adolescence or young adulthood (Herzog, 1982). Many patients currently in treatment report that they have engaged in repetitive binge and purge cycles for several years. Foods consumed often are high in carbohydrates, and the periods of overeating are generally added to normal eating at regular mealtimes. Some patients, however, report episodes of excessive dieting or fasting fluctuating with binges that lead to purging.

Physical features. The physical difficulties associated with bulimia in normal-weight patients are predominantly those caused by repetitive purging (Lippe, 1983). Patients who induce vomiting may have calluses on the backs of their hands; they may have parotid swelling and epigastric distress associated with chronic esophagitis. Episodes of mild to moderate gastrointestinal bleeding may be caused by excessive vomiting. All patients with significant repetitive vomiting have some degree of tooth enamel erosion as a result of chronic irritation by gastric acid. The major medical complication of bulimia is hypokalemic alkalosis, which may result in cardiac arrhythmias. Patients who use laxatives excessively may become dehydrated. Bulimic patients also may have a history of drug or alcohol abuse and it is important to identify and treat physical signs associated with these difficulties.

Psychological features. Bulimic patients know their problem and are quite distressed by their symptoms. They report that the bulimic symptoms are habitual and outside of their control. Their binging is usually done secretly; they are generally ashamed of their symptoms and reluctant to admit them. Many patients say that the binges are planned; others will describe periods of overeating that occur almost involuntarily. They also describe a point in eating when they are sure that they have eaten too much and therefore will purge after finishing eating. This decision then leaves them free to continue to eat as much as they would like. Caloric intake during a binge often exceeds 2500 calories (Mitchell, Pyle, & Eckert, 1981).

Patients describe a battle with themselves to gain control over their symptoms and prevent future binges, but their continual failure leads to worsening of the symptoms. Increase in binging frequency, coupled with the need to maintain secrecy, may lower the patients' self-esteem and increase their social withdrawal and isolation (Johnson & Berndt, 1983). Still, many bulimic patients report successful work or school performance, describe themselves as having friends, and may even have somewhat successful heterosexual relationships. Many patients say their binges occur during periods of loneliness, boredom, anxiety, or anger and that eating and purging may be used as ways to dissipate disturbing emotions (Gwirtsman, Roy-Byrne, Yager & Gerner, 1983).

Psychologically and behaviorally, then, bulimia occurs in a cycle in which psychological distress leads to eating behavior, which leads to anxiety, which leads to purging by vomiting or laxative abuse, which then relieves the anxiety but also may lead to worsening of self-esteem because the patient has again engaged in this distressing pattern. This, in turn, increases the frequency of eating because of the depression and distress caused by the syndrome itself. Depressed mood and bulimic symptoms are mutually reinforcing, each leading to a worsening of the other. Most patients describe the purging as something they learned to do as a way of controlling their weight. The entire experience of overeating and purging also is physically and psychologically consuming and exhausting. Patients then experience a period of quiet and relaxation which distracts them from the environment that caused their disturbing emotions.

Subtypes of bulimia. There is no agreement in the current psychiatric literature concerning subtypes of bulimic patients. Individual reports (Boskind-White & White, 1983; Pope, Hudson, Jonas, & Yurgelun-Todd, 1983) emphasized selected patient populations who responded to different treatment approaches and who had different levels of symptomatic behavior and psychological adjustment. Our impression from clinical experience is that the syndrome of repetitive bulimic behavior may be present in normal-weight individuals who are at significantly different levels of psychosocial functioning.

One group consists of young adults who have made a good overall adjustment, are functioning well in school and work, have adequate social relationships, and have some control over the symptoms and limited evidence of other impulse disorders. A second group includes patients who have a long history of depressive response to environmental stresses, exceedingly poor self-esteem, and who describe themselves as being depressed before the development of bulimic symptoms. There may be strong family histories of depression in near relatives. In the third group are individuals who have made poor psychosocial adjustment throughout adolescence and adulthood, who have significant difficulties with work and school adjustment, and marked problems in social relationships. Among these individuals the bulimic symptoms are usually erratic, impulsively pursued, and often life-threatening. Although these differences in bulimic patients have not been confirmed by extensive research, we believe strongly that a complete assessment of the individual's psychosocial functioning, emotional responsiveness, and degree of symptoms is essential at the point of initial evaluation and diagnosis.

Differential diagnosis. As with anorexia, the diagnosis of bulimia is made by confirming the presence of symptoms by history and elimination of organic causes for the vomiting by physical examination. Causes of repetitive vomiting, such as Addison's disease, need to be considered; however, the self-induced nature of the purging and the excessive caloric intake in episodes of binge-eating are not present in other organic diseases.

Eating Disorders and the Family

Eating disorders are powerful interpersonal phenomena. A person single-mindedly refuses to care for his or her body in an obvious way by becoming dangerously thin, or by overeating and purging, denies other problems, and resists the entreaties of family and friends to stop. When challenged, the individual may become defiant, secretive, and highly emotional. The individual's behavior is both beyond others' control and also highly compelling and engaging to people involved with the patient. The family is an individual's primary social context and an eating disorder in a family member becomes a focal point for family concern. Family behavior may reinforce the symptoms of anorexia or bulimia, or the family may interact in a way that diminishes the symptoms while encouraging more adaptive behaviors in the patient and other family members.

The Family with an Anorectic Member

Writers on anorexia and its treatment (Bruch, 1973, 1978; Crisp, 1980; Selvini Palazzoli, 1978; Sours, 1980) have uniformly described difficulties within the family. Bruch described the family as functioning as if members could read each others' minds. Yager (1981) described the family as focused on high achievement, communicating along narrow lines, and failing to recognize the anorectic child's individuality. Sours emphasized the family's need to maintain harmony and disavow distress or upset. These findings were derived primarily from clinical observation and retrospective analysis.

Minuchin and colleagues (Minuchin, Baker, Rosman, Liebman, Milman, & Todd, 1975; Minuchin et al., 1978) investigated the interaction of families with an anorectic member at the time the symptoms were present by having the family participate in a standardized series of tasks and a diagnostic stress interview. They identified five predominant characteristics of family interaction as excessively present and detrimental to overall family functioning: enmeshment, overprotectiveness, rigidity, lack of conflict resolution, and involvement of the sick child in unresolved parental conflict. These characteristics are not static pictures of family relationships, but they create a matrix of current behavior for all family members.

Enmeshment refers to a tight web of family relationships in which family members are highly sensitive to one another. They often infer moods and needs of others and submerge individual interests for the good of the whole. Overt criticism is rare. Although appropriate for the relationship between parents and young infants, enmeshment is inappropriate for spouses or parents and adolescents or young adults. Overprotectiveness describes a relationship in which autonomy is sacrificed and highly nurturant interactions predominate. Family members have a strong sense of vulnerability. The anorectic patient is often as protective of her parents and siblings as they are of her. In these families, the interactions of enmeshment, protectiveness, and conflict avoidance are rigidly preferred. Even during periods of stress or necessary developmental change, one observes the family to use, repeatedly and ineffectively, a narrow range of behaviors. In dealing with the anorectic child, the family responds as they would to a much younger child. Families with anorectic members have marked difficulty allowing for and encouraging the resolution of disagreement or conflict. One member of a disagreeing pair may abandon the conflict or other family members may enter, preventing mutually satisfying agreement. As these disagreements remain, a chronic state of tension and stress develops. Mutually reinforcing characteristics create a family organization that is fragile and unable to respond effectively to the symptoms of anorexia.

A final common feature of these families is involvement of the symptomatic child in unresolved parental conflict. By joining one parent in a stable coalition against the other parent, by providing a focus for common concern and action through her symptoms, or by having been caught between her parents in a loyalty conflict, the patient and her symptoms play a role in maintaining family integrity. Meanwhile, the family characteristics listed by Minuchin et al. provide the context in which the anorectic symptoms develop and are maintained.

Because of rigidly preferred family interaction patterns, the parents may be more concerned with the rightness of their own actions rather than their effectiveness. They may try, one parent by pleading, the other by demanding, to help the patient to eat, but when they fail, each parent recoils and leaves the anorectic patient alone and without support. Because they do not resolve conflict well, they do not compromise and work together. In the family, there may be either significant overcontrol so that everyone behaves in a rigid, controlled way, or an allowance for frequent loss of control which then leads to excluding that person from family life for a time. In overcontrolled families, small deviations in temper, relaxation, or achievement orientation tend to cause significant upset and are avoided. This pattern of parental behavior tends to be seen more frequently with the young anorectic person who diets actively and is obsessive herself. On the other hand, the older anorectic individual involved in frequent binging and purging cycles and loss of impulse control through substance abuse and sexual promiscuity more often belongs to a family that tolerates significant loss of control in a family member, including frequent behavior disorder, alcohol abuse, or other types of impulse disorder in a parent. The parents' concern with each other and their behavior in either case tends to leave them less available and less flexible in response to their child's eating disorder. These difficulties compound the families' enmeshment, overprotectiveness, and inability to resolve conflicts.

In this context the primary psychological features of anorexia described by Bruch (1973, 1978) fit and are adaptive. If the family is highly overinvolved with the anorectic person, she need not perceive her own sensations. Others may recognize them first or deny their presence. The child must also be vigilant to see and respond to signs of distress from others. In a family in which everyone is vulnerable and protection is necessary, interpersonal trust does not develop. When conflict and distress are denied or not resolved, the child does not develop a sense of competence, and her problem-solving skills are underutilized. Thus the demands of family interaction reinforce developmental lags that make adaptation to the extrafamilial world more difficult. This magnifies the importance of the family and acts to maintain the symptoms. As the symptoms worsen, they tend to deepen involvement and overprotectiveness of family members. The anorectic child's vulnerability inhibits challenges to her to act in a more mature fashion.

Finding it difficult to collaborate because of their unresolved marital conflicts and mutual distrust, the parents may counteract each other. This reinforces their opposing positions. Family hierarchy and leadership, which could lead to conflict resolution and better self-definitions, are absent, as are effective boundaries between family subsystems, while the boundary that separates the family from the outside world is too restrictive. The family system fails and the symptoms of anorexia persist and worsen.

The Family with a Bulimic Member

In many ways, interaction in families of bulimic individuals is similar to that of families who have an anorectic. Enmeshment, rigidity, and poor conflict resolution are frequently present, but there are some important distinctions. Bulimic patients are usually older than those who have anorexia nervosa, and they may live outside the home to attend college or to work. The patient maintains an independent stance, acting as though she were responsible for herself. However, as Stanton and Todd (1982) have found in their work concerning the family and drug abuse, the patient is actually pseudoindependent. She and her parents are in frequent contact. She also continues to depend on her parents when stressed and, although she may support herself at least some of the time, she often acts like a child with her parents, encouraging their concern with and involvement in her life.

A major area in which this occurs is in her bulimic disorder. Although many patients say that the symptoms are secret, the secret usually is known by family members and worries them. The family fluctuates between attempting to stop the behavior by injunctions and cajoling, and retreating when these are ineffective. The family becomes angry, blames the patient, and abandons her. After a while the cycle starts again. Alternating between overinvolvement and abandonment is characteristic of families with bulimic members; it happens concerning the symptoms of bulimia and in other areas of family life. Conflict is apparent in these families but unresolved. Perhaps the parents have not been happy together for many years; their sequence of argument, retreat, and reconciliation is stabilized by concern for the bulimic child regardless of where the child lives. These families may have other overt difficulties with impulse control. Schwartz, Barrett, and Saba (1984) described them as constantly taking "all-or-nothing" positions on behavior and relationships. One or both parents may have explosive tempers. There may be a history of substance abuse, especially of alcohol, and concern that one or both parents may become depressed and incapacitated. The family may also have a history of incest which reflects abuse of women, lack of impulse control, and the failure of limits on personally destructive behavior.

The family may approach treatment of the bulimic patient with the same impulsiveness. Treatment begins with an energetic commitment. The patient may begin to improve, and then her impulsive behavior or that of one or both parents may bring about a retreat from treatment, leaving the problem unresolved. The family of a bulimic patient is likely to be more outgoing, more expressive, and more chaotic than the family of an anorectic patient. As a whole, the family will take one side of an unresolved difficulty, stick with it for a while, and then switch abruptly and take the other side so that there is little consistency and no effective problem solving. The patient's symptoms also allow the family to be concerned with her as a dependent child, which stabilizes unresolved family conflicts. Anger is more apparent and more easily expressed in these families, and relationships are tinged with ambivalence. We have also treated several families in which an older child developed anorexia nervosa during adolescence and a younger sibling later developed bulimia, reflecting the family's concern with food, control, and body shape, as well as their ineffectiveness in managing their children's transition through adolescence to adulthood.

Primary-Care Assessment of Eating Disorders

A family's eating habits reflect parental nurturance, parental control, and the meaning of food and meals in that family and its culture. In addition to being times when food is consumed for nutrition, meals give families the experience of being together. Parents may regard their children's body shape and the nutritional adequacy of their diet as an indicator of their effectiveness as parents. Their adequacy as providers is demonstrated by the quality and quantity of food available at meals. Mealtimes may give family members the opportunity to interact with mutual support, encouragement, and respect; they may be the scenes for disclosing difficulty with parental authority or disagreements between spouses. In families in which there is concern about a parent's weight or health, mealtimes are an occasion to deal with these worries. An overweight family member will either demonstrate difficulties with control at that time or practice self-denial while other family members are eating. If a family member's health problem requires a special diet, other members may express concern for that individual's health and attempt to control her or her eating. Thus, families demonstrate their adequacy or reenact problems of organization and function at meals.

Children growing into adolescence increasingly want to choose their own foods and diet. If this challenges parental authority, the parents may try to control undesired external influences on the adolescent's behavior during meals. Adolescent girls may become concerned about their diet because of the importance they attach to body shape and physical attractiveness in gaining peer acceptance. Families may discuss and resolve these issues. If they do not deal with them, problems with eating, family relationships, and self-esteem persist and worsen.

When both parents are overinvolved with their own lives and not available to the children, haphazard eating may reflect a lack of cohesiveness and responsiveness within the family. The children may develop eating problems because of lack of supervision and parental authority. Mealtimes, then, may be especially tense experiences, leading family members to be self-conscious and unable to eat in a relaxed fashion. Problems with eating may be further reinforced by the parents' inability to either impose or relax control according to the child's needs.

The family physician should attend specifically to eating habits, dietary practices, and family behavior at mealtimes. Questioning family members about these issues, the physician will note eating behaviors that may be significant problems and special difficulties in encouraging family members to eat a proper diet without undue attention or guilt. A complete dietary history, including questions concerning dieting behavior and the existence of binging or purging, should be part of the physician's routine evaluation of an adolescent's health. The physician should monitor the adolescent's sense of self-esteem, autonomy, and personal control. Finally, the physician needs to be attentive to the ability of the family to respond effectively to the adolescent's need for supervision and direction, for autonomy, and for privacy.

The diagnosis of an eating disorder is a positive diagnosis based on the presence of disturbed eating patterns and disturbed conceptions about one's weight and body shape. It is extremely important for the physician to learn to identify aberrations in eating and dieting behavior as early as possible in their course and to help families reverse troublesome situations quickly before the symptoms of the eating disorder become established and self-perpetuating. Early in the course of these disorders extensive physical evaluations and laboratory studies may be unnecessary, because the diagnosis of an eating disorder is based on the history of the symptoms. As the physician notes a family's difficulties concerning eating-related behavior, he or she can assist the patients in helping the young person with her concern about her body and her ability to control food intake. At the same time, the parents, with the physician's guidance, can attend to difficulties the adolescent may have with self-esteem and personal control.

THE TREATMENT OF EATING DISORDERS

Evaluation by the Physician

The physician's evaluation of an eating disorder should include complete determination of the patient's physical status and an assessment of the family, especially in relation to the symptoms of the eating disorder. This evaluation should be completed during the physician's examination of the patient's medical condition. The physician's efforts with respect to the physical symptoms and medical difficulties related to the eating disorder must be coordinated with responses to the psychosocial and familial problems that occur simultaneously. The treatment approach, whether carried out independently by the physician, or by the physician in collaboration with a therapist experienced in treating eating disorders, must be one in which the body and mind of the patient are dealt with in concert and the patient is treated in relationship to her family. The medical evaluation, diagnosis, and recommendation must be made with the family and not only the patient in mind (Liebman, Sargent, & Silver, 1983). The goals of the medical evaluation of a patient with an eating disorder are: 1) to identify any underlying disease processes present at the time of the referral and ascertain that no physiologic process explains the weight loss; 2) to clarify the patient's physiologic condition and the nature of any metabolic difficulties resulting from the patient's symptoms that require immediate remediation; and 3) to prepare the patient and family for resolution of the physical, psychosocial, and familial difficulties associated with the eating disorder.

The physician's evaluation can be performed on an outpatient basis. The presence of all parental figures is required and underscores the need of parents and all family members to be involved in the treatment; it emphasizes the seriousness of the symptoms and enables the physician to obtain initial data concerning family interactions. The parents' presence ensures also that all relevant physical concerns can be raised at the time of initial evaluation. As the evaluation proceeds, the physician can gather a history of the development of the symptoms, methods used to achieve weight reduction if this has occurred, current dietary practices, and information concerning the use of self-induced vomiting or exogenous substances to achieve further weight loss. The physician should also obtain history concerning other physical symptoms including weakness, faintness, muscle cramping, loss of concentration, periods of dehydration, and difficulties with fluid retention. For female patients, menstrual history should be established accurately and other medical difficulties noted. In particular, the physician will want to pay attention to the presence of symptoms not generally associated with either anorexia or bulimia, such as frequent diarrhea or bloody stools indicative of possible inflammatory bowel disease, neurologic signs or symptoms associated with central nervous system tumors, or evidence of an endocrine disorder. The patient's report that she is actively dieting, although she is underweight, or that she is purging after eating is a positive indication of the presence of an eating disorder.

The physician should attempt to obtain the perception of each parent independently and to discuss the symptoms with the patient in the parents' presence. The physician should inform the patient that the frequency and severity of eating-related symptoms cannot be kept secret because of the seriousness of the symptoms and because all family members will be involved in the treatment of the eating disorder. The physician will want to ask the patient directly concerning her weight goal and her feelings about her body shape, and ask each parent how he and she have tried to resolve the eating-related symptoms. This information should be obtained in some detail so that the physician will know what happens at home either when the patient refuses to eat, or when it becomes apparent that the patient has overeaten and vomited.

Information concerning the patient's psychosocial adaptation, the family medical history, recent changes in the home, and other current family stresses will be useful. The physician should ask the patient about emotional difficulties and suicidal ideation or behavior. The patient's level of functioning should be determined, including school or work attendance and performance, peer relationships, social activity, career interest, level of self-esteem, and sense of competency. While assessing the patient, the physician will obtain an impression of her relating ability and her ability to work with him or her as they begin the process of resolving the eating-related symptoms. The physician will want to form an impression of the patient's ability to achieve impulse control, especially when anxious, and her ability to be expressive and direct, to make choices and act on them, to be assertive and to disagree. Finally, the physician will want to note the patient's ability to accept disappointment and acknowledge painful emotions.

In questioning the patient, the physician should attempt to help the parents to remain silent and listen. If the physician finds one or both parents interrupting frequently, correcting the patient, offering an alternative explanation, etc., this will demonstrate their level of overinvolvement. The physician will also want to develop an initial assessment of the family system by noting whether or not the parents act together and show respect for each other during this meeting. This helps the physician to form an impression of their ability to collaborate in times of stress. By noting each parent's individual impression of the weight loss and the family's previous efforts to remedy it, the physician will also note the family's attempts at conflict resolution in problematic situations. The family's evaluation will include an assessment of family leadership, the boundaries between family subsystems, the commitment of the family as a whole to effective problem resolution, and the importance the family places on maintaining harmony and stability even if that stability permits extremely problematic behavior.

The physican will need to carry out a thorough physical examination and appropriate laboratory studies to be certain of the medical diagnosis and the patient's physical condition. Our strong impression is that the diagnosis of anorexia or bulimia is achieved by recognition of symptoms and history taking. We routinely perform a complete blood count, including sedimentation rate, urinalysis, chemical profile, and electrolytes. For patients who have significant weight loss or electrolyte abnormalities, we perform a cardiogram; any patient whose neurological condition is of concern receives a skull radiogram; and, in selected worrisome situations, computed tomography studies of the brain are done. Patients who describe significant gastrointestinal symptoms that would not be expected in either bulimia or anorexia should have X rays of the gastrointestinal tract, and barium enema. If there is sufficient concern about the patient's endocrine status beyond that expected from weight loss, thyroid and cortisol studies may be helpful. These tests are usually normal, however, in uncomplicated cases of anorexia or bulimia. The anorectic patient's estrogen levels will be low purely on the basis of starvation-induced hypothalamic dysfunction.

Most patients with mild to moderate symptoms have normal physical examination and laboratory findings. The severely underweight patients' pulse and blood pressure may be significantly lower than normal. A pulse of 120 and blood pressure of 110 to 120 over 85 to 90 may indicate significant dehydration in a patient who is severely underweight and whose pulse is 50 and usual blood pressure 80 to 90 over 40. Worrisome laboratory results in patients with eating disorders include leukopenia indicating potential compromise of the immunological system, hypoglycemia, and elevated hemoglobin, hematocrit, and blood urea nitrogen indicative of dehydration. The patient's electrolytes deserve special attention. Hypokalemic alkalosis may be seen in patients who repetitively vomit. The absence of ketones in the urine of a patient in acute starvation may indicate the total utilization of fat stores for energy and is a disturbing sign. Abnormalities in liver enzymes usually occur after severe and chronic malnutrition. Any unusual laboratory results or unexplained physical signs on examination require further evaluation.

The Physician's Role in Treatment

The physician will now have identified the patient's diagnosis, physical condition and medical status, her developmental level, and the family's organizational and functional status. The presence of acute medical complications (such as dehydration or electrolyte abnormalities) requires immediate hospitalization and appropriate physical treatment. Medical hospitalization and the patient's participation in behavior modification programs have also been used to encourage weight gain (Collins, Hodas, & Liebman, 1983).

We recommend psychiatric hospitalization for patients who have eating disorders and whose weight is dangerously low (although it may not be causing acute medical complications), and whose symptoms are so out of control as to seriously compromise the patient's functioning in other areas of her life. Suicidal ideation or behavior, or psychotic behavior also necessitates the patient's psychiatric hospitalization. A hospital psychiatric program may be used to demonstrate the severity of the symptoms to the family and to augment outpatient treatment that has been ineffective (Liebman et al., 1983; Rosman, Minuchin, Liebman, & Baker, 1976; Sargent, Liebman, & Silver, 1984). Our family-oriented, hospital-based program is described below. Medical or psychiatric hospitalization is required in 15-20% of patients who have anorexia nervosa or bulimia to deal with acute complications or crises in treatment.

All anorectic or bulimic patients and their families will require outpatient treatment that addresses the patients' physical and psychosocial problems and the families' problems of organization and interaction. Treatment is a collaborative endeavor of family, patient, physician, and therapist. It is possible for the physician to carry out treatment of an eating disorder independently. Should the physician choose to do this, however, he or she will need to attend to the patient's physical and psychological difficulties in a unified way, while integrating the approach to the patient with the approach to her family. Whether the physician chooses to treat the eating disorder independently or to encourage the family and patient to work in psychotherapy with a family therapist, he or she will have to remain available to monitor the patient's physical condition, reinforce the treatment goals for the patient, including goal weight and expected rate of weight gain, and provide dietary information as needed. Patients who purge either by vomiting or laxative abuse will require medical evaluation to be certain that the patient's physical condition is stable, to reinforce improvement, and to be certain that outpatient treatment remains safe for the patient.

The decision of whether to treat an eating disorder independently depends on the physician's assessment of the patient and family. Treating patients for chronic eating disorders of longer than one year's duration is more difficult than treating patients whose symptoms have been present for a shorter period (Minuchin et al., 1978; Rosman et al., 1976). Rigid, denying families, families whose relationships are fixed and apparently unchanging, and families in which impulse disorder is a significant problem (like families with a history of alcohol abuse or significant obesity) are more difficult to engage in treatment, and treatment, in turn, is more difficult to carry out. Patients who do not form an effective relationship with the physician, who are extremely withdrawn, or who demonstrate stubborn denial and have great difficulty controlling their behavior also present more problems in treatment. It is unusual for a physician to treat such patients independently, even if he or she is comfortable working with an entire family and knowledgeable about adolescent development. In general, we recommend that the physician refer these difficult-to-treat patients to a family therapist experienced in treating eating disorders.

In many other circumstances, however, the physician might pursue treatment independently. These include young patients aged 12 to 14, who have moderate developmental delays and a relatively short duration of the eating disorder symptoms; families whom the physician knows from previous experience and on whom he or she has significant influence; and situations in which the symptoms of bulimia are infrequent or the weight loss of anorexia is mild. In these circumstances, the physician should tell the diagnosis to the family and encourage them to determine ways of limiting the eating disorder so that it does not become chronic or life-threatening. The physician can do this by helping the parents to reinforce the anorectic child's weight gain. For families of a bulimic patient, the physician can encourage the parents to determine ways of helping the patient to eat moderate amounts of food regularly and to tell the family before she vomits when she feels upset because she has overeaten. At the same time, the physician will want to encourage both patient and family to talk freely about their difficulties. These family meetings in the office should promote communication and conflict resolution, sometimes raising issues and problems the physician can help the family deal with in future meetings.

The physician should strongly encourage the father's closer involvement with the patient and encourage both parents to work together to provide emotional support to the patient and set limits concerning the eating disorder symptoms. Perhaps noting that the parents find it difficult to collaborate, the physician will need to encourage them to resolve differences and actively support one another as the child's symptoms improve. The physician, while monitoring the patient's weight, should keep a check on her participation in peer-group activities, her assertiveness and self-acceptance, and the degree to which the family encourages the patient's development of self-monitoring and autonomy. The physician should not engage in power struggles with the patient concerning her symptoms. The physician will state his or her goals concerning the symptoms of the eating disorder and then encourage the family as a whole, parents and patient, to work out a way to meet these goals. He or she then provides the necessary encouragement, support, and interventions to assist them in the process.

Referral for Family Therapy

Families who fail to improve with the physician's intervention, or those who will require psychotherapeutic attention after the initial assessment, should be referred to a therapist. The therapist should be experienced in treating patients for eating disorders, capable of working successfully with adolescents and their families, and willing to collaborate with the physician concerning the medical aspects of treatment. The therapist should also be able to use the physician's information and his or her determinations of the patient's condition to foster improvement of the family and patient. The physician should inform the therapist of his or her impressions, the physician's availability to monitor the patient medically and desire to collaborate in treatment.

The physician's referral for psychotherapy should be made in a positive fashion; the family should be informed that treatment will focus on what is necessary to improve the situation. Families of patients with eating disorders often will deny the severity of the symptoms or the presence of psychological difficulties and, therefore, the need for psychosocial improvement. They may wish the patient to work individually with the therapist who is expected to resolve the problem. The physician should help the family to understand that psychotherapy is necessary and that the entire family needs to participate. We suggest that the physician encourage everyone living with the patient to become involved in treatment because no one living with the patient is unaffected by willful starvation or repetitive binge eating and purging. By expressing concern about the patient's physical condition, the physician can emphasize the need for the whole family to participate in treatment. If the family fails to follow through with the referral and the physician is certain that treatment is necessary, he or she may need to insist that the family follow the recommendation just as they would if a family member had appendicitis and were referred to a surgeon.

If the parents are separated or divorced, we suggest that both natural parents participate in treatment. If the physician is aware of a serious physical or emotional difficulty of one or both parents, he or she will need to inform the therapist of this, as well as provide the parents with guidelines concerning how to maintain their own health while they participate in treatment. If there is a possibility or actual occurrence of sexual abuse, the physician must report this to appropriate authorities, notify the therapist, and encourage that parent to participate responsibly in treatment to resolve the problem of both the eating disorder and the sexual abuse or incest.

After referring the family for psychotherapy, the physician should arrange a follow-up meeting to ensure that the family has begun therapy and to discuss their first impressions. At that time the physician can reiterate the expectation that the family will continue treatment and encourage them to resolve any problems of treatment with the therapist. The physician and therapist should communicate regularly and work actively to resolve any areas of disagreement either concerning impressions of the patient or family, therapeutic approach, or treatment goals. In some situations, it will be necessary for both physician and therapist to meet with the family either to complete the process of referral successfully, to emphasize the seriousness of the patient's physical symptoms and condition, or to demonstrate a collaborative and united approach to the problem that will model effective conflict resolution, negotiation, and collaboration for the parents.

A brief description of the psychotherapeutic approach to eating disorders is presented below. Our approach is based on the techniques of structural family therapy developed by Minuchin and colleagues (Liebman et al., 1983; Minuchin, 1974; Minuchin & Fishman, 1981; Minuchin et al., 1978; Sargent et al., 1984). The physician must be aware of the therapist's approach to treatment so that he or she can reinforce the therapist's efforts through his or her own contact with the family during and after treatment.

Hospitalization for Eating Disorders

The hospital's treatment plan should allow for evaluation of family interaction and should center on treatment goals for the family even though only the patient with the eating disorder is hospitalized. These goals include encouragement of parental leadership, collaboration, and mutual support to help the anorectic or bulimic patient become more autonomous in caring for her body and psychological well-being, and to challenge the family's sense of helplessness or denial by helping them to acquire new problem-solving skills and communication patterns.

Hospitalization centers on establishing and achieving concrete behavioral goals for the patient and the family. The therapist assists the family in developing these goals by focusing attention on the patient's behavior and by encouraging the parents to decide together what changes they require before they are willing to have the patient back home. As the parents set goals in collaboration with the therapist and physician, enmeshment, parent-child coalitions, and poor conflict resolution in the family are challenged.

The parents' concern for their child is stressed and they are told that they need to change to help the patient. Family therapy meetings are held two to five times per week as the forum for reviewing, altering, and intensifying the treatment plan.

The patient earns the right to influence parental decisions by demonstrating her ability to take care of her body and showing social competence in relation to other patients in the unit. Our inpatient milieu includes patients with eating disorders as well as those with other behavioral and emotional difficulties. The daily routine includes individual therapy, group therapy, art and recreational therapy, nutritional instruction and assistance. Daily activities are task-oriented and usually involve collaboration with peers. Assertiveness and direct resolution of disagreements are encouraged. Psychotropic medications are used only if necessary for acute organic psychosis. We have found being with other patients with differing social backgrounds and difficulties to be very helpful for patients who have eating disorders. The patient can learn that, beyond her ability to lose weight, she has special talents and attributes that are valued and respected by others.

Outpatient Treatment of Patients with Anorexia Nervosa

The therapist's first goal is to establish a therapeutic relationship with all family members. Families confronted by a child's willful starvation are usually tense and distraught. They have attempted to get the patient to eat without success and may feel helpless. The parents may be confused and startled by the patient's problem. Often parents feel guilty or threatened by the occurrence of this problem in their family. The family system is out of control, yet family members frequently maintain a facade of normalcy, stating that everything would be fine if only the patient would eat normally.

The initial treatment contract will be concrete, specific, and problem-centered. The therapist will highlight concern for the patient's emotional and social difficulties in addition to the eating disorder symptoms, and treatment goals should reflect psychosocial issues as well as those of maintaining normal weight and eating habits. Treatment is defined as a learning process for the patient and family. The treatment contract will involve all family members, outlining clearly the parents' and siblings' roles in helping the patient.

The treatment contract will specify provisions for consistent weight gain by the patient. The therapist suggests to the family that the patient can and should gain one to two pounds per week. The patient's responsibility is to gain weight. She will gain freedom of activity and increased autonomy from her parents as she pursues weight gain successfully. The patient may choose how, what, and when to eat. The parents are then instructed to allow the patient to eat food of her choosing, and her performance is to be measured by weighing before the next therapy session. The patient's weight is one measure of the family's response to treatment and is used by the therapist to help the family to review their problem-solving skills as a unit. Steady weight gain by the patient will allow the therapist to prevent the patient's eating symptoms from focusing and directing family activity and maintaining enmeshment and overprotectiveness.

Family lunch sessions (Liebman, Minuchin, & Baker, 1974; Liebman et al., 1983; Liebman, Minuchin, Baker, & Rosman, 1975; Rosman, Minuchin, & Liebman, 1975) are a specific method of identifying family interactions concerning eating and of helping the patient to eat in the presence of her family, thus beginning the process of disengaging the patient from her parents. If the family has difficulty ensuring that the patient gain weight early in treatment, the therapist may need to call on the physician to reiterate the dangers of anorexia and the patient's capacity to eat normally and gain weight consistently.

While the patient is gaining weight (even if slowly), the therapist will help the family address the patient's psychosocial developmental difficulties and the family's unresolved conflicts. The therapist helps the family identify stresses that might have led to the patient's weight loss. Once these are identified, parents and patient are challenged to find alternative methods of coping with stress other than weight loss for the patient and predictable recurring enmeshed relationships of parents and patient.

At this point the therapist is particularly attentive to content that can be used in the therapy process to further the therapeutic goals of mutual support and conflict resolution between the parents and increased autonomy and self-respect for the patient. Often, as the patient begins to gain weight, she begins to feel ineffective again. The therapist helps the patient to speak for herself, to disagree with her parents, and to express in her own words the difficulties she is experiencing. The therapist helps the family recognize that disagreements between parents and children are part of family life, that separation is a painful process that must be undertaken by parents and children, and that increased autonomy for the patient requires that she demonstrate responsibility and earn parental trust. At the same time, the therapist helps the parents accept their increasing distance from the patient, the futility of trying to prevent her pain, and their need to encourage her in her life and her choices even though they may not always agree with her.

The therapist should also begin to explore the personal concerns of each parent. As the patient's symptoms improve, often the parents become increasingly aware of individual and marital concerns. Difficulties at work, problems with their own parents, issues of redirecting their energies away from parenting towards increased involvement in their own lives, and intimations of marital discord are added to the therapeutic agenda. Resolution of these issues becomes part of the therapeutic contract. The therapist may then shift to marital therapy for the parents and individual therapy for the patient (Liebman et al., 1983; Sargent et al., 1984). Group sessions may also be scheduled for the siblings.

Individual therapy with the patient focuses on maintaining the patient's disengagement from parental conflicts and encouraging her development of self-care, self-esteem, and interpersonal trust. The therapist maintains a supportive stance with the patient and slowly helps her to identify features of her experience that she can change and to develop strategies to change them. The therapist challenges the "all-or-nothing" logic associated with the patient's perfectionism, strongly supporting her competence and success while helping her to accept mistakes and disappointments. The patient can then be encouraged to attend more to external sources of enjoyment and satisfaction for their own sake as she learns to supervise herself and become truly autonomous.

Marital therapy for the parents centers on the couple's need to attend to themselves, their future, and their relationship. The therapist develops and maintains a focus on negotiation, compromise, and the possibility of mutual support and respect in the marriage. Past resentments and perceived injustices must be identified. The husband and wife then negotiate forgiveness for these past resentments with the therapist's support. The therapist monitors spouse interactions to encourage true agreement and commitment and does not allow one parent to capitulate. The therapist strongly discourages the spouses from involving the patient or siblings in their disagreements at home.

Termination of treatment occurs at different times for different family subsystems. We generally hold follow-up sessions monthly with the patient and the family for two to four months when the patient, spouses, and entire family are functioning effectively, and we sometimes maintain phone contact with patient and family for some time after that. We try to help family members to experience their own resources in dealing with stresses and transitions. We decrease our therapeutic involvement as these stresses are negotiated by family members with little disruption in other family members or subsystems.

Outpatient Treatment of Bulimic Patients

Much of outpatient psychotherapy of bulimic patients and their families will be similar to treatment for anorexia nervosa. The therapist will identify family relationships and determine when the symptoms occur, what events precipitate binges, and the role of family members in bringing on episodes of binging and purging. The treatment plan will identify the need for all family members to collaborate in resolving the symptoms and alternative means for the patient to respond to the stress and emotional upset that have led to the episodes. Supporting family collaboration, the therapist will resist the patient's often expressed desire to work on resolving the symptoms independently without her parents.

The therapist will identify positive features of the symptoms for the patient and her family and help them to establish and encourage alternative methods of satisfaction and release of tension. Together the family and the therapist will help the patient to eat when she is physically hungry and manage her diet appropriately to reduce episodes of weight gain and periods of anxiety that lead to purging behavior. Perhaps, as a first step, the therapist will suggest data collection concerning the symptoms (i.e., a record of what the patient eats and what she is feeling and doing when she eats). During this time the parents are instructed not to interfere with the patient's behavior. Restraining the family from trying to change rapidly reduces everyone's anxiety that the symptoms may be gone before positive change has occurred in family behavior and family relationships (Schwartz et al., 1984). Throughout the treatment the therapist actively supports the patient's individuation and independent control as he or she encourages parents to establish for the patient a foundation of self-acceptance and appropriate response to food and weight. Patient and family members learn to express and resolve conflict, while the parents learn to provide genuine support to the patient. Other difficulties with impulse control are addressed directly.

The major problems in treating bulimic patients include abrupt cessation of symptoms which may lead to premature termination of treatment, and the tendency of family members to become frustrated if the symptoms do not diminish rapidly. The therapist will persuade the family to participate in a gradual process and encourage their support as well as differentiation and development for both patient and parents. Like treatment for anorexia, therapy proceeds from family sessions to individual therapy for the patient and marital therapy for the parents. The development of themes and issues to be pursued occurs as described above. Recent reports (Pope et al., 1983) show that the use of antidepressant medication may be quite promising in the treatment of bulimic patients. Our impression is that antidepressant medication may be of great help to the patient in dealing with depressed affect and anxiety that lead to repetitive episodes of binging and purging. We believe strongly, however, that this medication should be used only when patient and family are actively engaged in the therapeutic process.

Cultural Intervention: The Physician's Role in Preventing Eating Disorders

Physicians can take an active role in the prevention and early identification of eating disorders. Many advertisements suggest that anyone can be thin. Especially for women, our culture implies that one's physical appearance is a sign of one's worth as a person and that discomfort with one's physical appearance can and should be remedied directly through appropriate dieting. This view, when taken to extremes by vulnerable individuals in vulnerable families, may lead to the development and reinforcement of the symptoms of an eating disorder. Family physicians can work with all families to support the development of a moderate approach to physical appearance and dieting behavior as they provide primary care. Physicians should be particularly attuned to adolescents' and young adults' difficulties in developing effective control and autonomy. As physicians work with families they will encounter parents who find it very difficult to encourage a young person's individuation and sense of personal responsibility. Regardless of the type of symptoms they have developed, these families will need the physician's assistance.

Physicians can also work with school nursing personnel to identify students whose dieting and eating-related behavior have become problematic. Working with schools and community organizations, physicians can encourage early identification and treatment of these patients as well as encourage other young people to be satisfied with their physiological characteristics and accept the limitations of their bodies. This includes advocating a more thoughtful and patient, less impulsive and moralistic approach to food and diet. If physicians also encourage alternative means of expression, appropriate and adequate family relationships, including mutual respect and support between male and female members of the family, and an increased acceptability of varieties of body shape, the incidence and the severity of eating disorders can be reduced, while their symptoms can be treated in an effective and humane manner.

Case Examples

Case History #1

Karen is a 12-year-old girl who had been treated by her family physician since birth. The second of three children, she lives with both parents in a small town near both her grandparents. During the preceding year, her paternal grandfather died and her grandmother began to eat dinner each evening with Karen's family. Karen's mother and 15-year-old sister were overweight. The family enjoyed eating and were proud of their cooking. Soon after her twelfth birthday, Karen began fasting for Lent, refusing to eat sweets and desserts. Devout Catholics, her parents saw this as a positive reflection of Karen's religious beliefs. Karen had always been thin and had been identified by the family as the determined child most likely to succeed at something difficult.

Karen continued fasting during the next six months, giving up more and more foods. Her parents alternated between talking about her eating habits and ignoring them in the hope that she would begin to eat more normally. During these six months, Karen at first stopped gaining and then her weight began to decrease. Her weight dropped from 80 to 60 pounds almost without the parents' notice. She had no physical symptoms and was proud of her weight loss. At school the nurses noticed Karen's eating habits and her growing thinness, checked her weight, and notified the family's physician and her parents. When the physician evaluated Karen she freely admitted active dieting and said she wanted to lose more weight. She was quite withdrawn and could not explain her behavior further than that. Her school work had remained excellent, but she had become socially withdrawn, spending less time with friends and playing less actively with her siblings. She was also noted to be increasingly irritable at home.

The physician's physical exam and routine laboratory studies indicated that Karen was significantly underweight for her age and height, but otherwise physically stable. After talking to both parents, the physician diagnosed anorexia nervosa and referred Karen to one of us for psychotherapy. At the first meeting, the parents were obviously concerned about Karen's thinness, guilty about their own lack of attentiveness to her dieting, and described meals as times of turmoil, confusion, and doubt for all family members. The therapist agreed with both parents that Karen needed to eat regularly and gain weight. He noted that the mother would become upset about Karen's eating but was unable to encourage her to eat more normally. Then the father would become involved and yell at Karen, becoming in the mother's eyes too intense and harsh with her and the mother would defend Karen. Karen's eating remained unchanged.

The therapist encouraged the father to take charge of dinner with the mother's support, while the mother was instructed to help Karen eat breakfast consistently. Both parents were encouraged to involve the school nurses, if necessary, to reinforce Karen's eating at school. The therapist also helped Karen to identify her need for support and encouragement and her need to be different from her mother and sister. Karen stated in a therapy session that she did not want to become overweight and was supported in this by both parents. The father was instructed to ask his mother not to become involved with Karen's eating at dinner. He was also able to restate his admiration of Karen's determination and ability to achieve and to resume paying attention to Karen's obvious strengths and skills in areas aside from her eating.

Karen gained weight consistently, first monitored by the therapist, then by the family physician twice monthly. In three months, Karen returned to normal weight with marked improvement in her behavior and eating habits. The family as a whole became more relaxed; grandparents were able to participate in the family, while the parents reestablished their position as the primary authorities for their children's development and behavior. After six therapy sessions over three months, the family was referred back to the primary-care physician. The therapist and physician had talked regularly during Karen's treatment and maintained telephone contact to review her continued progress and development after the conclusion of psychotherapy.

Case History #2

Donna is 18, and the youngest of three children living with her parents in a rural area. For three years, her father had increasing problems at work. He also had become worried about his health and was concerned about his diet and daily exercise routine. At age 16, Donna had also begun dieting regularly and had learned from friends at school how to vomit when she felt she had eaten too much. Her parents found this out and told their family physician. By then Donna was vomiting once a week. The family physician found Donna was in good general health except for her abnormal eating behavior. Her weight had remained normal. Concerned about Donna's lack of self-confidence and social withdrawal, however, the physician recommended that the family seek psychotherapy. The family did not do this for 18 months, and Donna's overeating and vomiting became increasingly frequent and more problematic. During this time, the physician monitored Donna's electrolytes and, noting that she had repeated episodes of hypokalemic alkalosis, prescribed potassium supplements.

Ultimately, Donna required hospitalization for hypokalemic alkalosis and dehydration, and her physician strongly encouraged therapy. Although this was begun, the family discontinued therapy after two sessions. The therapist informed the physician that treatment had stopped and urged the physician to encourage the family to resume it. When Donna became dehydrated and required medical hospitalization once more, her physician reiterated to the family the dangerousness of her condition and the family's need to gain control of the problem through psychotherapy and to persist with the therapy even if it was difficult. Donna had done well in school but had become more socially immature and isolated.

In sessions with Donna and her family the therapist highlighted Donna's worries about her eating and weight and her need for more family attention and support. The therapist helped Donna to express herself when she became angry or upset with her parents' rules, while also encouraging the parents to be consistent in enforcing reasonable rules concerning her behavior. The therapist developed an increasingly supportive and warm relationship with Donna's father so that he was less afraid of therapy and more able to reduce his attempts to control Donna. Encouraged also to increase her independence, Donna improved significantly after a short time and the family again dropped out of treatment. Informed of this by the therapist, the physician contacted the family and urged them to continue treatment to avoid Donna's relapse.

Donna's physical condition had worsened during this period, reinforcing the family's return to therapy. When the family complained about the therapist's work, the physician encouraged them to resolve this directly with the therapist. Therapy continued with the family as a whole for six months and with Donna individually for three months more. Her symptoms decreased markedly and then disappeared, and she made plans to leave home to attend college. She was more socially active with peers. Her parents ultimately addressed their marital problems and began to plan for the years when their children would no longer be living at home. Effective collaboration with the therapist in this case helped the physician to identify eating disorders in other patients and obtain effective treatment for them.

REFERENCES

Boskind-White, M., & White, W.C. (1983). *Bulimarexia: The binge/purge cycle*. New York: Norton.

Brotman, A.W., & Stern, T.A. (1983). Case report of cardiovascular abnormalities in anorexia nervosa. *American Journal of Psychiatry, 140*, 1227-1228.

Bruch, H. (1973). *Eating disorders*. New York: Basic Books.

Bruch, H. (1978). *The golden cage*. Cambridge, MA: Harvard University Press.

Cauwels, J.M. (1983). *Bulimia: The binge-purge compulsion*. Garden City, NY: Doubleday.

Collins, M., Hodas, G.R., & Liebman, R. (1983). Interdisciplinary model for the inpatient treatment of anorexia nervosa. *Journal of Adolescent Health Care, 4*, 3-8.

Crisp, A.H. (1980). *Anorexia nervosa: Let me be*. New York: Grune & Stratton.

Feighner, J.P., Robins, E., Guze, S.B., Woodruff, R.A., Jr., Winokur, G., & Munoz, R. (1972). Diagnostic criteria for use in psychiatric research. *Archives of General Psychiatry, 26*, 57-63.

Garfinkel, P., & Garner, D. (1982). *Anorexia nervosa: A multidimensional perspective*. New York: Brunner/Mazel.

Gwirtsman, H.E., Roy-Byrne, P., Yager, J., & Gerner, R.H. (1983). Neuroendocrine abnormalities in bulimia. *American Journal of Psychiatry, 140*, 559-563.

Halmi, K.A., & Falk, J.R. (1982). Anorexia: A study of outcome discriminators in exclusive dieters and bulimics. *Journal of the American Academy of Child Psychiatry, 21,* 369-375.

Halmi, K.A., Falk, J.R., & Schwartz, E. (1981). Binge-eating and vomiting; a survey of a college population. *Psychological Medicine, 11,* 697-706.

Herzog, D.B. (1982). Bulimia: The secretive syndrome. *Psychosomatics, 30,* 75-83.

Hillard, J.R., & Hillard, P.J. (1984). Bulimia, anorexia, diabetes: Deadly combination. *Psychiatric Clinics of North America,* 7(2), 367-379.

Johnson, C., & Berndt, D.J. (1983). Preliminary investigation of bulimia and life adjustment. *American Journal of Psychiatry, 140,* 774-777.

Liebman, R., Minuchin, S., & Baker, L. (1974). An integrated treatment program. *American Journal of Psychiatry, 131,* 432-436.

Liebman, R., Minuchin, S., Baker, L., & Rosman, B.L. (1975). The treatment of anorexia. In J.H. Masserman (Ed.), *Current psychiatric therapies*. New York: Grune & Stratton.

Liebman, R., Sargent, J., & Silver, M. (1983). A family systems orientation to the treatment of anorexia nervosa. *Journal of the American Academy of Child Psychiatry,* 22(2), 128-133.

Lippe, B.M. (1983). The physiologic aspects of eating disorders. *Journal of the American Academy of Child Psychiatry, 22,* 108-113.

Minuchin, S. (1974). *Families and family therapy*. Cambridge, MA: Harvard University Press.

Minuchin, S., Baker, L., Rosman, B.L., Liebman, R., Milman, L., & Todd, T. (1975). A conceptual model of psychosomatic illness in children. *Archives of General Psychiatry, 32,* 1031-1038.

Minuchin, S., & Fishman, H.C. (1981). *Family therapy techniques*. Cambridge, MA: Harvard University Press.

Minuchin, S., Rosman, B.L., & Baker, L. (1978). *Psychosomatic families: Anorexia nervosa in context*. Cambridge, MA: Harvard University Press.

Mitchell, J.E., Pyle, R.L., & Eckert, E.D. (1981). Frequency and duration of binge-eating episodes in patients with bulimia. *American Journal of Psychiatry, 138,* 835-836.

Pope, H.G., Jr., Hudson, J.L., Jonas, J.M., & Yurgelun-Todd, D. (1983). Bulimia treated with imipramine: A placebo controlled, double bind study. *American Journal of Psychiatry, 140,* 554-558.

Powers, P.S. (1982). Heart failure during treatment of anorexia nervosa. *American Journal of Psychiatry, 139,* 1167-1170.

Rosman, B.L., Minuchin, S., & Liebman, R. (1975). Family lunch session: An introduction to family therapy in anorexia nervosa. *American Journal of Orthospsychiatry, 45,* 846-853.

Rosman, B.L., Minuchin, S., Liebman, R., & Baker, L. (1976). Input and outcome of family therapy in anorexia nervosa. In J. Claghorn (Ed.), *Successful psychotherapy*. New York: Brunner/Mazel.

Russell, D. McR., Freedman, M.L., Feiglin, D.H.I., Jeejeebhoy, K.N., Swinson, R.P., & Garfinkel, P.E. (1983). Delayed gastric emptying and improvement with domperidone in a patient with anorexia nervosa. *American Journal of Psychiatry, 140,* 1235-1236.

Sargent, J., Liebman, R., & Silver, M. (1984). Family therapy for anorexia nervosa. In D.M. Garner & P.E. Garfinkel (Eds.), *The treatment of anorexia nervosa and bulimia*. New York: Guilford.

Schwab, A.D. (Moderator). (1981). Anorexia nervosa. *Annals of Internal Medicine, 94,* 371-381.

Schwartz, R., Barrett, M.J., & Saba, G. (1984). The family therapy of bulimia. In D.M. Garner & P.E. Garfinkel (Eds.), *The treatment of anorexia and bulimia*. New York: Guilford.

Selvini Palazzoli, M. (1978). *Self-starvation*. New York: Jason Aronson.

Sours, J. (1980). *Starving to death in a sea of objects*. New York: Jason Aronson.

Stanton, M.D., & Todd, T.C. (1982). *The family therapy of drug abuse and addiction*. New York: Guilford.

Strober, M. (1983). An empirically derived typology of anorexia nervosa. *Anorexia nervosa: Recent developments in research* (pp. 185-196). New York: Alan R. Liss.

Swift, W.J. (1982). The long-term outcome of early onset of anorexia nervosa: A critical review. *Journal of the American Academy of Child Psychiatry, 21*, 38-46.

Willi, J., & Grossman, S. (1983). Epidemiology of anorexia nervosa in a defined region of Switzerland. *American Journal of Psychiatry, 140*, 564-567.

Yager, J. (1981). Psychological aspects of anorexia nervosa. In A.D. Schwab, (Moderator), Anorexia nervosa. *Annals of Internal Medicine, 94*, 371-381.

13

A SYSTEMIC APPROACH TO SEXUAL DYSFUNCTIONS

BARBARA J. HOEK, M.A., COLLIER COLE, Ph.D., and BERNARD L. ROSENFELD, M.D., Ph.D.

Several factors have kept physicians from including sexual counseling in their routine patient care. Among these are the limited opportunity to hold lengthy counseling sessions in a busy office setting, insufficient medical school or residency training for treating sexual problems, and the physician's discomfort or embarrassment in discussing and dealing with sexual topics. In the approach presented here, we attempt to address these problems, stressing that certain "systemic" elements underlie the majority of commonly encountered sexual problems. By understanding and focusing on these elements, we believe the physician will be able to treat, effectively and briefly, patients who have a wide range of complaints related to sexual function.

We will review the strategic model of problem formation, applying it to the development of sexual problems, discuss the assessment and management of such problems, and propose ways of dealing with "roadblocks" to treatment. In the last section, we discuss the referral process for difficult management problems, supplemented by a suggested reading list for patients.

Our primary focus is on sexual problems and concerns that arise, typically, from psychogenic factors (e.g., limited sex information, belief in sexual myths, ineffective patterns of communication, performance anxiety). By and large, experts believe these psychological factors are dominant in the etiology of sexual difficulties (Crooks & Baur, 1983). This is not to say that organic factors such as chronic disease states, certain medications, or various genital infections are insignificant. We assume that the physician has taken an appropriate and thorough history and done physical and laboratory examinations to identify possible organic causes. These topics will not be reviewed here; Green (1979) and Masters, Johnson, and Kolodny (1982) provide overviews on organic causes.

Development of Sexual Problems

Traditionally, two theoretical frameworks, the behavioral and the psychoanalytic, have dominated our thinking about sexual dysfunction. More recently, the family therapy model has been used to approach the subject from a systems perspective (Papp, 1983; Penn, 1982; Storm, 1982). Despite obvious overlaps among the three schools of thought, differences of opinion remain on an exact conceptualization of sexual problems.

According to *behavioral learning theory*, sexual dysfunctions develop after an upsetting, anxiety-producing sexual episode. Subsequent sexual encounters remind the person of the earlier negative experience and evoke a similar anxious response. Anxiety, in turn, triggers the development of a sexual dysfunction by blocking the sexual response cycle and/or by leading to patterns of sexual avoidance behavior. The avoidance of sex is reinforced and maintained thereafter by the reduction of anxiety.

From a *psychoanalytic* perspective, sexual symptoms originate in unresolved oedipal and pre-oedipal developmental tasks. According to this view, sexual problems arise from the activation of forbidden infantile sexual wishes whenever the person engages in sex. The sexual dysfunction protects the person from engaging in an activity he or she perceives (unconsciously) as dangerous.

Family systems theorists address the matter in a slightly different manner. *Structural* family therapists, for example, maintain that sexual problems serve a stabilizing function in a disrupted couple or family system. These therapists believe that all members of a system participate, at some level, in maintaining a sexual symptom and that the symptom will persist until a more adaptive way of organizing the family can be found. The *strategic* model, on which this chapter is largely based, suggests that sexual problems are created and maintained by the application of incorrect or unworkable solutions to troublesome situations. We believe the family systems approach, and the strategic model in particular, offers a useful method for conceptualizing sexual problems and a unique approach to their treatment.

The Strategic Model of Problem Formation

In discussing the strategic approach to family therapy, Watzlawick, Weakland, and Fisch (1974) stated that, "under certain circumstances problems will arise purely as the result of a wrong attempt at changing an existing difficulty" (p. 36). They defined "difficulty" as an undesirable but quite common state of affairs that can be resolved by some commonsense action or must simply be tolerated because no known solution exists. The authors defined "problems" as "impasses, deadlocks, knots, etc., which are created and maintained through the mishandling of difficulties" (p. 37). Thus, in the strategic approach, symptoms are seen as the unintended result of benign but misguided attempts to correct a perceived difficulty. The attempted solution then not only becomes part of the problem, but, if applied repeatedly, is likely to make the situation worse. Two ways of turning minor difficulties into problems warrant special mention.

The first is a method of problem solving by which an individual attempts to force a behavior that, by its nature, can only occur spontaneously. This creates an impossible state of affairs referred to as a "be spontaneous" paradox (Watzlawick et al., 1974). An often cited example is that of insomniacs who assure themselves a sleepless night by trying to will a state of natural and spontaneous sleep. Obviously, the situation is made worse by repeated applications of the same solution: Natural sleep can only be achieved by not trying so hard to fall asleep.

Solutions of the "be spontaneous" type are most frequently used to combat a wide range of problems, real or imagined, in areas of bodily function and performance. These include difficulties with bladder and bowel function, appetite, cognitive functions like memory and concentration, mood states of depression and anxiety, and, of course, problems of sexual function and performance (Fisch, Weakland, & Segal, 1982, p. 129). In most cases, attempts to resolve such problems forcibly will do little to restore natural functioning and may, in fact, make it more difficult to attain.

The second mechanism of problem formation particularly relevant to our topic is the "utopia syndrome" (Watzlawick et al., 1974). This condition may be brought about by individuals who believe that life can and should run virtually problem-free. They see everyday difficulties not as unavoidable human events, but as problems in need of swift and permanent correction. Rarely do they recognize the implausibility of ever attaining such a utopian goal, believing instead that failure or imperfections are their own fault, or the fault of others. Such a patient will say, "If only I (she, he, or they) would try harder, this trouble would disappear." Feelings of frustration, helplessness, and despair associated with the utopian syndrome arise from failing to recognize that one's belief system needs changing, not the inability to prevent the difficulties of life.

From a strategic perspective, sexual problems arise from the same self-defeating cycle of attempted solution and failure experienced by the insomniac. "Be spontaneous" paradoxes and utopian beliefs play a prominent role in this process, but they account for only a portion of the ways a sexual difficulty may be transformed into a sexual problem.

Origins of Sexual Problems: A Strategic View

Most, if not all, people occasionally feel unable to be sexually aroused or to achieve orgasm. McCarthy (1977) estimates that one of four males has an unsuccessful first intercourse experience, and that, by age 40, 95% of all men will have at least one episode of erectile failure. The noted sex therapist, H. S. Kaplan (1974), suggested that, for an otherwise responsive and orgastic woman, failure to achieve orgasm during coitus may be a normal variant of female sexuality. In a study by Frank, Anderson, and Rubinstein (1978), 100 happily married couples were asked about the frequency and quality of their sexual relations. More than 80% of the couples reported being satisfied with their marital and sexual relations, despite the fact that 40% of the men and 63% of the women reported a sexual dysfunction.

This suggests that, while most of us encounter periodic sexual difficulties, only some individuals and couples identify these as problematic (Cole, 1983). From a strategic perspective, the difference between those who do and those who do not may well lie in their capacity to take a "let-well-enough-alone" attitude to an occasional lapse in sexual functioning. Perhaps because of inadequate information about sexuality or adherence to some standard of sexual perfection, some individuals may embark on the road to trouble by assuming too quickly that a problem exists. To illustrate, consider the problem-forming mechanisms involved in the development of an erectile dysfunction.

Case 1: The Individual

A recently divorced man is eager to improve his masculine self-image by experimenting with different sexual partners. His first attempt at lovemaking, however, ends in disappointment when he fails to achieve an erection. Acutely embarrassed and humiliated, he apologizes and takes his date home.

His doubts increased, he approaches his next attempt with more apprehension than the first. As he watches himself closely for signs of an erection, he finds it difficult to enjoy the encounter. As soon as sexual foreplay begins, he becomes aroused and achieves a semi-firm erection. Doubtful of his ability to sustain the erection, he immediately initiates intercourse. The result is a lost erection following intromission. Determined to avoid another failure, he and his date work for nearly an hour before they admit defeat.

Subsequent encounters are similar. Occasionally the man sustains enough of an erection to reinforce his belief that he will eventually succeed. He attempts a variety of solutions—alcohol, marijuana, not masturbating, pornography, morning sex—all without result. More and more certain that his problem is real, he consults his physician. The physician may prescribe hormones and give advice, which result in improvement, but when this proves temporary, the patient becomes more deeply depressed. He does not return for a follow-up visit.

His relationships with women deteriorate. Although his partners are supportive, his conviction that they pity rather than understand him is humiliating to him. Eventually he decides the best solution is to avoid sex completely. Ironically, the less seductively he behaves toward women, the more they seem to pursue him. The attention, rather than providing relief, increases his anxiety that he will eventually be forced to reveal his secret. Finally, he stops his efforts altogether, believing that he will never have a satisfying sexual relationship.

Discussion. Belief in any utopian sexual myth may easily lead to a reaction short of panic at the first sign of sexual difficulty. If "normal" functioning does not resume spontaneously, scrutinizing usually increases and conscious attempts to force the desired result are begun.

Self-imposed pressures to perform do not work and, in fact, make matters worse. Sexual excitement and release are spontaneous reflexes that occur when an individual receives adequate erotic stimulation under relaxed and pressure-free conditions. These reflexes cannot be made to occur on demand. Women with orgasmic and arousal difficulties who obsessively watch their own erotic build-up succeed only in blocking sexual responsiveness. Similarly, transient episodes of delayed ejaculation are easily transformed into intractable situations by belabored coital thrusting. Men who attempt to improve their performance by grading the firmness and duration of each erection will inevitably ensure a less than satisfying score.

While many of the solutions used to resolve sexual problems fall into the "be spontaneous" category, others do not. Men who are rapid ejaculators, for example, frequently try to delay ejaculation by focusing on arousal-reducing thoughts during lovemaking (computing overdue bills, counting "strokes," etc.). As learning control of ejaculation requires an ability to cease penile stimulation just before orgasm, such techniques often perpetuate the problem by blocking awareness of important pre-ejaculatory cues. Alcohol and drugs continue to be sought as solutions to sexual problems despite widespread knowledge of the dangers of overuse. Like alcohol, sexual abstinence for brief periods may be beneficial in breaking a continual series of failures. Carried to extreme, however, avoidance of sexual contact reduces the opportunity for practicing sexual skills and intensifies the pressure to perform once sexual relationships are resumed.

Sometimes omission or avoidance of certain solutions is as troublesome as using incorrect ones. Women who have orgasmic dysfunctions are known to avoid behaviors that would increase their arousal and chances for attaining orgasmic release. Foremost among these are masturbation, sexual fantasy, cunnilingus, and making assertive requests for foreplay and effective clitoral stimulation. Many sexually dysfunctional men have equal difficulty allowing themselves to enjoy less goal- or performance-oriented sex. Their socially learned inability to adopt a passive-receptive role in lovemaking severely limits the amount of erotic stimulation they might otherwise receive.

A common thread in the failure to resolve most sexual problems is the individual's unawareness that the real problem is his repetitive use of wrong solutions, not a defect of his or his partner's. Such misperceptions are usually shared by a sexual partner who, by attempting to help, contributes equally to maintaining the problem.

Case 2: The Couple System

Stressed by the demands of a newborn baby, a young wife begins to lose interest in sex. Her husband, noticing his wife's unresponsiveness, wonders if there might be a problem. To assure himself that there is no real cause for concern, he increases his seductive overtures. Still disinterested, the wife avoids her husband's advances, but worries that her repeated refusals will cause him to feel personally rejected. Not wishing to displease or frustrate him further, she agrees to a sexual encounter despite a lack of real desire. Husband and wife enter the bedroom nervously, both anxious about disappointing the other.

The husband, preoccupied by his concerns, initiates foreplay in somewhat mechanistic fashion. At the same time, the wife intensifies her efforts to force an excited response. The final result is a loss of arousal and pleasure for both. Afterward, they do not discuss the experience because they do not wish to hurt or embarrass each other.

During the following weeks, the frustrating encounter is repeated often. Each time the wife fails to respond, the husband's need for reassurance grows, and their lovemaking becomes an unpleasant chore. As she resumes her distancing maneuvers, his insecurity and number of advances escalate. A well-defined cycle of mutually reinforcing and self-defeating interactions is now complete: The more he pursues her, the less likely is she to respond to his needs; and the less his needs are met, the more frantically he attempts to arouse her. The cycle may continue in this way until one or the other, or both, decide to seek help. At this point the physician may hear these common complaints: "She won't let me get near her!" and "I'd rather he'd just leave me alone!"

Discussion. According to family systems theory, problems exist largely in the interactions *between* individuals. This implies that partners in a couple system are equally responsible for maintaining a sexual difficulty. From a strategic perspective, sexual problems that occur in the context of a two-person relationship are created and maintained by the benign, reciprocal attempts of *both* partners to improve the situation. Through a series of circular interactions, the attempted solutions by one individual reinforce, and are reinforced by, those of the other. In a sexual context, this reciprocal process is likely to escalate rapidly because so many couples avoid open discussion of sexual matters and because performance pressures, once begun, are very difficult to stop. For this reason, a significant portion of time in couples' sex therapy is directed to developing or reintroducing more direct communication and more pleasure- rather than performance-based sexual behaviors.

The goal of a strategic-based approach to resolving a sexual dysfunction is to interrupt the reciprocal cycle of couple interactions that perpetuate the problem. The first step in treatment, for that reason, is identifying the couple's methods of solving their problem and discovering how these attempts prolong the dilemma.

Interviewing Patients About Sexuality

"Some physicians take a rather detailed sex history from every patient, while others never hear a sexual complaint," wrote Perry (1980, p.64). This difference among physicians comes from many factors, including time constraints and patients' willingness to discuss sexual matters frankly.

But the most critical variable is the physicians' comfort level with sexuality and their attitudes towards sexual health care. Physicians who inquire routinely about their patients' sexual functioning report two to five times more sexual problems in their practices than do those who feel ill at ease with such questions and rarely ask (Burnap & Golden, 1967). A dramatic illustration of the need for inquiry was provided by an outpatient clinic study in which 1,180 men were screened for erectile dysfunction (Slag et al., 1983). Although 401 men (34%) had an erectile dysfunction, only *six* had been identified as having that problem before being interviewed by the authors. Clearly, health care providers are as likely as consumers to have culturally based inhibitions about discussing sexual matters.

There are, of course, other highly sensitive and anxiety-producing topics (e.g., bladder and bowel function) that the physician must learn to discuss. Unlike these others, however, sexual functioning is related more to the quality of life than its prolongation (Leif, 1978). As a result, the breach of "propriety" required to discuss sexual concerns cannot be as easily justified as the need to rule out life-threatening illnesses. Fears of offending or embarrassing the patient, which are eventually overcome in other areas of medical care, remain a source of discomfort for physicians reviewing sexual issues.

Patients experience the same inhibitions and are quick to cooperate, therefore, by not bringing up sexual matters. These circular interactions of patient and doctor often reinforce one another, making it even more difficult to broach the subject. The physicians' responsibility is to break the cycle by simply asking about sexual concerns.

Although an open, nonjudgmental attitude in dealing with patients' sexual lives has been stressed countless times, one cannot always achieve this because one's own values, biases, and misbeliefs are often hardest to detect. They show up suddenly when a patient, assumed to be heterosexual, turns out to be homosexual, when the "nice young girl" asks for information about venereal disease, or when a personal friend or relative contracts herpes. These biases are natural and human but, once revealed, should be kept apart from treatment decisions. Later, one's approach and expectations can be altered consciously to fill in the discovered blind spots.

When to Inquire

The best time to ask about sexual activity is during the review of the patients' physical condition. For men, this is best done after discussion of the renal system and problems in micturition (Sharpe & Levay, 1980). In examining women, questions about sexual concerns can be integrated easily in a discussion of the female reproductive system, menstruation, and contraception. Questions about sexual functioning early in the physician-patient relationship will make it easier for patients to reveal problems later.

Although questions about sexuality are not appropriate during medical crises, convalescing patients *and their partners* must have an opportunity to ask and be advised about their return to sexual activity. This is equally true of surgical patients, especially when impairment of sexual function is expected.

Questions to Include

Kolodny, Masters, and Johnson (1979) have suggested a short series of questions they believe are likely to detect "more than 95% of sexual problems in a clinical practice" (p. 558). These questions are:

- Are you currently active sexually? If so, what is the approximate frequency of sexual activity?

- Are you satisfied with your sex life? If no, why not?
- (For men) Do you have difficulty obtaining or maintaining an erection? Do you have any difficulty with the control of ejaculation?
- (For women) Do you have any difficulty becoming sexually aroused? Do you ever experience pain during intercourse? Do you have difficulty being orgasmic?
- Do you have any questions or problems related to sex that you would like to discuss?

Obviously, the practitioner will want to phrase these questions in his or her own language to avoid sounding overly stilted. Most patients will respond readily if approached by the physician in a self-assured and relaxed manner. If, however, the physician detects strong resistance, the subject should be dropped and reintroduced at a later time when greater trust and rapport have been established.

Follow-up and Inclusion of the Sexual Partner

When the inquiry reveals a specific sexual complaint or when one is mentioned by the patient without prompting, a more thorough assessment will be needed. Even in abbreviated form, this will take a half hour or an hour, so that the patient should be scheduled for another appointment. If the patient is married or has a steady sexual partner, the partner should be invited to come along. His or her presence will be invaluable in the assessment process and expedite treatment.

Some patients will not like the idea that their partner is a part of the sexual problem. Evaluation and treatment of sexual difficulties are strongly enhanced by, but do not absolutely require, the participation of both sexual partners. If the patient strongly resists a conjoint session, he or she should be seen alone. Once the patient's fears are reduced, joint involvement can be discussed again.

Specific Sexual Problems

Evaluation of a sexual dysfunction begins with attempts to obtain a detailed description of the problem and its context, with a focus on the frequency and general quality of sexual interactions. Next, the interviewer inquires about the sexual partner's role, systemic factors other than sexual ones, and most important, solutions the patient and partner have attempted. The patient's goals for treatment need to be clarified and perhaps adjusted to be realistic.

Defining the Problem

The meaning of a woman's statement, "Doctor, I can't have an orgasm," may indicate a global complaint like "I've never had an orgasm" or the more specific, "I can't have orgasm during intercourse." Patients should be asked, therefore, to explain their experiences with the problem, when and how often it occurs, patients' and partners' response to its occurrence, and when the problem began or was first noticed. Emphasis is on what, where, how often, and when, not why.

For family therapists the focus of treatment is on changing current patterns maintaining a problem, not on exploring the past. Physicians, however, who must differentiate organic and psychogenic causes, need information about the onset, duration, and temporal sequence of a sexual disorder. According to Kolodny, Masters, and Johnson (1979), "Most organically induced sexual problems are persistent and progressively worsening, as opposed to psychogenic problems, which may more frequently be episodic or situational" (p. 590). There are notable exceptions, however, which are discussed thoroughly by Kolodny et al.

Sexual problems are relative. Rapid ejaculation may be far more disconcerting to the man whose wife is orgasmic only with sustained coital thrusting than to the man whose wife prefers short lovemaking sessions. The question "In what way is this a problem for you?" helps physicians avoid imposing their own values and expectations on patients.

The Sexual Context: Frequency and Quality of Sex

Once the patient's specific complaint is understood, the physician must inquire about the larger sexual system. How frequently does the individual or couple have sexual relations? Are there changes or patterns that may impede resolution of the problem? Too-frequent sex may, for example, indicate a lack of spontaneity and exaggerated efforts to force a response, while sex engaged in too seldom may prevent discovery of new solutions. Sometimes the problem itself is a disagreement over too much, enough, or too little, and physicians must point out that both partners contribute to initiation or refusal of a sexual overture. For example, initiation by one person usually follows a readiness cue given by the other, just as rejection can often be traced to the disinterest of *both* parties, not just one. Especially when partners disagree strongly, it is usually true that, on some level of awareness, each is maintaining a covertly agreed-upon frequency that fits their marital system best.

Sexual problems affect and are affected by the quality of the whole sexual relationship. Patients should be asked about the degree of pleasure they find in lovemaking because, once the cycle of attempted solution and failure begins, much of the joy and intimacy of sex disappears. The loss of pleasure inhibits full sexual arousal, which, in turn, perpetuates attempts to force an erotic response. In some cases, this escalating spiral can be interrupted by merely pointing it out to the patients. Others may have to be informed of special techniques to enhance sexual arousal, which are described in this chapter's treatment section.

The Partner's Role

A systemic assessment requires an examination of the partner's role, but without the interviewer's taking sides in trying to find the source of a sexual problem. This is difficult for the medical practitioner who is likely to hear only one version of a story.

A patient who blames his wife for his erectile dysfunction, might say,

> My wife is always pressuring me to perform. Oh, she'll try to help me get an erection, but after she gets tired, she wants to blame the whole problem on me! She says I'm not doing it right and that if I loved her more, I'd be able to get it up. I've told her it has nothing to do with how much I love her, but she just won't let it go!

If his wife could also be interviewed, the picture might balance out:

> My husband is so obsessed with getting an erection that he insists I spend hours stimulating his penis. I try to convince him we're working too hard at it, but he won't listen. Lately, he's become so preoccupied with his problem, he doesn't know I'm alive. Our sex life is a disaster! There's no tenderness or holding or even kissing anymore, just the constant push to get an erection. Once I even told him that if he would start acting like he loved me instead of treating us both like machines, he might be able to get that damn erection! I realize that I was wrong, but I just felt so frustrated.

Family physicians must be careful to avoid the normal tendency to sympathize with one spouse against the other. Collusion of this sort will not only restrict their perspective, but help reinforce a view of the situation the couple has already found unworkable.

In addition to asking about the partner's response to the problem situation, physicians need to determine whether or not the partner's sexual difficulties are being obscured by those of the identified patient. Women's sexual problems that may contribute to men's sexual difficulties include any physiologic or psychologic condition that decreases vaginal lubrication or makes sexual interaction painful. Ejaculatory problems may develop in men whose partners have difficulty reaching orgasm as a result of pressure (on the male) to prolong coital thrusting during intercourse (Steege, 1981). Similarly, male problems with ejaculation and erection may contribute to the development of anxiety-based arousal and orgasm difficulties in women.

Systemic Factors Outside the Sexual Relationship

Conflict or major change in the immediate or extended family network, stress caused by the illness of a family member, and fears of job loss are stressful situations that may influence the continuation of a sexual difficulty. The existence of a sexual dissatisfaction or complaint does not necessarily indicate trouble in the larger couple system, but the quality of dyadic interactions needs to be explored.

If physicians believe that the sexual problem may be secondary to a troubled marital relationship or another life circumstance, they should discuss this with patients. Physicians should be careful, however, to talk about it in a manner that respects the patient's definition of the problem. Some patients will breathe a sigh of relief at this signal of understanding, yet others will feel slighted, defensive, or misunderstood if the topic is not handled carefully.

"I know I get wound up a lot about my work, but if my wife would just let me have a little sex, everything would be fine" is a common complaint. Here the best strategy is to reverse gears quickly, apologize for the error in thinking, return to the patient's original formulation ("My problem is my wife"), and indicate agreement with it. "Now that I think of it again, Mr. Jones, I can see that your assessment of the situation is much clearer than mine. Your wife's reluctance to have sex is obviously the main problem. Let me give you the names of some competent sex and family therapists who I think can help her. I would recommend, however, that you join the first couple of sessions to let the therapist know just what her problem is." Physicians can then inform the therapist of their observations and intervention so that these may be incorporated into future treatment planning.

Attempted Solutions

In this phase of the interview process, questions about attempts to solve the problem will begin to reveal patterns of self-defeating and self-reinforcing behaviors in the individual or couple system. Is the patient concentrating so hard on success that he or she has fallen into the "be spontaneous" paradox? Are the partners caught in a repetitive sequence of interactions, each watching and reinforcing the other's lack of spontaneity? If so, they may not know that they are unwittingly precluding a natural physiological response.

Is the woman who has vaginismus or dyspareunia forcing herself to endure painful intercourse time after time to please her partner? Such efforts, though clearly well meant, perpetuate the cycle of anticipatory pain, followed by heightened anxiety and more pain. Undoubtedly the male partner will be caught in the same cycle and be progressively less able to provide her with the slow, pleasure-based approach she needs to relax fully.

Women whose desire and orgasmic functions are impaired should be asked about their experience and comfort with the more arousing forms of stimulation such as masturbation, cunnilingus, and sexual fantasy. Unproductive use of mental distracting techniques and avoidance of sexual stimuli with men who ejaculate rapidly need to be identified. Obviously, men who have erectile problems should be asked about attempts to use drugs or alcohol as aphrodisiacs or relaxants.

In discussions of such highly sensitive matters as masturbation and sexual fantasy, both physicians and patients will experience some anxiety. Useful methods for reducing discomfort are to preface questions with the rationale for introducing an embarrassing topic ("Masturbation is the easiest way for most women to achieve orgasm") and to emphasize the normality of the behavior involved ("Many people aren't aware that, according to Kinsey, most women try masturbation at one time or another"). It is neither necessary nor appropriate to ask a patient about the content of privately held sexual fantasies. Permission to use and enjoy sexual fantasy is sufficient intervention. (An often recommended book for women who wish to explore this area is *My Secret Garden* by Nancy Friday, 1973.)

Other Helpers

In addition to having talked to spouses, many patients will have consulted or compared notes with, for example, an intimate friend, sibling, parent, or minister about their sexual problem. The advice from such sources is sometimes wrong and may actually help to maintain the problem rather than alleviate it. "Trying harder" only increases pressures to perform, while simplistic formulations like "You just need to relax and it will go away" leave people feeling more demoralized than before. For these reasons, it is important to inquire what other people significantly involved with the patient have been doing to help with the problem (Fisch et al., 1975). An attempt to correct the effects of faulty advice may have to be made.

Setting Goals for Treatment

Encouraging patients to set clear, *modest* goals and commit themselves to a specific number of sessions or office visits will enhance the likelihood of treatment success. Discussing rules for goal setting, Haley (1976) wrote: "Problems, whether one calls them *symptoms* or *complaints*, should be something one can count, observe, measure, or in some way know one is influencing" (pp. 40-41). *Specific* sexual problems (those related to orgasm, erection, ejaculation) are relatively easy for patients to observe, count, and measure. More general complaints (those having to do with the quality of a sexual relationship) need to be translated into usable, that is, solvable, form.

Coached by physicians, patients must assume major responsibility for translating a general goal into a more specific one. Increased frequency of sexual activity, sometimes used as a measure of improvement, is not always an appropriate goal because frequency often has little to do with quality. (Boring sex is not made more interesting by simply having it more often.) If the sexual problem were solved, what would be different? And, for example, how would the sexual partner know that the problem had been solved? With these sorts of questions physicians will help patients establish goals that reflect their own situation and heighten their motivation for change.

Managing Sexual Problems

Since the publication of Masters and Johnson's *Human Sexual Inadequacy* in 1970, the literature on therapeutic techniques has become vast. We shall not repeat here what has been discussed thoroughly elsewhere (see reference list).

The majority of techniques physicians need in order to manage their patients' sexual concerns fall into three categories: giving reassurance and information about sexual normalcy; maximizing sexual pleasure; and minimizing pressures to perform. The first two are covered comprehensively in other publications. The third—pressure to perform—is a common thread in most sexual problems. For this reason, the largest part of our discussion on treatment will be devoted to the strategic handling of commonly encountered obstacles to reducing performance anxiety.

Giving Reassurance and Information About Sexual Normalcy

Regardless of how lightly patients may broach the subject, physicians should deal seriously with all questions about sexuality. The fact that the topic has been raised at all indicates that the patient or someone in the patient's family considers it important. Factual information should always be followed by an effort to identify the motivation and context of an inquiry.

Who actually needs the information sought, and what created the need? Careful investigation may reveal that changes in the sexual behavior of a family member, especially that of a child, may not be related to sex at all. Children may use sexual outlets to relieve anxiety brought about by changes in the family system (e.g., the recent loss or addition of a family member, a protracted illness, hospitalization, or change in job status). Increased masturbation and attention to sexual stimuli can be normal means of reducing stress in family members of all ages.

The question patients ask most frequently is: Am I (or is my spouse, child, older parent) sexually normal? Although physicians need not be experts on sexuality to handle such questions, they should be familiar with normal sexual behaviors and concerns at all stages of the developmental life cycle. One needs to know, for example, that intercourse before marriage, masturbation, and occasional attraction to same-sex peers are so common as to be considered normative for both sexes during adolescence. The need for sex education is not, however, restricted to the young. Adults of all ages need accurate information from their physicians about changes in the sexual response cycle associated with such events as pregnancy, major illness, the taking of various forms of medication, menopause, and others. Older adults require information and counseling about normal changes in sexual functioning associated with aging. Failure to transmit this information to them can be attributed to the older adults' embarrassment and to physicians' discomfort in talking about sex to patients who may be as old as their own parents. Being aware of these factors will help physicians to care more effectively for their older patients.

Most of us tend to gauge what is sexually normal by generalizing from our personal experiences. Awareness of contemporary sexual practices reduces the possibility that professional judgments will be biased by personally held value systems. Statistics from the work of Kinsey and his collaborators (Kinsey, Pomeroy, & Martin, 1948; Kinsey, Pomeroy, Martin, & Gebhard, 1953) are still valuable guidelines for counseling adults:

1) More than 95% of men and about 62% of women practice masturbation at one time or another.

2) The average woman reaches orgasm in 95% or more of her masturbatory attempts, which suggests that this may be the technique most likely to produce orgasm in women.
3) A man usually achieves orgasm within about four minutes of intromission, while a woman who is orgasmic during intercourse requires from 10 to 20 minutes.

In practice, effective handling of sex-related questions often has as much to do with the way in which physicians respond as the exact answers they provide. An open, unbiased attitude and a willingness to be candid about areas of speculation or ignorance will reassure patients that the information is based on solid ground. Physicians should know where to obtain needed facts and have this information available to patients.

Techniques to Maximize Sexual Pleasure

Couples who complain of low sexual desire and dull or overly goal-oriented sex lives have a particular need for outside direction in revitalizing their sexual relationship. A wealth of techniques has been developed for this purpose (McCarthy, Ryan, & Johnson, 1975; Munjack & Oziel, 1980; Schover, 1982; Stuart, 1980). The intent of most of these is to increase sexual arousal by fostering greater attention to the sensual rather than performance aspects of lovemaking. Best known are the "sensate focus" exercises developed over a decade ago by Masters and Johnson (1970). These homework assignments incorporate a graduated hierarchy of desensitizing touching—not necessarily sexual—experiences to reduce performance anxiety and improve nonverbal sexual communication. Other techniques, such as keeping a daily journal of sexual feelings and thoughts, and making lists of sexual likes and dislikes, are used to increase awareness of sexual arousal and its precipitants (Schover, 1982). Permission to use sexual fantasy, and suggestions to engage in brief necking and petting sessions without intercourse or orgasm, and to initiate sex in never-before-tried ways, are other examples. Some couples respond well to contracts which stipulate sexual or nonsexual favors to be exchanged daily.

Techniques to increase sexual arousal are useful in treatment of most sexual problems. Participation by the couple as a unit in treatment is advantageous but not required. Our major precautionary advice is to consider the patients' unique sexual attitudes, feelings, and experiences before assigning homework exercises to them. If a person is reluctant to try certain behaviors, it is best to yield to his or her preferences. The physician might say,

> I can appreciate your reluctance to try this next step. It's important not to go too quickly, and I think you are wise to be cautious. In treating sexual problems, we always seek to match the homework assignments to the patient's readiness to try a new behavior. Let's back up and see if there aren't some steps in between the exercise you and your wife did last week and the one I just suggested.

Guidelines for Minimizing Pressures to Perform

The key to successful resolution of most sexual difficulties is to persuade patients to forego useless attempts to force a response that can only occur spontaneously. Generally speaking, cooperative, well-motivated patients will readily comply with suggestions to take a less goal-oriented approach to sexuality, and they will report back good results at their next visit. For a small percentage of patients, however, matters will not improve so rapidly because these patients are unwilling or unable to abandon the notion that good things come to those who "try harder." Sometimes not only the patient has difficulty switching gears, but someone in the patient's life, usually the sexual partner, will have the same stubborn problem. Professional helpers in such situations often end up feeling as frustrated as their patients. No matter how well disguised or convincingly stated, the bottom line in repeated suggestions to "let go," "enjoy yourself more," or "loosen up" is always the same: You *should* work harder at becoming spontaneous. One frequently ends up in the ironic position of pressuring people to stop pressuring themselves!

The following is a discussion of two classes of interventions used by strategic family therapists to manage problems of the "be spontaneous" variety.

Change through restraint. To quote the master hypnotist, Milton Erickson, "Whenever you start depriving anyone of anything, they are going to insist that you give it to them" (Haley, 1973, p. 70). This observation is the basis of restraining maneuvers, techniques used in strategic psychotherapy to inhibit, restrain, or forbid change (Weeks & L'Abate, 1982). All forms of strategic restraining are variants of the same theme: To achieve change, discourage it (Tennen, 1977). Restraining techniques involve encouraging people to change slowly or to stay the same. Aiming for a small positive change in the affective tone of a couple's lovemaking will, for example, do more than a hurried attempt to correct their specific sexual problem. In a similar vein, rapid change is discouraged to prevent a setback.

Techniques that attempt to achieve change by actually forbidding it were first made famous by Masters and Johnson (1970). Their use of a ban on intercourse and orgasm to reduce pressures to perform has led to the widespread application of the procedure to every form of sex therapy. Beginning with nongenital sensate-focus exercises, sex therapists assign couples to engage in mutual pleasuring of one another's bodies. Touching the partner's genitals or proceeding to orgasmic release is, however, strictly prohibited. In successive assignments, patients are gradually "allowed" to undertake the behaviors they wish to engage in. This step-by-step approach not only reduces performance anxiety but enhances sexual desire by explicitly forbidding its expression. Just as stolen apples taste better than bought ones, illicit sex can be more exciting than that fully licensed.

Restraining maneuvers need not be limited to sensate-focus exercises, as they can be easily extended to fit a variety of situations in the treatment of sexual problems. Couples may be asked to "stay the same" for the first week of treatment to collect further baseline data about the frequency and nature of their difficulty. To do so, they will need to avoid changing their problem in any way and take careful written or mental notes about when the problem occurred and under what circumstances. Rapid change is often achieved by this simple assignment. To ensure continued good results, however, the couple should be followed up for several weeks.

Instructions to avoid change are particularly useful with single male patients who do not have steady partners with whom to practice the pleasuring exercises. For example, a young single man, who complained of difficulty in achieving and maintaining firm erections, was instructed to engage in normal sexual relations with his favorite girlfriend, but to stop when he noticed the smallest sign of an impending erection. He was to resume sexual activity only after being certain his penis had returned to a nonerect state. Finally he was advised to tell his girlfriend beforehand that the sudden change in routine had been prescribed by his doctor so that additional data could be gathered on his problem. During the second session, the patient confessed sheepishly that he had been unable to do his homework. Despite his best efforts, he could not prevent an erection. After expressing mild disappointment, the therapist collected the patient's observations and issued the same assignment. The young man called two weeks later to say he no longer needed treatment because his problem had disappeared. The therapist reacted with surprise and invited him to call back any time he needed further help.

The same technique is effective for rapid remission of *transient* episodes of prolonged or delayed ejaculation. At first, the man is asked to engage in normal sexual activity but to prevent ejaculation under any circumstances. This is slightly different from simply advising an individual to cease self-induced pressures to "force" an ejaculation. As in the case above, an unequivocal *ban* is placed on experiencing even one episode of the desired behavior until the next visit. To ensure success, the patient is told he must proceed slowly, switch from a performance- to a pleasure-based sexual style, and guard against the certain setback that would follow a too rapidly (i.e., prematurely) achieved ejaculation. If the symptom does not remit in one to two weeks, the practitioner may prescribe a nongenital and then a genital pleasuring exercise (McCarthy, Ryan, & Johnson, 1975). Gradually, the ban on ejaculation is applied only on occasions selected by the couple for performing the pleasuring homework. The majority of cases will be resolved successfully by this intervention.

A variation of the technique of encouraging patients to "stay the same" is to ask them to make their symptom or problem worse to feel a greater sense of control over it. Although this is a complicated maneuver, to be used with care, the principle is to reduce the excessive anxiety that sometimes accompanies completion of certain homework assignments. The approach, referred to as *symptom prescription*, was used with a couple referred for treatment of the wife's sexual anxiety.

The couple's previous therapist had prescribed a nongenital pleasuring exercise as a first step to reducing the woman's fears. Her husband reported that she had been so nervous during the assignment that she had "lain there like a stiff board through the whole ordeal." Both partners were acutely embarrassed by their inability to complete such a simple task and were clearly steeling themselves for their new therapist's first suggestion.

To prevent this couple from having another and even more demoralizing "failure," they were asked to repeat the pleasuring homework but with an amendment. To learn more about her symptom and gain better control over it, the wife was instructed to spend the first 20 minutes of the exercise trying to amass as much tension and anxiety as she possibly could. At no point was she to give in to the desire to let herself go until she had completed *at least* 20 minutes of sustained tension. Prescribing the very behavior she found so difficult to eliminate reduced the possibility of failure. An additional benefit came from a contingency suggestion, similar to suggestions used to induce a hypnotic trance ("Only *after* you sit in that chair will you be able to fully relax," or, "Only when your hand touches your face can you go completely asleep" (Erickson & Rossi, 1979). The result for this patient was a successful pleasuring experience with her husband, quite unlike their previous encounter.

Reframing: Increasing options for change. People often find it difficult to resolve a sexual problem because they define their situation in such narrow terms that only one or two solutions seem possible. Reframing, as the term is used here, refers to the act of providing individuals with more options for change by altering their view of the problem or some aspect of the situation. Occasionally, a problem is reframed or redefined in such a way that the person loses the need to change because he or she no longer believes that a problem exists (Fisch, Weakland, & Segal, 1982). This was apparently the case in the following example given by Haley (1973) about Milton Erickson, who was a master at relabeling couples' problems.

One of Erickson's patients was a newly married man who had a playboy reputation but became impotent on his wedding night. His bride felt disappointed, bitter, and rejected. Erickson relabeled his impotence as a compliment. He told the couple that the husband was so overwhelmed by the beauty of his bride that he felt (and had become) incompetent (reported in Weeks & L'Abate, 1982, p. 109).

As this demonstrates, most attempts at reframing are designed to replace a negative frame of reference with a more positive one. It may seem impossible at first that a positive connotation could be found for problems as unpleasant as low sexual desire, erectile dysfunction, vaginismus, and others. When one recalls, however, that sexual symptoms often result from benign but misguided efforts to restabilize a couple system, the possibilities for positive reframing become more apparent. Reframing is particularly useful in treating women for low sexual desire, which is perhaps the most commonly heard sexual complaint today.

As Watzlawick et al. (1974) pointed out, there is no therapeutic advantage in the typically held view that low sexual desire in women is evidence of a withholding, hostile attitude toward the male partner. This belief encourages rather than discourages feelings of helplessness and resentment in both partners and ignores the interactive nature of this problem. As in the case cited earlier of the woman who tried to will a state of arousal to protect her husband, problems of this sort generally originate from one or both partners' desires to prevent trouble, not create it. When such efforts fail, hurt and doubt on both sides can often be dealt with effectively by reframing the woman's sexual difficulty as an artifact of her admirable, though misguided, attempt to spare her husband's feelings. Viewed like this, the problem ceases to be defined as one of an angry wife's acting punitively toward her spouse. She can now, in fact, be praised for her sensitivity and caring and told that, while these qualities may have contributed to the development of her problem, they also lie at the heart of resolving it.

Then the practitioner can present a new solution to the patient's dilemma. He or she can tell the wife that it will be temporarily impossible for her to satisfy her husband sexually, because erotic feelings cannot be forced and always take a long time to reappear. As an intermediate step, however, she can begin to work on the problem by transferring the energy she had spent on worrying about her husband's sexual needs to helping him feel special and cared for in nonsexual ways. Might she prepare a delicious meal for him this week and give him a warm, tender smile when he comes home? With simple prompting, the woman will usually be able to offer her own ideas as she, of course, is the expert on her husband.

With the situation framed in this manner, women will often agree with these suggestions and begin acting on them immediately after the first session. The predictable result is an improved attitude by the husband, less urgency to pursue his wife, and a more romantic, sensitive approach when he does make sexual overtures. In a relatively short time, the increased affection and intimacy between the two will often lead to spontaneous resumption of the wife's sexual appetite.

But rarely can long-standing cases of low sexual desire be treated so rapidly. The identified patient is often unable or unwilling to consider this plan because of fear that the partner will misinterpret any kindness as a sexual invitation. A strong negative reaction to the above intervention usually indicates that the sexual problem serves an important function in maintaining the couple's relationship. In such cases, it is wise to consider referral for sex or marital therapy.

In a type of intervention we call *medical reframing*, a physical symptom with clear psychologic origins—in this case, a sexual dysfunction—is described to the patient as possibly having an organic cause. The purpose of relabeling a psychologic problem as physiologic in nature is to give the patient a definition of the problem that places it out of his or her conscious control. This has several treatment advantages. First, the individual is blocked in further use of "be spontaneous" measures to force symptom resolution, since the problem is now defined as one that is not responsive to such efforts. Second, the patient is more likely to cooperate with a prescribed course of treatment when the problem is placed in a traditional medical framework. Obviously, this technique is most appropriate and effective for patients who have defined their problem accurately as psychological but who have, as a result, compulsively employed a set of self-defeating solutions.

After giving the problem a medical frame, the physician can redirect the patient's attention and energies from trying to achieve sexual perfection to following "doctor's orders." A typical prescription would include instructions to avoid unnecessary stress (such as that associated with coitus and orgasm), to obtain regular relaxation on a daily basis, and to follow a carefully outlined diet. Directions for a nongenital sensate focus exercise can be offered as an alternative form of physical contact during this phase of treatment. Presented in this manner, many patients will readily accept their physician's advice and will report unexpected improvement of the sexual problem in several weeks.

Finkle (1978) gave an example of medical reframing. In counseling older men who complain of erectile dysfunction, he begins with an assessment designed to rule out neurovascular urologic defects, then examines the patient's prostate gland. He wrote:

> Rectal examination may identify prostate enlargement or boggy texture of a chronically congested gland due to unrelieved sexual needs. Urinalysis may show a few leukocytes. The expressed prostatic secretion will probably contain several or many leukocytes. Chronic congestive prostatitis, an organic disorder, is mentioned to the patient when the findings are explained at the end of the interview. Specifically, he is told that a physical condition, beyond his control, has been found by the doctor. Prostatitis is explained to the patient as being involved in, rather than being the sole cause of his sexual difficulty. As a therapeutic ploy to relieve him of the psychologic onus of "having it all in his head," a program of treatment is prescribed for the congestive prostatitis. . . . A drug such as methenamine mandelate is prescribed to remind him, as he takes the pill four times daily, that treatment has begun "to help soothe the irritated gland." For the same soothing effect, he is to drink at least one glass of water every two hours throughout the day, and to abstain from sexual activity, alcohol and spicy foods for the next seven days. (p. 457)

Finkle explains to the patient the multicausal nature of sexual problems and cites the role of performance fears in perpetuating and escalating the patient's difficulties. To underscore the point, Finkle tells a brief story that illustrates how striking out at bat in one inning may lead to similar results in the next. Finally, he reminds the patient to not attempt intercourse "to rest the gland." In another kind of reframe, he compares the prostate problem to a sprained wrist. If the patient's wrist had been injured, the physician would be able to apply a cast to immobilize the joint until it heals. As splinting a gland is impossible, the patient must create the same effect by following the aforementioned instructions. Finkle concludes with suggestions for several 15-minute follow-up visits, and he reports that most patients improve by the third visit.

Medical reframing may well be most useful with older adults who are accustomed to and likely to expect a medical-model approach. We adapted Finkle's method successfully in treating a patient in his mid-sixties who had made little progress in many months of sex therapy. All that eventually proved necessary was to prescribe a two-week abstention from all sexual relations because of the patient's "need to physically rest his penis." Given this medical-sounding framework, the patient was able to cease his coercive efforts and regained erectile function.

Medical reframing is most effective for treating minor, uncomplicated sexual difficulties. A careful history should always prevent the application of techniques recommended by the patients' former practitioners. Too often sex therapists encounter patients who have put off needed psychotherapeutic help for a long time because they hoped that their sexual problem had an organic cause. Medical reframing should be avoided with such patients to prevent unnecessary prolongation of their sexual difficulties.

Years of experience in applying the techniques described above lead us to the following observations. Prohibiting and restraining techniques seem to yield most dramatic results when applied to performance complaints in men, that is, problems with erection and ejaculation. The same techniques in treating similar problems in women, those concerning orgasm and arousal, have yielded more variable results. The female sexual response is so closely tied to the woman's emotional state that treatment of women seems to go better when the focus is on relationship factors. That is why reframing techniques, especially those that seek to emphasize and enhance the positive qualities in a couple's relationship, may prove most useful to physicians working with female patients.

When to Refer a Patient

The traditional indicators for referring a patient for psychiatric or sexual counseling are many and varied. Kaplan (1975) indicated that such factors as significant medical illness, use of narcotics, alcoholism, and major active psychopathologies (e.g., paranoia, depression, thought disorders) suggest that professional mental health expertise is needed. Witkin (1977) suggested that brief sexual counseling techniques may not be sufficient to produce change in partners who lack caring and cooperation.

Physicians can, however, be effective "change agents" in helping individuals improve their sexual relationships (Group for the Advancement of Psychiatry, 1974). The brief office counseling strategies described in this chapter can in most instances influence a couple's relationship significantly and positively. After all, Masters, Johnson, and Kolodny (1982) continue to emphasize that accurate sex education and information, opportunities to lessen fears and to practice sexual activities, and supportive professional help are the major ingredients in improved sexual functioning. This is true for many problems physicians encounter in their practices. Indeed, much evidence has shown that short-term, intensive counseling approaches can produce significant and lasting change (Chesney, Blakeney, Chan, & Cole, 1981; Kinder & Blakeney, 1977).

We have found that six to eight counseling sessions are sufficient in most cases to bring about measurable change and improvement in the patients' presenting problems. When symptoms do not change or the relationship seems to deteriorate (as shown by patients' failure to keep appointments, not carrying out assignments, the partners' increased tension or strain), physicians should refer the couples to a professional sex and family therapist. From a systemic viewpoint, these conditions suggest that the presenting sexual problem may serve to maintain homeostasis in the overall relationship.

Physicians wishing to locate an appropriate specialist may contact the American Association of Sex Educators, Counselors, and Therapists (AASECT) or the American Association for Marriage and Family Therapy (AAMFT) in Washington, DC. Both organizations publish directories of qualified professionals practicing throughout the country. The same information for specific communities is available from departments of urology, obstetrics and gynecology, and psychiatry in major medical centers.

Referring a patient for sex or family therapy requires the same time and effort as recommending surgical or other specialized treatment to a patient. The physician should contact the specialist to discuss how best to initiate and accomplish the referral. To a couple the physician should indicate that, although progress has been made in addressing their problem, a professional sex and family therapist can help them achieve even better results. This kind of approach, which emphasizes a couple's strengths and assets, will go a long way toward keeping them from assuming that their difficulties are permanent and too difficult to change.

REFERENCES

Burnap, D.W., & Golden, J.S. (1967). Sexual problems in medical practice. *Journal of Medical Education, 42*, 673-680.

Chesney, A., Blakeney, P., Chan, F., & Cole, C. (1981). The impact of sex therapy on sexual behaviors and marital communications. *Journal of Sex and Marital Therapy, 7*(1), 70-79.

Cole, C.M. (1983). Sexual disorders and the family therapist. In J.C. Hansen, J. Woody, & R. Woody (Eds.), *Sexual issues in family therapy*. Rockville, MD: Aspen Systems Corporation.

Crooks, R., & Baur, K. (1983). *Our sexuality* (2nd ed.). Menlo Park, CA: Benjamin-Cummings.

Erickson, M.H., & Rossi, E.L. (1979). *Hypnotherapy: An exploratory casebook*. New York: Irvington.

Finkle, A.L. (1978). Genitourinary disorders of old age: Therapeutic considerations including counseling for sexual dysfunction. *Journal of the American Geriatrics Society, 26*(10), 453-458.

Fisch, R., Weakland, J.H., & Segal, L. (1982). *The tactics of change*. San Francisco: Jossey-Bass.

Fisch, R., Weakland, J.H., Watzlawick, P., Segal, L., Hoebel, F.C., & Deardorff, C.M. (1975). *Learning brief therapy: An introductory manual*. Palo Alto, CA: Mental Research Institute.

Frank, E., Anderson, C., & Rubinstein, D. (1978). Frequency of sexual dysfunction in "normal couples." *New England Journal of Medicine, 299* (3), 111-115.

Friday, N. (1973). *My secret garden: Women's sexual fantasies*. New York: Trident Press.

Green, R. (Ed.). (1979). *Human sexuality: A health practitioner's text*. Baltimore: Williams & Wilkins.

Group for the Advancement of Psychiatry (1974). *Assessment of sexual function: A guide to interviewing*. New York: Jason Aronson.

Haley, J. (1973). *Uncommon therapy: The psychiatric techniques of Milton H. Erickson*. New York: Ballantine.

Haley, J. (1976). *Problem-solving therapy*. San Francisco: Jossey-Bass.

Kaplan, H.S. (1974). *The new sex therapy*. New York: Brunner/Mazel.

Kaplan, H.S. (1975). *The illustrated manual of sex therapy*. New York: Times Books.

Kinder, B., & Blakeney, P. (1977). Treatment of sexual dysfunction: A review of outcome studies. *Journal of Clinical Psychology, 33*, 523-30.

Kinsey, A.C., Pomeroy, W.B., & Martin, C.E. (1948). *Sexual behavior in the human male*. Philadelphia: Saunders.

Kinsey, A.C., Pomeroy, W.B., Martin, C.E., & Gebhard, P.H. (1953). *Sexual behavior in the human female*. Philadelphia: Saunders.

Kolodny, R.C., Masters, W.H., & Johnson, V.E. (1979). *Textbook of sexual medicine*. Boston: Little, Brown.

Leif, H.I. (1978). Sex education in medicine: Retrospect and prospect. In N. Rosenzweig & F.P. Pearsall (Eds.), *Sex education for the health professional: A curriculum guide* (pp. 23-26). New York: Grune & Stratton.

Masters, W.H., & Johnson, V.E. (1970). *Human sexual inadequacy*. Boston: Little, Brown.

Masters, W.H., Johnson, V.E., & Kolodny, R.C. (1982). *Human sexuality*. Boston: Little, Brown.

McCarthy, B.W. (1977). *What you still don't know about male sexuality*. New York: Crowell.

McCarthy, B.W., Ryan, M., & Johnson, F. (1975). *Sexual awareness: A practical approach*. San Francisco: Boyd & Fraser.

Munjack, D.J., & Oziel, L.J. (1980). *Sexual medicine and counseling in office practice: A complete treatment guide*. Boston: Little, Brown.

Papp, P. (1983). Comment on "interminable sex therapy." *Journal of Marital and Family Therapy, 9*(1), 11-13.

Penn, P. (1982). Multigenerational issues in strategic therapy of sexual problems. *Journal of Strategic and Systemic Therapies*. *1*(3), 1-13.

Perry, J.A. (1980). Commentary on: Bravesen, R.G., How do you get patients to talk about sexual problems? *Medical Aspects of Human Sexuality, 14*(11), 64.

Schover, L.R. (1982). Enhancing sexual intimacy. In P. Keller & L. Ritt (Eds.), *Innovations in clinical practice*, Vol. 1. Sarasota, FL: Professional Resource Associates.

Sharpe, L., & Levay, A.N. (1980). The sexual history: Part 2. *Sexual Medicine Today, 4*(11), 18-23.

Slag, M.F., Morley, J.E., Elson, M.K., Trence, D.L., Nelson, C.J., Nelson, A.E., Kinlaw, W.B., Beyer, H.S., Nuttall, F.Q., & Shafer, R.B. (1983). Impotence in medical clinic outpatients. *Journal of the American Medical Association, 249*(13), 1736-1740.

Steege, J.F. (1981). Female factors which contribute to premature ejaculation. *Medical Aspects of Human Sexuality, 15*(1), 73-74.

Storm, C.L. (1982). Sexual problems: An opportunity to work strategically. *Journal of Strategic and Systemic Therapies, 1*(3), 14-23.

Stuart, R.B. (1980). *Helping couples to change: A social learning approach to marital therapy*. New York: Guilford Press.

Tennen, H. (1977). Perspectives on paradox: Applications and explanations. In M. Rohrbaugh (Chair), *Paradoxical strategies in psychotherapy*. Symposium of American Psychological Association, San Francisco.

Watzlawick, P., Weakland, J. H., & Fisch, R. (1974). *Change: Principles of problem formation and problem resolution*. New York: W.W. Norton.

Weeks, G.R., & L'Abate, L. (1982). *Paradoxical psychotherapy: Theory and practice with individuals, couples, and families*. New York: Brunner/Mazel.

Witkin, M. (1977). Sex therapy as an aid to marital and family therapy. *Journal of Sex and Marital Therapy, 3*(1), 19-30.

APPENDIX: BIBLIOGRAPHY FOR PATIENTS

Barbach, L. (1976). *For yourself: The fulfillment of female sexuality—A guide to orgasmic release*. Garden City: Doubleday.

Barbach, L. (1982). *For each other: Sharing sexual intimacy*. New York: Anchor Press/Doubleday.

Bing, E., & Coleman, L. (1977). *Making love during pregnancy*. New York: Bantam.

Broderick, C. (1979). *Couples: How to confront problems and maintain loving relationships*. New York: Simon & Schuster.

Butler, R., & Lewis, M. (1976). *Sex after sixty*. New York: Perennial Library Harper Row.

Castleman, M. (1980). *Sexual solutions*. New York: Simon & Schuster.

Friday, N. (1973). *My secret garden: Womens' sexual fantasies*. New York: Trident Press.

Kaplan, H. (1975). *The illustrated manual of sex therapy*. New York: Times Books.

McCarthy, B., Ryan, M., & Johnson, F. (1975). *Sexual awareness: A practical approach*. San Francisco: Boyd & Fraser.

Scheingold, L., & Wagner, N. (1974). *Sound sex and the aging heart*. New York: Human Sciences Press.

Zilbergeld, B. (1978). *Male sexuality: A guide to sexual fulfillment*. Boston: Little, Brown.

14

FAMILY INTERVENTION IN THE PSYCHOSES: THE ROLE OF THE FAMILY PHYSICIAN

WILLIAM R. McFARLANE, M.D. and C. CHRISTIAN BEELS, M.D., M.S.

Psychosis and the Family Practitioner's Dilemma

When facing patients who have a major psychiatric disorder, family practitioners often find themselves in the midst of a disconcerting contradiction. Like the patients' clergy, attorneys, employers, friends, and families, they are being implicitly asked for help. They know that the most appropriate help is psychiatric treatment, but they may also sense that to suggest such help may mobilize a nascent tendency to refuse that treatment outright. In the most emotionally charged situations (for example, in the case of a paranoid person), the dilemma can be agonizing for those in the patient's immediate social network, including the family physician. The risks of referral and nonreferral seem almost equal. Most family physicians have been through this experience and found many potential solutions unsatisfactory or even counterproductive.

Families and patients have reasons for resisting psychiatric treatment, some of which we discuss. They include social stigma, guilt, mystification and fear of incarceration—fear, in short, of entering a humiliating social status. Education, empathic understanding, and a good referral from the person first consulted—often the family physician—are important steps to overcoming the problem of a psychosis. The main purpose of this chapter is, therefore, to guide the doctor in providing those essential services.

Earlier theories about the etiology of the psychoses, especially schizophrenia, seem to have contributed to families' resistance to treatment. Although Freud's conception that the psychoses are predominantly neurophysiologic disorders is now shared by most contemporary researchers, psychoanalytic and family-dynamic concepts gained wide popular circulation and acceptance during the 1945 to 1975 period. One implication of these ideas is that the families, and especially the mothers, of psychotic patients may be viewed, or even view themselves, as the cause of the condition. Given the catastrophic nature of these disorders, it is small wonder that many patients and their families will initially seek help from nonpsychiatric physicians in an attempt to avoid the implicitly accusatory message that has been inherent in psychiatric diagnosis and treatment. The family would like to hear a medical or neurologic diagnosis, if only to know that they did not cause the patient's extreme distress. Thus, one aspect of the dilemma arises from a discrepancy between popular and scientific understanding of the disorders themselves.

Later in the chapter we will describe several new treatments for schizophrenia, mania, and major depression. These therapies, if applied competently and comprehensively, have at least the degree of efficacy physicians have come to expect from treatment of many chronic medical illnesses. Under optimal conditions, it now seems possible in many cases to arrest an acute episode, prevent major deterioration in functioning, and reestablish a large measure of normal existence. The hitch is that these treatments are complex, time-consuming, somewhat challenging personally, require the contributions of several disciplines, and are best carried out by a team of well-trained clinicians. In other words, these new approaches are not well-suited to the constraints of the individual family physician's office practice. Thus, at present, it is even more imperative than before that the patient and his or her family reach a competent but specialized clinical service.

The notion that family physicians may not be the best long-term therapists for psychotic patients may seem overly pessimistic, but it is rooted in recent views of the social processes that tend to accompany the psychoses. Unlike minor psychiatric conditions, these disorders induce massive disorganization in patients' lives and their social networks. From a systems point of view, schizophrenia *is*, basically, disorganization at the neurophysiological, psychological, family, and social-network levels. That disorganization often leads to several deficiencies: of information, of the capacity to handle stress, of the personal resources to provide the necessary support, and of the ability to find more adaptive responses to the situation. The same is more or less true of major affective disorders. Our view is that treatment of psychotic patients requires a set of widely differing skills that one psychiatrist rarely possesses. Solo treatment, even the most skilled, has great disadvantages. A team of therapists can create much more support simply in terms of shared problem-solving effort. The family physician is not only at a technical disadvantage, but at a numerical disadvantage as well.

Nevertheless, the family practitioner is likely to have the initial contact with many psychotic patients simply because so many of them live in the community. Given the widespread inadequacies in treatment services for deinstitutionalized or never-institutionalized mental patients, these patients tend to have more medical problems that have gone untreated for a long time period, and they may not be able or inclined to find their way to or through the often fragmented system of psychiatric services. Instead, they seek help in a nonpsychiatric setting. The previously institutionalized patients may be avoiding psychiatric clinics for fear of being rehospitalized, given the negative associations of several years or even decades of hospital life. Finally, like their nonpsychotic peers, many patients may see the family doctor as a benign, fatherly, or even magical figure, who is not likely to punish them with involuntary commitment.

The contemporary family practitioner, then, exists at the confluence of several seemingly contradictory trends: the often unsuccessful attempts at deinstitutionalization; the continued stigmatization associated with psychosis; a widespread acceptance of a family-blaming psychodynamic notion about the cause of these conditions; the massive disorganization attendant on a long-standing mental disorder; and the emergence of newer, more effective, but more complex treatments that usually require an organization of specialized personnel for their implementation. The outcome of all of these phenomena is a tendency for the psychotic person and his or her family to appear in the family practitioner's office and to avoid a referral, while, at present, they will be much more likely to benefit from referral to a multidisciplined psychiatric service.

What follows is a review of the family processes that tend to accompany schizophrenia, so that physicians may know what to expect when meeting with patients' families, and some suggestions of preferable means of talking to families about the illness and treatment options, to expedite a successful referral. Note that involving the patient's family is taken for granted, because we believe that successful treatment will involve the family and it is likely that referral will be successful only if the family assists in the process. Clearly, if services are lacking or referral is steadfastly refused by all concerned, the practitioner's problem will be confounded. In the section on guidelines for management by the family physician we shall give some guidelines for situations in which family physicians may be forced to manage a case themselves.

Contemporary Concepts of Schizophrenia

During the past decade new concepts of the nature of the psychotic mental disorders have emerged, concepts that are at once more specific and more comprehensive than those that preceded them. These models have come from basic research and from insights gained from clinical experience with new drug and social therapies. Although the basic pathophysiology of these disorders and the psychosocial contributions to their causes and course are still imperfectly understood, it seems possible now to describe with some confidence a general paradigm that is congruent with the more reliable findings and observations. In simplest form, this concept is a psychosomatic model, in which biologic factors are seen as the prerequisite for the development of the syndrome, but in which some social and interactional processes mediate both initial onset and long-term course. Thus, there is reciprocity (positive feedback) between brain function and various, often quite specific, processes in the social environment. The relative power of the brain dysfunction and psychosocial influences may vary considerably among affected individuals and in a given individual may vary over time. In broad outline, such a concept bears striking resemblance to the evolving view of coronary artery disease and diabetes, whose apparent determinants are interacting genetic, physiological, dietary, psychological stress, and social factors. (See Sergio Henao's discussion of the biopsychosocial medical model in Chapter 2.)

In this section, we will pay special attention to the family, which is the most significant part of the social environment for the majority of patients with a major psychiatric disorder. We will also describe the present understanding of the pertinent biological and psychological processes. These latter aspects are emphasized here, because an accurate picture of contemporary research findings is one of the major underpinnings of an effective and empathic approach to patients and their families. To be aware, for instance, that most psychotic disorders, especially the chronic forms, are now seen as having primarily biologic origins casts a rather different light on the nature of family interaction, both past and present. We believe that, on the basis of little evidence, the family has for too long been considered a major etiologic factor in the psychotic illnesses, and that this bias has had severely negative effects on family morale and coping capacity. By simply communicating to the family that the patient is as truly ill as patients with more clear-cut medical conditions and by explaining some of the basic physiology of psychotic illnesses, the family physician can provide a major service to all concerned, even if the patient is referred ultimately to a psychiatric service or clinician. As will be seen in the section on family intervention, the more effective family therapies involve just this kind of basic education.

A. Diagnostic Criteria

Schizophrenia, a disastrous illness that has been the subject of both endless theorizing and clinical despair has recently been more rigorously defined by the *Diagnostic and Statistical Manual of Mental Disorders, Third Edition (DSM-III)* of the American Psychiatric Association. To be sure of the diagnosis, the patient must exhibit at least one of the following symptoms:

- Bizarre delusions
- Somatic, grandiose, religious, nihilistic, other delusions without persecutory or jealous content
- Delusions with persecutory or jealous content if accompanied by hallucinations of any type
- Auditory hallucinations with a running commentary on the individual's thoughts or two or more voices conversing with each other
- Auditory hallucinations with content of more than two words having no relation to depression or elation
- Incoherence or other marked thought disorder if associated with one of the following:
    - blunted, flat, or inappropriate affect
    - delusions or hallucinations
    - catatonic or other grossly disorganized behavior*

Other criteria are: deterioration from a previous level of functioning and continuous duration of the illness for at least six months.

These criteria specifically exclude the multitude of brief atypical psychoses that either do not recur or, if they do, are not accompanied by a major loss of social or vocational functioning.

Of equal importance is the exclusion of patients with affective or mood alterations (mania or depression) that *precede* the onset of schizophrenic symptoms and/or with a strong affective component in their initial presentation, in spite of their "schizophrenic" symptoms. These patients are now seen as having a major affective disorder, a view that has profound therapeutic and prognostic implications. Beyond strict diagnostic criteria, the so-called negative or deficit symptoms—apathy, social withdrawal, flat affect, lack of initiative, limited tolerance for pressure or stimulation, and specific attentional deficits—have come to be seen as both more reliable secondary criteria and as perhaps the core of the illness as a life-long incapacitation.

Research Perspectives

Brain dysfunction. Basic research has been focused on a number of areas, but two seem especially promising (for a recent review see Wyatt et al.,

---

*Adapted from American Psychiatric Association *Diagnostic and Statistical Manual of Mental Disorders* (Third Edition). Washington, D.C., American Psychiatric Association, 1980. Used with permission.

1982). The first involves advanced brain scanning and other neuropathological methods to elucidate subtle but significant alterations in neural activity in schizophrenic patients. For instance, computerized EEG studies have found major differences in levels of neural activity between patients and controls (Morihasa, Duffy, & Wyatt, 1983). CAT-scanning has disclosed a large subgroup of patients who have enlarged brain ventricles and widened sulci, which suggests cortical atrophy or underdevelopment (Rieder, Donnelly, Herdt, & Waldman, 1979). Rigorous pathological examinations have disclosed that, at autopsy, many patients have areas of chronic inflammation and gliosis near the base of the temporal lobes and in perilimbic areas, suggestive of old infectious or autoimmune processes (Stevens, 1982). Thus, the use of more sensitive methods seems to demonstrate a range of abnormalities in the cortical areas most involved in attention, abstract thought, foresight, initiative, and cerebral integration of thought and emotion.

The other fruitful research area involves the role of synaptic transmission. The effectiveness against psychosis of neuroleptic medications correlates with these agents' dopamine blocking capacities. This suggests that dopamine plays a major role in at least the acute phase of the illness. The prevailing wisdom is that hyperactivity in dopaminergic tracts, especially those linking limbic, hypothalamic, and frontal cortical areas, plays a central role in mediating the positive symptoms of agitation, confusion, hallucinations, and perhaps delusions (Wyatt et al., 1982). Other neurotransmitters, primarily serotonin and norepinephrine, seem to be implicated as well, but in ways that are far from clear.

An aspect that has received much recent attention is the variability of the course of schizophrenia. Long-term retrospective study of patients, particularly in Europe, has suggested that as many as one-half of them have "good" or "moderate" courses, with recovery of minimal capacities for independent living by middle age. American experience with well-designed and -implemented rehabilitation programs has demonstrated that optimal treatment can materially affect long-term outcome in many, if not the majority, of patients.

At the psychological level, the data point to deficits in the schizophrenic patients' ability to maintain and control their focus of attention and to regulate arousal of central and autonomic nervous systems (Venables, 1978). These problems seem to be related: Poor attentional focusing leaves the patient susceptible to being flooded by external and internal stimuli, producing excessive arousal, which in turn seems to interfere further with concentration and cognitive tracking. The psychological effect of phenothiazines is to enhance attentional capacities (Corbett, 1976): Many schizophrenics describe the therapeutic effects as feeling their "heads clear" or their "thoughts slow down." The attention-arousal model is the centerpiece of recent educational efforts to help families and patients understand the condition by which they are all so much affected.

Thus, a cursory survey of recent developments in physiological, pathological, and psychological research provides a more precise and yet multivariate concept of schizophrenia as a set of diseases with differing etiologies but certain final-common-pathway psychological effects that occur in the acute phases of several or all of them. This model is reminiscent, of course, of new knowledge concerning mental retardation, in which a supposed unitary syndrome has turned out to consist of perhaps a hundred different diseases. Schizophrenia is probably even more complex, in that environmental factors seem to play a major role in determining at least the course if not incidence. One recent study underlines the complexity. Sedvall and Wode-Helgrodt (1980) measured cerebrospinal fluid levels of dopamine and serotonin metabolites. Abnormalities correlated significantly with a family history of schizophrenia, but the finding held equally for patients and controls, suggesting that genetically determined abnormal neurotransmitter metabolism is not, independently, a sufficient cause to bring on a clinical syndrome.

Family Interaction

As is true of our biological knowledge, our understanding of family processes in the schizophrenic disorders is incomplete but developing. Significant progress has been made in distinguishing social processes that seem to exacerbate or protect against morbidity. It has become clear that, with the partial exception of oddities of parental communication, none of the family factors of interest are either specific to the syndrome (therefore, present in all affected families) or independent etiological factors. It does seem, however, that when present in excess and in combination certain family factors have a strong bearing on the short-term course and possibly onset of the illness. We have emphasized four discrete, interacting factors.

Stigma and burden. Many families seem to experience shame and a sense of stigma when one of their members develops schizophrenia or an affective disorder, although in the latter the family's feelings seem to be not as strong. In part, this reflects the general society's attitude: Even recent surveys show a persistent negative attitude towards the mentally ill. The growing evidence that patients are the victims of neurochemical disorders not of their own making seems to have had no discernible effect on stigma. Recent attempted and successful assassinations by deranged individuals and the clamor to eliminate the insanity defense seem to have turned public opinion more solidly against mental patients.

Most families have not reported *feeling* stigmatized, although the variation in research samples has been wide. Nevertheless, loss of friends and decreased contact with relatives after first episodes have been reported. Further, many families attempt to conceal the fact of their offspring's condition from friends and even relatives. Thus, there is a contradiction in the literature: Family members tend not to confirm that they carry a sense of stigma, but their behavior and that of members of their social networks suggest that mutual avoidance and withdrawal seem to occur.

At the same time, families with patients living at home or nearby carry a large extra burden of responsibility, anxiety, confusion, and exasperation in response to the schizophrenic relative's inability to manage his or her own affairs. It is remarkable that so few patients are actually rejected or abandoned by their families. Common problems include disruption of daily routine, loss of sleep, extra expenses, tension secondary to the unpredictability of the patient, strained family and marital relationships, and difficulties in communication. Parents often become partially enslaved by the process. Most families accept these extra burdens with remarkable grace, but the toll is often high in terms of their general health and quality of life.

The overall effect of stigma and burden is often demoralization and a sense of confused helplessness. The peculiar combination of effects of the illness on the family often leaves members with a sense that no one will be able or want to help them. The family physician is likely to have to address these feelings in the process of evaluating the situation and making a referral. It is not unusual for family members to present exacerbations of chronic medical conditions, which they may relate to stress induced by their schizophrenic relative. Families need to know that help is available, that most families experience these reactions, and that avoiding treatment will only amplify their problems. It should also be remembered that these reactions may well be translated into blame and anger directed at the patient. Such a tense atmosphere, as we will discuss in the section on expressed emotion, will, in turn, have serious negative effects on the patient. The need for intervention, then, is not related solely to providing family support but to preventing further exacerbations of the patient's psychosis.

Communication deviance. A highly specific but circumscribed family phenomenon, termed communication deviance (CD), was originally reported by Singer and Wynne (1965). (For a thorough review see Singer, Wynne, & Toohey, 1978.) The observations are that most parents of schizophrenics communicate with each other in ways that are more subtly amorphous or fragmented than normal, creating a communication style that is similar to the thought disorder that is a core symptom of schizophrenia. The relatives often use odd, ambiguous, idiosyncratic language in which the focus of attention tends to drift, rather like tangentiality. It has been speculated that this process serves a psycho- or family-dynamic function (e.g., to avoid conflict), but the possibility remains that it is a subclinical expression of a common underlying heritable disorder. There is some reason to think communication deviance may be of etiologic significance, since in prospective studies of psychosis (Doane, West, Goldstein, Rodnick, & Jones, 1981), CD in families precedes overt symptoms in the patient in a small but significant number of cases.

Many other forms of communication difficulty can be found in families with a disturbed member, but they may be as much a result as a cause of the problem. They include compulsive blaming and criticism, double messaging, speaking for others, failing to listen, and interrupting. Although these communication problems do not appear to be specific to the psychoses, they clearly predispose to confusion, poor task performance, and high levels of emotional reactivity, all of which will tend to aggravate a psychotic disorder.

Family physicians should not be surprised, therefore, if the family members of schizophrenic patients are difficult to understand. Nevertheless, recent experience with multiple family (McFarlane, 1983a) and behavioral family therapies (Falloon & Liberman, 1983) suggests that significant improvement can be induced in both specific and general forms of communication problems. Interviewing families with these difficulties requires patience and gentle but firm reminders about staying on the topic. In severe instances, physicians may find that they have to structure the conversation, to maintain a focus. Perhaps the simplest but most effective technique is to assure that everyone, patient included, has a chance to be heard for his or her perspective on important issues, without being interrupted by "helpful" relatives. This strategy often has surprising beneficial effects, while it expresses the interviewer's confidence that each family member is competent and has a significant role to play in understanding and ameliorating the overall situation.

Family isolation. Deficiencies in the family's social support systems are neither specific to the psychoses, nor are they always found in families of patients. A clinical cliché for many years was that the families of schizophrenics are socially isolated, but some research data now partially confirm that observation. While studying expressed emotion (see below), Brown and his colleagues (1972) noted that families showing the highest degree of criticism, hostility, and overinvolvement with the patient also were markedly cut off from social contact with friends and non-household relatives. Closer examination of their social networks revealed that: (a) patients whose relatives are known to their friends tend to have their networks survive the first hospitalization; (b) the social networks of schizophrenics are already smaller and more family-based at first admission; (c) the average size of those networks is about one-half of normal; (d) many network characteristics correlate with level of psychopathology; and (e) having a schizophrenic in the family seems to induce network contraction.

The assumption that having a smaller, family-based network is less adaptive depends on certain ideas about the function and value of those social connections. Especially in coping with a major mental illness, social networks seem to provide a number of crucial influences. These include emotional and instrumental support, access to other useful people who are not so intensely involved, access to more varied resources and information, and the imposition of helpful constraints and demands. While these supports are of objective benefit during an *acute* episode, families actually report feeling more needful of help in dealing with *chronicity* and its associated day-to-day exhaustion and anxiety.

Particularly since the advent of deinstitutionalization, schizophrenic patients have become much more dependent on their families. Thus, the family's lack of social supports has become especially critical, because, as has been proposed, many of the family's internal difficulties—including those that predispose patients to relapse—are a secondary effect of inadequate social support. These findings are the principal arguments for multiple family groups. Such an artificial social network makes it possible for clinicians to arrange for affected families to provide for each other what may be missing in an individual family.

This discussion implies that family physicians will need to take an inventory of those who might be available to the psychotic patient's family for support, guidance, relief, and sometimes financial assistance. Since family members may have cut themselves off from, or been rejected by, many members of their own networks secondary to the onset of the illness, some encouragement and persistence may be required in reestablishing the needed relationships. The objective is to establish many connections of low intensity and obligation to assure a continued variety of supports over the long run. It is often useful to meet with or interview by telephone those whom the family so identifies, both for information and to obtain commitments to bolster family members in ways that seem realistic and appropriate. Such moves may be necessary even if the goal is only a successful referral, because these more peripheral network members may help to overcome the family's reluctance or noncompliance during the transfer interval. In addition, many areas of the country now have well-organized self-help groups composed of families of the mentally ill; participation may be especially helpful as part of the long-term treatment plan. At the very least, such groups can guide the practitioner in compiling a list of available resources.

Enmeshment and expressed emotion. Curiously, the most solidly documented family factor in schizophrenia is also the *least* specific. This factor has been called "expressed emotion"—a high degree of criticism, hostility, and overinvolvement, directed towards the patient by a relative in close contact with him or her. It is associated with a much higher tendency to relapse (Brown, Birley, & Wing, 1972).

The effect is significant enough that many patients from *low* expressed emotion (low-EE) families not only have lower rates of relapse, but the patients seem not to require maintenance medication, except as protection from the effects of disruptive life events. It appears, then, that benignly indifferent families who also provide basic support and encouragement may actually be protecting their patient members against relapse. Given the growing evidence that tardive dyskinesia, a frequently irreversible side effect of neuroleptics, is related to total lifetime dose, it has become especially important to capitalize on that seemingly preventive potential in families. It is also noteworthy that the same sort of effect of EE on relapse has been found in depression.

Although many psychodynamic explanations have been proposed to account for the predominance of high-EE (70% of families with a schizophrenic member, in some studies), we find it more parsimonious and useful to suggest that these reactions are, at least in part, prompted by the very nature of chronic psychotic illnesses. On the one hand, the patient appears helpless and confused, leading to an overprotective stance and overattention from parents. On the other hand, psychotics, even in remission, are usually exasperating and often *appear* to be lazy, hostile, and even manipulative, provoking relatives' criticism and hostility. Further, it seems plausible that these reactions may be a displacement onto the patient of disappointment and resentment derived from experiences with the inadequate results of psychiatric treatment. The picture is complicated by the observation that in many families the overprotectiveness (or enmeshment at the family level) seems to predate the onset of the overt syndrome. The overall process, then, seems to consist of positive feedback interactions between family characteristics and the disorder itself, each amplifying the other.

Anderson, Hogarty, and Reiss (1980) elaborated the concept of reciprocal feedback by citing the abundant evidence that the core psychological deficits in schizophrenia are dysfunctions of attention and arousal. High levels of EE are seen as provoking physiologic arousal, which in turn leads to exacerbation of attentional deficits, provoking withdrawal and/or symptomatic relapse. Sturgeon, Kuipers, Berkowitz, Turpin, & Leff (1981) have actually measured autonomic arousal via galvanic skin conductance in the presence of key relatives. The entrance of a high-EE relative provoked gradually escalating galvanic skin-response fluctuation rates in the ill family member, while low-EE relatives elicited gradually decreasing rates. The authors concluded that *low*-EE relatives had a measurable *calming* effect on the patient, suggesting that optimal emotional responses by family members could actually be a deterrent to relapse.

Most of the new family therapy approaches that we will review in the section on major affective disorders have as a primary objective the reduction of family EE. Suffice it here to say that reducing the level of criticism and overinvolvement has become both feasible—through focused family intervention—and as effective in preventing relapse as would be predicted from the EE research.

Interactions of family factors. Some studies describe interactions between the four factors reviewed above. For better or worse, these interrelationships make the picture significantly more complicated.

Brown and his colleagues (1972) found that social isolation of the family unit correlated with the level of expressed emotion. Likewise, it seems that EE and deviant communication have a strong correlation and predate the onset of the disorder (Doane et al., 1981). Although it has been suggested that communication deviance and social isolation could be expected in the same family, no direct data support the contention so far. One can extrapolate the EE-isolation and EE-CD correlations, and speculate that isolation and CD would tend to coexist, at least statistically. As for stigma, there is some evidence that being stigmatized promotes family isolation.

We have proposed that, in the lives of schizophrenic patients and their families, these correlations translate into a pattern of reciprocal interaction, creating an evolving spiraling feedback process that results in clinical deterioration. Consider the following example. After an acute episode, as friends and extended family withdraw, the patient and the nuclear family spend more time together: Overinvolvement becomes almost inevitable with semi-enforced isolation. The patient's residual symptoms assume greater importance to family members, simply because they are less distracted by other relationships. As time passes, the increasing impatience of family members with these residua leads them to be more insistent on normal functioning, which is out of the patient's reach. They begin to be more critical, especially of deficit symptoms like oversleeping, withdrawal, lack of initiative and responsibility. As the level of tension rises, the patient's recovery becomes impeded by the extra attention and the burden of expectation and criticism. Tendencies towards idiosyncratic communication will be exacerbated by the tense atmosphere and the family's isolation on one hand, and the increasing severity of the patient's thought disorder on the other. The usual outcome of this process is likely to be a symptomatic relapse, at which time family or patient will seek the aid of the family practitioner, emergency room, or psychiatrist. The family one sees at that point may well be cut off from friends and helpful relatives, anxious and agitated, highly overinvolved with the patient, perhaps hostile towards him or her and somewhat difficult to understand.

Let us turn now to recent developments in family therapy for this disorder, because what has been learned provides a great deal of guidance in choosing interventions effective in reversing the kind of spiraling deteriorations described.

Family Intervention in Schizophrenia

Essential Elements of the New Approaches

Some innovative treatment programs have been developed over the past decade. Two-year follow-up data from clinical trials of these programs are positive and suggest that we have found ways of working with families and patients that may influence the course of the patients' recovery from psychotic episodes. The changes are in the direction of better social function, less frequent relapse, and decreased family burden. One characteristic common to these approaches is an attitude that identifies the family as a major source of strength for the patient during the recovery process and seeks to help the family capitalize on strengths and skills which contribute most to the patient's recovery.

We include here just enough of a description of the common elements of these programs so that physicians can talk with families about what to look for in a referral, and how education, treatment, and family life can work together. These elements may also serve as a rough guide for managing a case, should that become necessary. Guidelines for physicians on management are included at the end of this section.

The core elements to be described below are derived from the following clinical research programs:

1) Psychoeducational family therapy (Anderson, Hogarty, & Reiss, 1980)
2) Behavioral family therapy (Falloon & Liberman, 1983)

3) Relatives' groups (Leff, Berkowitz, & Kuipers, 1983)
4) Crisis-oriented family therapy (Kopeikin, Marshall, & Goldstein, 1983)
5) Multiple family therapy (McFarlane, 1983a)

Physicians interested in using the specific techniques associated with these therapies are strongly encouraged to review these reports (McFarlane, 1983b). These therapies provide a framework for approaching many major psychiatric, psychosomatic, and even some medical disorders, and are not limited to the schizophrenic disorders. They have as their goals the amelioration of the course of the illness, not its cure. Most aim towards reducing relapse frequency beyond that achievable with good pharmacologic management, and most specifically attempt to enhance the psychosocial functioning of the patient. The means to achieve these goals include a small group of seemingly essential, specific, and targeted interventions, designed either to compensate for identifiable deficits in the patient (e.g., tendencies towards hyperarousal or attentional deficits) or to reverse common iatrogenic, culture- or illness-induced phenomena in the family, especially criticism and overinvolvement.

Joining with family members. Most of these new approaches begin with efforts to join with family members empathically, validating their despair, fears, confusion, and exasperation while mobilizing their concern and energy for the ensuing rehabilitation effort. The objective is to create a strong, task-oriented organization of staff-family-patient. Issues of blame are openly discussed, with assurances given that there is little evidence to substantiate a parental responsibility for the illness; usually, family members are explicitly recruited as vital partners in the treatment.

Family education. Education of family members is the core of most of these therapies. Ranging from orientation to the seriousness of the acute psychotic episode to lectures on neurochemistry and the mechanism of action of neuroleptics, these educational programs attempt to demystify symptoms, clarify various aspects of the treatment process, and sensitize the family to the reality of the patient's subjective experience and to the validity of his or her postpsychotic inability to function. They teach family members what the positive or negative effects of their behavior are likely to be on the patient's overall condition and course. In most families this kind of information raises morale, relieves guilt, enhances cooperation, and elicits a true sympathy for the patient's predicament.

Interactional change. The family's acquisition of a clear concept of the basic phenomena of schizophrenia facilitates their acceptance of a few crucial family-interactional interventions. These have three, highly specific foci: recognizing prodromal signs and symptoms and taking early action to forestall relapse; reducing expressed emotion, especially criticism and overinvolvement; and correcting specific but symptom-reinforcing family communication and behavior patterns. These interventions are central to these therapies' capacities to prevent relapse, because they address directly the most common and well-documented sources of recidivism. Combined as they are with education, they have the quality of training rather than psychotherapy.

Family structural intervention. Perhaps nothing illustrates the differences between earlier and newer approaches more clearly than the way in which power in the family is felt to be best distributed. The new therapies strongly validate the relatives as co-therapists and caretakers, with the patient temporarily placed in a structurally subordinate and age-inappropriate position. This strategy is a matter of principle for Haley (1980) and Madanes (1981), who have developed a family therapy model based on achieving a proper hierarchy in the family between parents and young adult offspring. For the education-oriented therapies listed above, the principle is a matter of common sense and pragmatism, the natural result of an illness-based approach. In practical terms it means that the family needs to be in charge of the patient to implement the rest of the treatment package and to reduce organizational confusion and emotional intensity in the family environment. It also puts the family in a position to foster a gradual and controlled resumption of responsibility by the patient.

Multiple family meetings. Bringing affected families into contact with one another is an intervention whose value has been suggested by research on the role of social support in reducing morbidity (Beels, 1981) and by the apparent effectiveness of multiple family groups. Multiple family, relatives', and self-help groups all expand the availability, variety, and flexibility of social supports for participating families. Perhaps the primary rationale for fostering relationships between families is the time-tested value of banding together to cope with major chronic illnesses and traumatic events. This is particularly true in schizophrenia, in which it is likely that stigmatization will tend to drive families into isolation. Beyond providing social support and empathy, families also are quite adept at pointing out to each other obvious interactional problems and holding each other responsible for making the necessary corrections. For all these reasons, many of the new therapies include multi-family meetings as the preferred format for altering interaction, providing education or enhancing family socialization. In addition, they seem to be effective in their own right in reducing relapse, while being economical and enthusiastically accepted by families (McFarlane, 1983a). They seem to inevitably foster the staff-family-patient partnership that is central to all the new therapies.

Guidelines for Management by the Family Physician

If, in spite of our recommendation to the contrary, you find yourself unavoidably the responsible manager of a patient suffering an episode of psychosis, here are some suggestions on ways of proceeding.

The keys to managing such a patient are medication, education, and control over the environment. Your role as the physician fits admirably with these approaches. We will not discuss specific medications and dosages here, because excellent texts are available on that subject. "Rapid tranquilization" may be achieved with a high-potency phenothiazine such as haloperidol. In this technique, frequent, small doses are given until certain target symptoms, such as agitation, are affected. This approach may be used either to avoid hospitalization or to make management of the patient easier in hospital. Once symptoms are under control, maintenance antipsychotic medication is chosen according to patient acceptance, absence of side effects, and other factors that may be idiosyncratic to a particular patient.

If this is a patient's first episode of psychosis, bear in mind that 10-30% of first episodes do not recur, and many that are indistinguishable from schizophrenia thus have to be reclassified after a brief illness as atypical psychosis (Ciompi, 1980; Huber, Gross, Schuttler, & Linz, 1980). There is also the possibility that the affective symptoms may be overlooked in what appears to be a first experience of schizophrenia. This is particularly true if the attack is an irritable manic episode with loose associations, ideas of reference, and manic distractibility. Antipsychotic medications such as phenothiazines will help these symptoms, and the whole affair may be misdiagnosed as a schizophrenic episode. The alert diagnostician who notes the manic quality of some of the patient's symptoms and prescribes a trial of lithium (rather than phenothiazine maintenance) after the acute symptoms have subsided will serve the patient and family particularly well, as the prognosis for good interval function and general lack of deterioration is much better in this illness than in schizophrenia.

For all these reasons, diagnosis and prognosis in a first episode should be approached with caution. The general term "psychosis" is the best one to use, and we emphasize that it is extremely important to *have* a word to call this illness. Families and patients are especially prone to denial in a first episode. The educational approach at this time (modified somewhat from Goldstein's—see Kopeikin et al., 1983) is to schedule a definite number of meetings (six is recommended) with the family immediately before or after the patient's discharge from the hospital, or if hospitalization has been avoided, as soon as convenient at home.

The educational family meetings proceed with a definite four-step agenda

1. Something Serious Actually Happened

Help the family to recognize the reality of the experience and abate their very common and understandable tendency to denial. Introduce the word "psychosis" and whatever other descriptive terms seem to be helpful. This is a good time to review with patient and other family members their detailed experience of prodromal symptoms such as change in sleep pattern, unusual irritability, peculiar recurrent thoughts, and others. Emphasize that these symptoms can be used as early warning signs which, if noticed early by the patient or others, would make it possible to get an episode under control with medication before more distressing full-blown symptoms appear (Herz, Szymansk, & Simon, 1982). All this is in line with the general philosophy of helping the family to be knowledgeable, to put a positive sense of expertise in place of their feelings of fear and inadequacy.

2. Stress Played a Part in It

Review with the family the stresses and strains the patient or other family members were experiencing at the time of the episode. Types of stress that may have special importance in a psychotic episode are those that accompany a change of status in which the patient is risking his or her acceptance in a new social setting. Examples include getting a job, engagement, moving, any change in level of intimacy with someone of the opposite sex, going to college. Family dissension of all kinds, especially when some new role is directly or indirectly expected of the patient, is a source of stress, as is the feeling of family members that the patient is not living up to expectations.

3. These Stresses Could Occur Again, and So Could the Psychosis

Introduce the family to the idea of the patient's vulnerability to this kind of stress, and the importance of being alert to a recurrence.

4. If the Stresses Do Reappear, There Are Things the Family and the Patient Can Do About Them

Some lowering of expectations for the patient's competitive achievements should be considered, at least temporarily. The family should come to understand that it is not a great loss if the patient gets ahead somewhat more slowly in life than they had expected. In particular, the family should be helped to identify noxious sequences of behavior that cause the patient anxiety. After an acute episode, it is better to err on the side of low expectations. If up to a year goes by without trouble, the patient will very likely begin to make his or her own move toward initiative and activity again.

In second or later episodes, especially if six months or more have elapsed since the prodromata of the first, the diagnosis of schizophrenia should be entertained, although consultation with a psychiatrist to rule out affective disorder is still advisable. At this stage, the family and patient are beginning to contemplate the possibility that they face a lifelong, perhaps recurrent or deteriorating illness, and this possibility must be faced in as positive terms as are available. (Recall that there is evidence that 20-50% of patients diagnosed as schizophrenic return to good social function much later in life, often after many years of poor adjustment [Ciompi, 1980; Huber et al., 1980].)

A number of approaches combining medication, education, and environmental control have been described in the literature (Anderson et al., 1980; Falloon & Liberman, 1983). The first step is to educate the parents and other responsible people, and after them, the patient, on management of the illness. In spite of the patient's tendency to retreat and withdraw, large areas of his or her intelligence, humor, and original personality may remain intact or return in a somewhat attenuated form. The important thing is the management of daily life while awaiting the return, a year to two years from the present exacerbation, of a reliable movement towards the responsibilities of the outside world.

Begin by teaching the family that the patient has an impaired ability to selectively edit and shut out stimuli from the environment. At times, everything seems important, significant, to be attended to. Phenothiazines help patients with this editing and ordering problem by raising the threshold of certain synapses in the brain's limbic system. But the family, and changes in social and physical aspects of the environment, can alleviate this problem as well.

The family can help by providing a minimum of confusing or conflicting or ambiguous instruction on what to do, and a maximum of consistent social and physical cues on what is expected. That is on the cognitive side. On the emotional side, sympathy, interest, and encouragement combined with a certain dispassionate tranquility are needed.

The best way to accomplish these objectives (since it is hard consciously to change atmospheres or attitudes) is to concentrate on the minimum requirements of maintaining the household, especially those the parents need to keep their lives practical and satisfying. Least attention should be given to the patient's decorum, initiative, or appearance of having a correct attitude toward the future. Concentrate on practical tasks and routines, and encourage consistent, regular duties like cleaning or washing the dishes.

If you will be sharing your responsibility for the patient with another agency, and you have a choice of agencies, there are a number of things to look for. The service's staff members should be pragmatic, friendly, and interested in their work, willing to talk to and educate family, friends, and you, their medical consultant. They should be activity- and home-oriented (as opposed to expecting visits to be only in their office, by the patient alone). They should have the sort of lifelong perspective on chronicity and its dilemmas and suffering that we have described. You can identify these characteristics of a treatment organization only by visiting it and talking about cases with the staff. Do not rely on the reputation of the agency with local "experts"—see for yourself what the atmosphere of the place is like. Atmosphere is almost always more important than professional paper qualifications.

Major Affective Disorder

Research Perspectives

In shifting our attention from schizophrenia to major affective disorder, that is, bipolar manic-depressive disorder and unipolar depression, we see a different picture of social-biological interaction. Affective disorder is now considered to be primarily a metabolic disorder, specifically of the physiologic mechanisms that control mood and, probably, sleep-wake cycles. There is much less evidence that psychosocial factors contribute to manic relapse, while there is some such evidence for depression, but much controversy as well. It is safe to assume at present that manic and many depressive patients exhibit a pattern of cyclical relapse that is not determined by the vicissitudes or qualities of social relationships of life in general. Further, a growing body of research data and clinical experience suggests that lithium maintenance is remarkably protective against both manic and depressive relapse (far more so than neuroleptics in schizophrenia), and that the major psychosocial variable associated with relapse is the patient's choosing to discontinue medication and the family's inability to ensure compliance (Prien, Caffey, & Klett, 1973). Many, if not most, patients with bipolar illness are able to lead essentially normal lives, with adequate medication compliance, so that one should not assume that residual disability will persist, as it will for schizophrenic patients. The picture is not quite so sanguine for patients who have unipolar depression, but the range of outcome is much closer to that of bipolar illness than of schizophrenia. In many patients depressive relapses clearly are precipitated by uncontrollable and overwhelming life events, but the factors that separate cyclical from crisis-induced depressions are not clear at present.

The family picture in these disorders is also different. Most patients who have an affective disorder are older, independent, and many are married, so that one is less likely to be dealing with patients who still depend on their original families. Research and clinical observation of the marital relationships of bipolar patients suggest a wide range of variation—from patients being fully functional to markedly disturbed. Those in the latter group tend to present a distinct pattern. Their spouses seem to be quite fearful of and preoccupied with relapse; helpless in improving their marital relationship; committed to controlling affect and avoiding intimacy, largely by denial of hostility and anxiety; and preoccupied with feelings of early parental loss and/or deprivation (Ablon, Davenport, Gershon, & Adland, 1975).

Severely dysfunctional couples tend to assume a configuration of overfunctioning by the well spouse in a way that suggests an underlying investment in the continued underfunctioning of the depressed spouse. One sees excessive protectiveness, willingness to assume many, if not all, household, economic, and social responsibilities, reluctance to shift them back to the depressed partner as he or she recovers, and simmering but often overcontrolled resentment compensated for by a false cheerfulness. The result of this skewed alignment is that there is little incentive for the patient to improve and few areas in which to experience competence, which prevents the return of self-esteem. In severe cases, the well spouse may become depressed and dysfunctional upon the antidepressant-induced recovery of the unipolar patient.

Even in the absence of long-standing and severe marital problems, the marital relationship during or shortly after an acute manic or depressive episode will be temporarily quite disturbed. The well spouse of the manic patient is likely to be profoundly exasperated, even panicked by the patient's profligate behavior, angry, demanding, and irritable affect, and the cascade of social and economic consequences of the last episode. Mania may leave in its wake enormous debts and major disruptions of work, family, and peer relationships. The manic individual, even when recovered, rarely understands the lingering wrath and/or fear he or she has provoked in close friends, relatives, children, and spouses. The spouses of patients are as likely to be angry and resentful—given the almost total withdrawal of affection and support towards others that is a nearly universal consequence of a major depression—but they feel a great need to suppress these reactions because their ill spouse is so clearly despondent, helpless, and hypersensitive to criticism.

They feel abandoned, exploited, inadequate, lonely, guilty, and sexually rejected. Spouses of manic and depressive patients may complain of having gotten a "bad deal" by marrying the affectively ill patient, as most first episodes occur after the usual age of courtship and marriage. Those who knowingly marry a manic or depressive person may, consciously or not, have a caretaking role as part of their plan for married life; these marriages often assume the over- and underfunctional pattern noted above. The possibility of divorce often hangs over the case: previous separations and divorces are not uncommon. Because the patient rarely understands the basis for the spouse's postepisode irritability and unresponsiveness, the couple may continue to be out of phase after recovery, but with the roles reversed.

Therapeutic Intervention

As in the section on schizophrenia, we leave the important discussion of drug management of affective disorders to the many excellent texts on the subject. In terms of psychotherapeutic intervention, many of the core elements of the new therapies for schizophrenic patients will be highly effective in affective disorders, with specific modifications. We focus here on the management of couples with a healthy or only mildly conflictual relationship, because they may be treated by family practitioners after the patient is stabilized and asymptomatic on lithium or antidepressants.

The approach is really a variant of the sort of counseling one might do with any family in which a member has a chronic but manageable disease. The approach should include thorough education regarding the nature of the disorder; its course; methods of prevention of relapse; the action of medication and side effects; and extensive exploration of the patient's and spouse's feelings regarding the impact of the illness on each other. Of special importance is the framing of their reactions as "normal under the circumstances," thereby leaving as little basis as possible for protracted blame and guilt. Planning for the future should include: a) ready access to a psychiatrist for maintenance medication and clinical assessment (or consultation about these); b) agreement about continuing the medication as prescribed; c) patience in and commitment to reestablishing harmonious marital relations; and d) maintaining, enhancing, or repairing the social-network relationships that were there before onset of the last episode. Practical considerations for manic patients might include establishing a separate bank account for the spouse (to protect family resources in the event of a relapse) and including in the treatment plan a sympathetic co-worker or supervisor, at the patient's workplace, who can support the medication regimen, provide emotional support, and serve as an additional monitor of incipient symptoms of relapse.

Couples who have a more pathologic, symbiotic relationship will require intensive marital therapy—of no mean difficulty—as an adjunct to the patient's lithium maintenance. They will be best served by a psychiatrist especially competent in couples therapy. Considerable evidence shows couples *group* therapy is the preferable alternative, so that one factor in referral may be the availability of that modality (Davenport, Adland, Gold, & Goodwin, 1979). Patients who have major affective disorders and are still living at home with parents beyond the usual age of emancipation will probably be involved in the enmeshed processes described in the section on schizophrenia. They will be likely to require intensive intervention; we recommend psychiatric referral for these patients to a service that offers the package of interventions developed for these more severe cases.

Summary

Outcome evaluation of the new approaches to treating psychotic patients is only partially complete. As we have written elsewhere:

> Conclusive, longer-term results will not be available for a few years. . . . What does seem well supported is the general principle that the family of the mentally ill adult has an untapped therapeutic potential. This potential can be realized if family members are approached with the proper attitude and technique, and the probability is good that there will be an improvement in the course of the illness and that a more stable, knowledgeable, and resilient family will result in the long term. At this time, the results of these therapies are sufficiently positive that judicious application in clinical practice seems justified. Even incremental improvements of these disorders, if achieved economically, are worth the effort, given that a more definitive treatment still seems frustratingly beyond our grasp. (McFarlane, Beels, & Rosenheck, 1982, pp. 252-253)

REFERENCES

Ablon, S.L., Davenport, Y.B., Gershon, E.S., & Adland, M.L. (1975). The married manic. *American Journal of Orthopsychiatry*, *45*, 854-866.

Anderson, C.M., Hogarty, G., & Reiss, D.J. (1980). Family treatment of adult schizophrenic patients. *Schizophrenia Bulletin*, *6*, 490-505.

Beels, C.C. (1981). Social support and schizophrenia. *Schizophrenia Bulletin*, *7*, 58-72.

Brown, G.W., Birley, J.L.T., & Wing, J.K. (1972). Influence of family life on the course of schizophrenic disorders: A replication. *British Journal of Psychiatry*, *121*, 241-250.

Ciompi, L. (1980). Catamnestic long-term study on the course of life and aging of schizophrenics. *Schizophrenia Bulletin*, *6*, 606-618.

Corbett, L. (1976). Perceptual dyscontrol: A possible organizing principle for schizophrenic research. *Schizophrenia Bulletin, 2*, 249-265.

Davenport, Y.B., Adland, M.L., Gold, P.W., & Goodwin, F.K. (1979). Manic depressive illness: Psychodynamic features of multi-generational families. *American Journal of Orthopsychiatry, 49*, 24-35.

Doane, J., West, K.L., Goldstein, M.J., Rodnick, E.H., & Jones, J.E. (1981). Parental communication deviance and affective style. *Archives of General Psychiatry, 38*, 679-685.

Falloon, I.R.H., & Liberman, R.P. (1983). Behavioral family interventions in the management of chronic schizophrenia. In W.R. McFarlane (Ed.), *Family therapy in schizophrenia*. New York: Guilford Press.

Haley, J. (1980). *Leaving home*. New York: McGraw-Hill.

Herz, M.I., Szymansk, H.V., & Simon, J.C. (1982). Intermittent medication for stable schizophrenic outpatients—An alternative to maintenance medication. *American Journal of Psychiatry, 139*, 918-922.

Huber, G., Gross, G., Schuttler, R., & Linz, M. (1980). Longitudinal studies of schizophrenic patients. *Schizophrenia Bulletin, 6*, 592-605.

Kopeikin, H.S., Marshall, V., & Goldstein, M.J. (1983). Stages and impact of family crisis therapy in the aftercare of acute schizophrenia. In W.R. McFarlane (Ed.), *Family therapy in schizophrenia*. New York: Guilford Press.

Leff, J.P., Berkowitz, R., & Kuipers, L. (1983). Intervention in families of schizophrenics and its effects on relapse rate. In W.R. McFarlane (Ed.), *Family therapy in schizophrenia*. New York: Guilford Press.

Madanes, C. (1981). *Strategic family therapy*. San Francisco: Jossey-Bass.

McFarlane, W.R. (1983a). Multiple family therapy in schizophrenia. In W.R. McFarlane (Ed.), *Family therapy in schizophrenia*. New York: Guilford Press.

McFarlane, W.R. (Ed.). (1983b). *Family therapy in schizophrenia*. New York: Guilford Press.

McFarlane, W.R., Beels, C., & Rosenheck, S. (1982). New developments in the family treatment of the psychotic disorders. *Psychiatry Update, 2*, 242-262.

Morihasa, J.M., Duffy, E.H., & Wyatt, R.J. (1983). Brain electrical activity mapping (BEAM) in schizophrenic patients. *Archives of General Psychiatry, 40*, 719-728.

Prien, R.F., Caffey, E.M., & Klett, C.J. (1973). Prophylactic efficacy of lithium carbonate in manic-depressive illness. *Archives of General Psychiatry, 28*, 337-341.

Rieder, R.O., Donnelly, E.F., Herdt, J.R., & Waldman, I.N. (1979). Sulcal prominence in young chronic schizophrenic patients: CAT scan findings associated with impairment on neuropsychological tests. *Psychiatry Research, 1*, 1-8.

Sedvall, G.C., & Wode-Helgrodt, B. (1980). Aberrant monoamine metabolite levels in CSF and family history of schizophrenia. *Archives of General Psychiatry, 37*, 1113-1116.

Singer, M.T., & Wynne, L.C. (1965). Thought disorder and family relations of schizophrenics: IV. Results and implications. *Archives of General Psychiatry, 12*, 201.

Singer, M.T., Wynne, L.C., & Toohey, M.L. (1978). Communication disorders and the families of schizophrenics. In L.C. Wynne, R.L. Cromwell, & S. Matthysse (Eds.), *The nature of schizophrenia*. New York: Wiley.

Stevens, J.R. (1982). Neuropathology of schizophrenia. *Archives of General Psychiatry, 39*, 1131-1139.

Sturgeon, D., Kuipers, L., Berkowitz, R., Turpin, G., & Leff, J. (1981). Psychophysiological responses of schizophrenic patients to high and low expressed emotion relatives. *British Journal of Psychiatry, 138*, 40-45.

Wyatt, R.J., Cutler, N.R., DeLisi, L.E., Jeste, D.V., Kleinman, J.E., Luchins, D.J., Potkins, S.G., & Weinberger, D.R. (1982). Biochemical and morphological factors in schizophrenia. In L. Grinspoon (Ed.), *Psychiatry 1982*. Washington, DC: American Psychiatric Association.

Venables, P.H. (1978). Cognitive disorder. In J.K. Wing (Ed.), *Schizophrenia: Towards a new synthesis*. New York: Academic Press.

15

CHRONIC ILLNESS: A SYSTEMS PERSPECTIVE

NELLIE P. GROSE, M.D., M.P.H. and THELMA JEAN GOODRICH, Ph.D.

Surveys in the United States and in Britain report that 7-10% of all children under 18 years of age suffer from a chronic physical illness (Mattsson, 1972). These percentages represent an estimated 3.3 to 4.8 million children who are affected by such conditions as asthma, diabetes, leukemia, and seizures (Isaacs & McElroy, 1980). Ten percent of the patients treated in pediatric practice are chronically ill children. As for adults, the 1979 National Health Interview Survey indicated that 26.5 of 1000 persons needed help in the home because of a chronic health problem and that 5.5 of 1000 stayed in bed most of the time because of their ill health (Advanced Data, National Center for Health Statistics, 1983).

Obviously, with prevalence at these levels, chronic illness merits serious attention. Our purpose here is to examine several aspects, first addressing some issues of definition, then presenting a systems view of chronic illness. This view entails an examination of the interaction among several elements—the characteristics of the illness, those of the patient and the patient's family, the characteristics of health care providers and of society. One part of such a system, a family with one child diagnosed as suffering from a chronic illness, will be described in detail. Finally, we shall discuss the ways in which family physicians can act as therapeutic agents in the system that includes them.

Definition

The Commission on Chronic Illness (1956) defined chronic disease as comprising "all impairments or deviations from normal" which have one or more of the following characteristics: They are permanent, leave residual disability, are caused by nonreversible pathological alteration of the patient, require special training of the patient for rehabilitation, and require long periods of supervision, observation, or care.

"Permanent" implies that there is no reasonable hope of restoring the body to its earlier state and that the impairments will last until death. It is a pessimistic definition and therefore tends to promote a pessimistic view of chronic illness.

Other definitions of chronic illness use dimensions such as duration, degree of incapacity, degree of severity, progression, prognosis, and the type of care required. Thus, chronic illness can be defined as

> a disorder with a protracted course which can be progressive and fatal or associated with a relatively normal life span despite impaired mental and physical functioning. Such a disease frequently shows periods of acute exacerbations requiring intensive medical attention. (Mattsson, 1972)

Yet, using these factors in the definition leads to some odd categorizations. For example, arthritis, diabetes mellitus, and hypertension, usually thought of as chronic diseases, sometimes cause only minor disability, while hay fever, which is not a standard chronic disease, may be totally incapacitating during seasonal exacerbations. Recurrent low back pain, sinusitis, and irritable bowel are further examples of this latter point.

Perhaps it would be more useful to view chronic illness not as an entity but as an umbrella. In deciding what fits under the umbrella, we combine the long-term aspect of the chronic "condition" with the functional disability of the handicap and add the concept of disease as an active process. In a primary-care setting, all illnesses that are recurrent and problematic for the patient may well be considered chronic illnesses. The umbrella then covers such conditions as rheumatism, arthritis, cancer, heart conditions, and mental disorders, as well as everyday troubles such as backache, asthma, bronchitis, dermatitis, and obesity.

A Systems View of Chronicity

These attempts at definition contain hints of another idea: that it is not the disease that determines classification; rather, in a social context of belief and behavior, the patient and physician decide whether or not a disease is chronic. No illness exists in a vacuum. Many factors contribute to its chronicity: the patient's personality, the reaction of family members and physicians, situational stress, definition of the event, available resources, and so on. These components are so interrelated with one another and with the disease process that "to contrast 'organic' with 'psychogenic' in etiological importance is both outmoded and a dangerous over-simplification" (Pinkerton, 1971, p. 257). Convalescence also is continually affected by psychological, social, and physiological factors. Not acting one at a time and unilaterally on a static illness, these factors add up in cumulative fashion. Their complex interaction creates, and continues to create, something new, so that the evolving system moves through time.

To view chronicity from a systems perspective is difficult because the identified illness is so powerful an organizing principle. It is almost irresistible to regard the patient as a passive respondent to influences of the family (and other important components of the situation, including the disease and the physician). But this view is far from accurate, for the patient "is not only continually interacting with the family system but he is an active participant in the interaction. He is not only affected by the system, but is simultaneously affecting the system" (Meissner, 1967, p. 156). Let us consider some of the ways in which an illness comes to be seen as chronic.

The Role of Illness Characteristics

Certain characteristics of an illness—its reversibility, permanence, and the degree of resulting disability—define it as chronic. Variations in these and other characteristics affect the patient's and family's response to the illness and, in turn, the characteristics of the illness are affected by that response.

Consider, for example, a patient who has a malignant cerebral tumor that produces neurological deficits versus a patient with Berry's aneurysm that can be corrected surgically. The onsets as well as prognoses and treatments differ sharply. Thus each of these physiological conditions introduces a distinctive situation into the patient-family-physician system and creates very different contexts for interaction. Of course, the same illness would likely be different in different patients, as would the response of two different family-physician-patient systems.

Taking the symptom of pain as an example, suppose the patient believes pain is God's punishment and must be endured, and therefore does not seek treatment. That patient is less likely to be labeled chronic, given medications, and reacted to as chronically ill than is someone who believes pain is unwarranted and intolerable, demands medications, and comes for treatment repeatedly.

The sort of an illness, whether it is congenital or acquired, the expectations regarding it, the area of the body it affects, the types of symptoms it produces, the types of clinical procedures it requires—these are active elements in the system, as are the family physician and the patient. In the circularity of systems, it is difficult to predict how any one element will fare in the sense of "if this, then that." Our point is that illness characteristics play an important role, even though they are not the sole determinants of the development of chronicity, and may be modulated or exacerbated by the response to them.

For example, Susan T. is a 26-year-old emergency room nurse who has symptoms of fatigue and malaise and has experienced parasthesia of her right hand intermittently for about six months. Her neurological evaluation produced no diagnosis. Her colleagues and physician eventually suspected depression and began to interact with her accordingly. They constantly asked her why she was depressed and they all recommended psychotherapy. Her supervisor transferred her to work in a "slower and less demanding ward." Eight months later, she was confirmed as having multiple sclerosis. Multiple sclerosis with its vague and inconsistent symptoms will cause a system to organize in a different way from, say, a heart attack which has clearer symptoms.

The Role of the Patient

> However serious the handicap, however exasperating its capriciousness or restrictive its treatment schedule, none has any meaning in isolation from the patient himself. (Pless & Pinkerton, 1975, p. 174)

A patient's age and hence the quality of the protoplasm help to maintain or disrupt chronicity. At extremes of life, the ability to resist infection and to heal is more critical than during the middle phases of life. Perhaps as important to the response to the illness are the individual's personal characteristics and stage of development. This point is well-illustrated in cases in which a high level of cooperation, maturity, healthy attitude, and understanding play a significant role in health maintenance.

An example is Sherry, a-17-year-old adolescent diagnosed as having insulin-dependent diabetes mellitus at age 15. During the next two years, she was admitted to the hospital many times, usually in severe ketoacidosis. The doctors, nurses, and social workers were puzzled because she seemed to understand the illness and the dietary regimen that would keep her from having ketoacidosis. Concerned, the physician urged her family and teachers to watch her closely. At one point, a member of her family even followed her to school to see if she stopped by the candy store. Nothing seemed to help; she continued to require frequent hospitalizations. At the time this history was obtained, she was in the hospital for the tenth time. In the stereotypically rebellious response of adolescents to any sort of restriction, she often said: "I hate everything and everyone. Why should I care? Everyone tells me what to eat and not to eat. Since I am going to die anyway, I will do what I want."

The physician and other health professionals viewed Sherry's rebellious refusal to follow her diabetes regimen as an indication of "badness," a character deficit in a very difficult adolescent. They failed to recognize that, in this particular case at this particular time, their direct educational efforts to press for good control were generating resistance in the interaction. Sherry's family, out of love and concern, acted in the same way as the health professionals, pressing for adherence to the regimen by constant questioning and vigilance. The more they all pushed Sherry to follow her protocol, the more she pushed back, disregarded the recommendations, and "did her own thing," thus escalating the chronicity of her relapses.

In Sherry's case, the family therapist requested the health professionals as well as Sherry's family to continue their efforts to get Sherry to cooperate with treatment by observing her closely for a two-week period. They were not to let her know she was being observed, however. This instruction required that they avoid asking her questions or correcting her or advising her during this period. The reason given for this request was that it was important to gather data to help diagnose the depth of Sherry's self-destructiveness. The effect of the task was to change the nature of the interaction. Sherry now felt on her own and, having nothing to fight against, decided with the help of the therapist that "her own thing" might include taking care of herself. Subsequent hospitalizations were not necessary.

The Role of the Family

How does the family contribute to chronicity? Such factors as lack of resources, attitudes of embarrassment and guilt, and difficulty with life transition may be involved. We suggest that the critical factor is the family's interaction with the identified patient. Well-intended actions of loving family members may work contrary to their hope of helping the patient get better.

James B. is a 55-year-old "never been sick" executive who suffered a severe myocardial infarction. He was discharged home after three-and-a-half weeks of hospitalization with instructions for rehabilitation. His wife and two daughters, who loved him dearly, made sure he "never overexerted" himself. As James said, "In the early days at home, I could not even go to the bathroom without telling my wife." Whenever his doctors approved increasing physical activity, his wife cautioned him against it. She explained, "I just don't want you to be sick again; I want you to be around a long time. I love you, and I think it's better for you to go more slowly." Increasingly depressed, James became an invalid. He had been cast in a sick role and, even though well-intended, his family's love, care, and concern were maintaining the chronicity of his illness. Watzlawick and Coyne (1980) eloquently describe a similar case of a stroke patient.

The Role of Health Care Professionals

Health professionals, especially physicians, play a large role in establishing and maintaining the notion that a given condition is chronic. As Balint (1957) describes it, this role begins with history taking. When a person is first seen by a physician, the initial complaint is usually ill-defined, nonspecific, and unsophisticated: "I have a pain," or "I have a headache." The patient and physician then begin a joint project of defining the problem. The physician will probably ask questions based on his or her training in a specialty. A complaint of headache, for example, will lead a neurologist to emphasize questions pertaining to a space-occupying lesion; a family physician will ask questions about lifestyle; a psychiatrist will probe for depression; a systems therapist will stress questions concerning family dysfunction.

If the patient responds within the offered framework, the symptoms become organized into a named illness, and patient and physician have an "it" to discuss, ponder, prove, or disprove. If the patient cannot fit answers into that framework, the patient is referred to another specialist who begins the process anew, but with a difference: The patient has picked up some of the physician's language. In time, as the patient sees more health professionals, the language gains sophistication and the formulation becomes objectified: "I have stress-related migraines."

The point is not that history taking should be done differently, but that the process helps produce the outcome of the work. When symptoms seem to be recurrent, when they have been understood as representing a named disorder, and when the disorder carries the known designation of not being self-limiting, it becomes reasonable for all parties to use shorthand labels. One consequence is that these labels help the health care provider make assumptions about the meaning of the language used. If the diagnosis is accepted as presented, without scrutiny of the phenomena behind that language or of the manner in which the diagnosis was made, there is a risk of contributing to the chronicity of the problem. For example, the diagnostic label itself may connote helplessness to the patient and family and deter them from examining adaptive changes open to them. Without careful discussion, the physician has no way of knowing if this is the case. A clinical example illustrates many of these points.

Mr. and Mrs. C. brought their 16-year-old son, Harry, to their family doctor because he was "acting strange at home and in school. He hears voices telling him to leave home and he stares blankly into space a lot, as if communicating with someone." His parents were afraid he had become schizophrenic because Mrs. C.'s aunt, diagnosed as schizophrenic, had behaved similarly. The family doctor concurred with their suspicion and referred Harry to a psychiatrist who subsequently hospitalized him for evaluation and treatment. He was diagnosed as having schizophrenia and was discharged after a month with a prescription of long-term medications.

Harry was disheartened when he returned to his regular routine. He complained that his friends, family, and teachers all treated him with "suspicion and overconcern." Within six months, he relapsed and was hospitalized for two days, this time in a public hospital because his parents could not afford private care.

Over the next three years, Harry saw two other psychiatrists, both of whom accepted the diagnosis of schizophrenia without reevaluation. Thus, the changes Harry had experienced during that time were not taken into account. His parents had divorced and he was living with his mother, holding a part-time job as a grocery checker.

During a subsequent relapse, Harry was seen by a family therapist who gave the problem a fresh beginning by calling it a "variant of schizophrenia." That relabeling released Harry and his family from their expectations associated with "regular" schizophrenia, i.e., a mental illness on a steady downhill course with repeated hospitalizations and continuous medication. As long as they believed they were up against such an invincible force, they could only help fulfill the prophecy, not alter it. When the therapist relabeled the diagnosis to be a "variant of schizophrenia," he opened the possibility for them to change their views and behavior. The new label stayed close enough to the old one to avoid directly challenging the family's previous experience and former ways of responding, yet it injected enough confusion and doubt about the certainty of the course of the disease to permit some new interactions in the family. Within a brief period of time, Harry was able to live on his own and return to college.

Although this example concerns a disorder that involves mainly mental symptoms, a similar point can be made for illnesses that manifest mainly physical symptoms.

Billie N., a 43-year-old former nurse, consulted one of us (NG) because she had "difficulty with her bowels." She had seen many other specialists before one had been of help to her. She was visibly frustrated and angry with the medical profession. At age 20 she had been diagnosed as having ulcerative colitis. The news was devastating because to her it meant "early death, poor health, and inability to fulfill motherhood as I would like to."

Depressed for years, she moved to another city and became established with another physician who took her diagnosis at face value and treated her "ulcerative colitis." Her depression continued, although her gastrointestinal pains were never severe.

After another move, she began to consult a family doctor who reviewed her history and symptoms carefully and told her she had "irritable bowel syndrome." She was immensely relieved, but felt she had missed many years of enjoying life. Whether or not her "ulcerative colitis" was truly present at first, whether or not it healed miraculously is not the issue; the point is that the labels we affix to patients' illnesses can contribute to the chronicity of a problem.

Another way physicians may contribute to chronicity is by mistaken actions based on good intentions of doing no harm. One example is the case of a 15-year-old Chinese student brought to the emergency room by his friends who thought he had had a seizure. The ER physician admitted him to the observation ward overnight because the boy's parents were out of town. Next morning the neurologist admitted him to the hospital for evaluation. He was discharged as having had "possible seizure" and sent home without medications but to be watched closely. The young man resented the sick role, and his family was under much stress. At 18, he had difficulty obtaining a driver's license although there had been no episodes for three years. For years, the notation "possible seizure" may cause problems for him in whatever situations his medical records are relevant.

The biases of physicians may contribute to the chronicity of certain illnesses, of which alcoholism is the prototypical example. Low-back pain, recurrent vaginitis, depression, and tension headaches are others. When these disorders are suspected, physicians tend not to listen for the importance of the symptoms to the family and other systems significant to the patient, and tend to limit interventions to pharmacological agents.

The Role of Society

We use the term "society" to mean anything beyond the family unit—health institutions, agencies, community, and public opinion. What in interactive terms contributes to chronicity? We quote a newspaper article to illustrate an extreme case: "A Chinese immigrant who was confined for 31½ years to a series of state mental hospitals, apparently because he couldn't speak English, has finally gained his freedom. . . . When Tom began acting strangely during treatment for tuberculosis and nobody could be found who understood his Chinese dialect, the state apparently decided he was psychotic and had to be institutionalized. Tom is barely mentally competent now and needs constant care" (*Houston Chronicle*, December 30, 1983, p. 7). Based on the details given about this person, one must ask whether society has turned an individual who had a cultural and language disadvantage into an incompetent, chronically dependent person.

The social stigma still attached to mental illness, alcoholism, and drug abuse in many cases prevents early intervention and optimal rehabilitation. Many people who sense that they or their relatives need to be in the care of a psychiatrist or a substance abuse program delay in order to avoid the stigma associated with such treatment. In the meantime, further deterioration occurs at every level, from the cellular to the social.

Our existing health care systems bar the chronically ill from optimal care. Currently we have two forms of medical care, a sophisticated personal system for private patients and a disjointed, impersonal one for the poor. One result is that the private patient has easier access to the network of remedial services needed by the chronically ill and in fact crowds the chronically ill, poor patient out of existing services. Although some services are available to the poor, public programs are fragmented, difficult to enter, and discontinuous. The practical problems created by fragmentation are especially detrimental to the care of the chronically ill, especially children. Responsibility for children's long-term care rests with their parents, who may be caring for other children as well. Long-term illness in a family often exacerbates the family's psychosocial problems, which, in turn, interfere with the parents' ability to care adequately for the chronically ill child.

Families who have a chronically ill member often appeal to community agencies for help. In many communities, however, services are compartmentalized and do not deal with the whole family as a unit. Communication between agencies is usually inadequate and family members may receive conflicting advice. Such situations can only lead to the families' alienation from health and welfare agencies.

Moreover, the physical facilities of many health or welfare agencies often are ill-suited to the needs of chronically ill persons. Their low energy, mobility problems, and strict medical regimens make it difficult for them to travel to offices and clinics at institutionally scheduled times. If they do, they may not be able to handle admission procedures that resemble an obstacle course.

We have been discussing ways that society exacerbates chronicity, but the larger point is to emphasize the role of society's institutions and attitudes. These may, of course, contribute to the amelioration of chronic illness. There are community services for early detection, rehabilitation, and for reducing the stigma of certain illnesses, including hypertension, cystic fibrosis, sickle-cell disease, cerebral palsy, coronary artery disease, diabetes mellitus, and muscular dystrophy.

THE FAMILY WITH A CHRONICALLY ILL CHILD

A child's chronic illness has far-reaching consequences for the patient, family, and physician. The situation has some distinctive features that make it quite challenging to manage. First, overprotectiveness, which retards development and progress in a patient of any age, is most likely to be present when the patient is a child. Second, it is more socially acceptable for an ill child than an ill adult to give free rein to the expression of upsetting emotions and behaviors. Although regarded as permissible, these may be very troublesome to the family and physician. Third, the chronically ill child may become a "lightning rod" for marital or family problems, thereby complicating the child's and the family's adjustment to the illness and complicating the physician's role as well. We will focus on these and other problems in the hope of fostering plans for early detection and prevention. We cannot, of course, predict outcomes in the complicated contexts being described. Our scenarios are mostly poor ones for purposes of emphasis. We will look at situations first from one point of view, then another, but the web of interactions in the system must be kept in mind.

The Child's Experience

As mentioned earlier, a significant minority of our children are chronically ill: " 'Halfway children' they are called; their existence is precariously contingent on a complex system of hospital care, pharmacological additives, surgical corrections, and artificial devices all designed to rehabilitate broken bodies or prolong condemned lives" (Geist, 1979, p. 8). There are significant effects on the child's intellectual, emotional, and social development, not so much from the disease itself as from the restrictions it and its treatment impose on the child's physical activity, social interaction, and expectations about life's promises (Blom, 1968; Katz, Kellerman, Rigler, Williams, & Siegel, 1977; Klein, 1976; Mahaffy, 1965; McAnarney, Pless, Satterwhite, & Friedman, 1974; Pless & Roghmann, 1971; Reddihough, Jones, & Richard, 1978; Voeller & Rothenberg, 1973). We will explore these issues from the perspective of the ill child (or, rather, from the perspective of those who have observed and written about the ill child).

Emotional turmoils. Children sometimes experience their illness, its symptoms, or its treatment as punishment for unacceptable thoughts or behavior. The children's interpretation may have a variety of sources, even admonitions by parents like "Don't eat so much candy," or "Don't play in the rain." Although these are necessary warnings from parents, children may draw on them mistakenly to make sense of the experience of chronic illness.

Afraid, then, that the illness is caused by misconduct, the child becomes reluctant to discuss its origin (and parents often believe causes are too complicated to explain). Thus the child has no chance to correct misconceptions. The resultant guilt increases the child's discomfort and may contribute to inhibition, withdrawal, and excessive self-restraint (Maddison & Raphael, 1971).

The child may also have fears of death and abandonment, although he or she may not express these directly. Avoidance of such painful subjects by parents and medical caretakers further discourages the child from talking about them, but constant crying or compulsive behavior may become their expression. The child's inability to speak of fears explicitly and have them addressed properly may lead to poor cooperation with treatment regimens.

Loss of self-esteem is another reaction common among chronically ill children. Feelings about being different and looking different from other children often result in feelings of inferiority and worthlessness (McAnarney et al., 1974; Moore, Holton, & Martin, 1969). Such reactions, combined with the disturbing responses of others, produce withdrawal and isolation.

Physical activity. A child's intellectual development depends in part on active interchange with a sufficiently stimulating environment. To the extent that chronic illness limits the range of these interactions, it may interfere with certain aspects of intellectual development, yet favor others. The loss of many typical childhood activities may, for example, increase the value placed on excelling academically. Learning pursuits may be the only area still open to the child for gaining experiences of control and mastery and play. When normal play is limited, play may come to be redefined as the development of cognitive skills because these skills please adults and are rewarded by them (Anderson, 1981).

Restriction on the child's activity has still another consequence. Active play is an important way to express and resolve conflict. When active play is restricted by illness, what reaction do we most want to see in the child? It may well be that the child who resists and complains about restrictions is finding an alternate way to bypass and resolve conflict. Such a child is a difficult patient, but he or she is dealing with the situation in a beneficial way. More placid behavior, which may look like good adjustment, may actually represent apathy and withdrawal (Maddison & Raphael, 1971).

Social interaction. For chronically ill children, social interaction is characterized by regulation of activity according to a time schedule, relatively little participation in the world of peers, and socialization into the world of adults (Anderson, 1981). This pattern of interaction in itself differentiates these children from well children. In addition, the nature of the interactions, that is, the response of others to the ill child and vice versa, is markedly influenced by reactions to the illness. At school, for example, chronically ill children may be excluded from normal activities even though they could participate in them. These exclusions, along with others like being socially ostracized or required to use a different drinking fountain, are symptomatic of fears of contagion—fears that persist despite teachers' and pupils' knowledge that the illness is not contagious (Cyphert, 1973; Pearse, 1977). In addition, the ill child, like children who are different for some other reason, often suffers much teasing and ridicule from other children.

Expectations. The primary context for any child's life is, of course, the family, a context marked by a high degree of reciprocity. Each family member contributes to the distinctiveness, integration, atmosphere, and identity of the family. Even a baby occupies this position, and even a young child is aware of her or his special contribution. It is the loss of their accustomed contribution that chronically ill children experience most deeply. Adjustment to this loss means that the child must

> 1) experience a rebirth, as it were, of oneself as the same person with a different body-image, and 2) integrate one's self-conception into this new physical perception so as to perceive oneself as once again a contributing member of the family, and eventually of society at large. . . . (Geist, 1979, p. 8)

The impact of chronic illness on expectations about oneself and one's abilities depends on the developmental stage of its onset, and so does the response. Small children usually protest vigorously to restricted movement or loss of skills recently acquired. For adolescents, chronic illness impairs progress towards autonomy and may evoke rebelliousness. As mentioned, struggles over compliance with the treatment regimen may be expressions of independence (Heisler & Friedman, 1981). These age-appropriate responses are preferable to both extreme submissiveness, where the child seeks help from every possible source, and extreme rejection, where the child refuses even necessary help (Harding, Heller, & Kesler, 1979; Lowit, 1973).

The Family's Experience

The consequences of having a chronically ill child begin when the family hears the diagnosis. Grief and anger are common, natural reactions to any significant loss. In this case, what is lost is the previous image of a normal healthy child and of all hopes and dreams associated with that state (Heisler & Friedman, 1981). The parents may suffer such grief that they cannot be supportive to their child (Friedrich, 1977; Mattsson, 1972). Sometimes these feelings are so overpowering that they are replaced by denial. The parents' denial may take the form of misinterpreting the physicians' explanations, asking the same questions repeatedly (Maddison & Raphael, 1971), looking for other medical opinions (McCollum & Gibson, 1970), or refusing to accept the implications of the illness (Tisza, 1962).

Once the initial shock has passed, the family begins to reorganize to incorporate the care of the chronically ill child. This process is illustrated by Priscilla O.'s family.

A part-time secretary, Priscilla O., brought her 11-year-old son, Melvin, to the physician's office complaining of his increasing malaise, fatigue, weight loss, thirst, and poor school performance. Insulin-dependent diabetes was diagnosed after a five-day hospitalization. Priscilla's husband, Ray, also has diabetes with complications of kidney disease. Priscilla committed herself to caring for Melvin so that he would not "become like his father."

Priscilla left her job to stay at home and give her full attention to Melvin. She knew where he was at all times and watched everything he did and ate. His nine-year-old sister, Clara, was given Melvin's household chores in addition to her own. She never complained aloud because she knew that her brother was ill. Ray felt very much excluded by his wife: "You never give me the same attention for my diabetes that you do Melvin." Still, he did not complain much because he believed Priscilla was giving their son proper care.

The family members were seen over a period of time—Clara most frequently, for a variety of psychosomatic complaints; Ray for diabetes, which was not in adequate control; and Melvin for his illness.

The family's structure and function had obviously changed. The bond established between mother and son was a way of caring for the sick child, but it had other consequences as well. The father felt closed out by the twosome and cut off from his wife. Moreover, further interviews by the family therapist revealed that this present coalition was fueled by one in the past. Priscilla's mother had formed a similar bond with Priscilla's brother when he developed rheumatoid arthritis. This family realignment also affected the sibling subsystem. Common ways of acting out sibling rivalry were forsworn and perhaps "sibling rescue" took over (Hoffman, 1981). Clara, given her brother's chores, resented his special position and felt unloved, a common interpretation of parental neglect (McAllister, Butler, & Lei, 1973). This feeling certainly was a source of conflict between Clara and her mother, and was likely to be one of the stressors that contributed to Clara's frequent visits to the physician.

Siblings. Healthy siblings may become highly stressed by the family's reliance on them to remain "well," perhaps to survive for two, to take care of the parents and somehow fulfill the expectations the family has for the children (Penn, 1983). Resentment exists along with many other kinds of feelings and, indeed, well siblings have many reactions that are cause for concern. Healthy siblings of children who have cancer have been found to experience a sense of loss that may disrupt their relationships with parents, friends, or the ill child, distort their perception of the ill child's physical appearance, or lead to disturbances in the routine of family life (Iles, 1979). Siblings of children with congenital heart disease have been reported to have an unusually high number of problems and psychosomatic disorders (Apley, Barbour, & Westmacott, 1967). As many as half of the siblings of children with leukemia have been found to have significant difficulties ranging from enuresis to school phobia (Binger, 1973). These findings point up the need for a family approach to the treatment of one ill member.

Parents. The parent who has primary responsibility for the child's care cannot give the same amount of attention to the marital partner as before. Resentment and hostility may mount between the parents, robbing each of needed support. Frequently, they feel deprived of time and energy for leisure activities, time to be alone with the spouse, and time for oneself (Tisza, 1962). Parents often struggle with feelings of guilt about having somehow caused the child's illness (Harding, Heller, & Kesler, 1979). If the disease is genetic, such feelings are especially troublesome. Sometimes the reaction is to overindulge and overprotect the sick child (Harding et al. 1979). This reaction limits the parents' ability to maintain discipline and interpersonal boundaries in the family, and it increases the child's perception of herself or himself as highly vulnerable (Brantley, Stabler, & Whitt, 1981).

Indeed, two of the greatest problems families of chronically ill children have are finding the proper balance in discipline and helping the child develop maximum potential (Harding et al., 1979). If parents take a hopeless view of the child's dependence and helplessness, they protect too much and foster the child's perception of incompetence. Under these circumstances, the child fails to progress evenly. Yet there is also a danger if the child is protected too little, as happens when parents overestimate the possibilities and avoid seeing the limitations. The child reflects this view by acting with false bravado, taking risks, and trying to function along developmental lines far beyond actual capability. This is a critical area, for the parents' perception of the child and of the child's disability has greater impact on the child's self-concept than does the handicap itself (Harding et al., 1979).

Family strain. The ever-present need for medical care—and the ever-present possibility of crisis—may keep family routines disrupted and lead to troubles ranging from impaired social relationships to dissatisfaction with medical services. The latter is often well justified by long waits at clinics and pharmacies, high costs, and red tape. Social relationships become impaired from several causes: babysitters are difficult to find; procedures for care of the child may require privacy; behavioral problems are common (Harding et al., 1979).

The picture then is of a system under severe strain. The combined effects of poor health and an unfavorable family situation seem to be cumulative over time (Pless, Roghmann, & Haggerty, 1972). Not surprisingly, the rate of family breakdown in these circumstances is high (Bruhn, 1977; Livingston, 1957; Salk, Hilgartner, & Granich, 1972).

Even when the illness is in remission for a time, we find that the family is usually still under stress and may not shift responses quickly to handle a symptom-free period. In the case of Melvin and his family, Priscilla brought Melvin to the physician when Melvin turned 16, to discuss his wanting to leave home to set up an apartment with a friend. His mother was sure that if Melvin left home, his diabetes would become uncontrolled. "How could you do that to me?" she asked him. Still tied to the old family structure, Priscilla was holding on to patterns of interaction that now needed changing. Melvin, no longer a "sick" child, was ready to move beyond his dependent status, but his mother was not. Referral for family therapy brought good results and Priscilla accepted Melvin's moving out of the home within a year.

Family strength. With all the strains brought on by chronic illness, how does any family survive? Many families develop coping strategies that strengthen family functioning and allow successful management of these hardships.

One coping strategy is to share the burdens of the illness (Venters, 1981). This strategy involves strengthening family bonds by encouraging shared activities and emphasizing that all members are important contributors to the family. Family members should try to maintain meaningful outside contacts and to reach out for help from others.

Another helpful strategy is normalization (Anderson, 1981). The disease as defined by medical science may be perceived as a physiological abnormality, but parents may make a distinction between the abnormality and their own reactions to the child. If parents think of themselves as treating their child as a normal child, they will manage situations so that the child will not stand out as being different. The whole family may, for example, change eating habits so that the child who has diabetes mellitus will not feel strange. Sometimes whole families do physical therapy with the ill child as part of a family exercise program. Other normalizing tactics include giving siblings vitamin pills at medication time, buying wigs for the child with hair loss, and preparing school teachers and classmates for the ill child's altered appearance or activities (Krulik, 1980).

A third coping strategy is to endow the illness with a meaning (Venters, 1981). This approach has to do with locating the event of the child's falling ill in some larger context that lets the event be seen as making sense rather than being senseless. Some families draw on a religious explanation, others on a medical-scientific one. Being able to assign a meaning to their child's suffering allows families to focus on the best aspects of the hardship and find encouragement to seek solutions to their problems.

The Physician's Experience

Family physicians bear special strains when treating patients with chronic illness. Often they feel ill-prepared by their training to cope with the complexities of long-term management required by such patients. Lacking, too, is the customary expectation of working toward cure, which could otherwise undergird the enormous expenditure of effort. Faced with feelings of hopelessness, helplessness, and inadequacy, physicians sometimes attempt to compensate by increasing their activity or by blindly adhering to medical regimens that may be only marginally helpful. The physician's long, close relationship with the patient and family, which is so necessary for accomplishing all that *can* be done, makes the physician vulnerable to an unusual amount of suffering in response to the trials brought on by chronic illness. (For additional comments on this point, see Chapter 16.) All this adds greatly to the risk of burnout, an emotional exhaustion characterized by cynicism and a dehumanized view of patients (Maslach, 1978).

Yet, along with the special strains, the potential for special rewards is great. Personal contact with families, the opportunity for intimacy, admiration for the courage of patients and their families, the belief in comprehensive care, the sense of serving in a way few people wish to do—these are reasons for persevering in such difficult work. Indeed, since family physicians in the main see patients who have *self*-limited illnesses, they often find their influence more surely felt in chronic illness than in any other circumstance.

Obviously, whether the physician will be strengthened rather than immobilized by the challenge of treating the chronically ill patient depends on her or his capacity to cope with difficulty (Pearlin & Schooler, 1978). The following are ways to increase that capacity as it applies to chronic illness:

1) Conducting research that is expected to advance knowledge about causes or treatment provides a sense of doing something about the distressing circumstances.
2) Careful planning helps to incorporate chronically ill patients into a primary-care practice. Some physicians have found helpful a half-day clinic reserved for the chronically ill. Besides adding focus and efficiency, this scheduling permits school nurses, social workers, family therapists, and medical specialists to attend, thus enhancing comprehensive management. Like scheduling, keeping track of information requires extra attention. Flow sheets like those described by Schmitt (1973) are essential for following a patient's changing symptoms, medication, laboratory results, and consultations.
3) Using all available resources increases the physician's sense ofcompetence and decreases the sense of isolation. One example already mentioned is working with an interdisciplinary team. Others are the establishment of good communication with subspecialists involved with the patients, attending specialty clinics, and participating in courses about the management of chronic illness.
4) Some recommendations have arisen from research on burnout among health professionals (Maslach, 1978). Support groups and retreats may turn out to be restorative because they help physicians to recognize the existence, legitimacy, and power of their own feelings.
5) Specialists in the treatment of chronic illness have reported that they have been rescued from despair by drawing on the strength of the patient or family. Of course, physicians have the responsibility not to be a burden to their patients, but the capacity for reciprocity fosters continuing commitment to one another and to the task.

The Physician as a Therapeutic Agent

Successful management of chronic illness depends upon the recognition that illness in one member of the family has a major influence on the mental health, relationships, and perhaps even the continued existence of the family, especially if the patient is a child (Steinhauer, Mushin, & Rae-Grant, 1974). The importance of the physician's role here cannot be overstated, nor can its enormity. Providing care for the psychological and physiological needs of patient and family for a long time offers significant challenge and may require significant changes in the physician's routine ways of managing.

Studies have shown that physicians are generally unaware of at least half of the psychological and social problems of their patients (Querido, 1963), and they usually overestimate how much their patients know about their illness (Boyle, 1970; Samora, Saunders, & Lawson, 1962). Patients may recall less than half of what their physicians tell them about the disease and its treatment (Joyce, Caple, Mason, Reynolds, & Mathews, 1969; Ley & Spelman, 1965, 1967). Only half the parents of chronically ill children know the correct diagnosis of their child's illness (Lau, Williams, Williams, Ware, & Brook, 1982), and even fewer expect the physician to help with the psychological and social aspects of their child's illness (Breslau et al., 1975; Pless & Pinkerton, 1975). If patients and families do not themselves mention their confusions and problems, and yet these factors have critical implications for compliance, the physician must be alert to observe, remark, and question.

The Doctor-Patient Relationship

More than any other type of patient, the chronically ill person must receive unconditional positive regard from the physician. This behavior has been described as "demonstrating to your [patients] that no matter what they may have done—or are continuing to do—you accept them as valuable human beings" (Herr & Weakland, 1979, pp. 29-30). To accomplish this stance, the physician must resolve personal conflicts about typical responses patients have to illness, such as dependency, egocentricity, and denial.

In their discussion of therapeutic effectiveness, Truax and Carkhuff (1967) concluded that "therapists or counselors who are accurately empathic, nonpossessively warm in attitude, and genuine are indeed effective—regardless of their training or theoretical orientation" (p. 100). We believe these remarks hold true for the doctor-patient relationship as well and that continuously available access to one particular physician is especially important for the patient with chronic illness in which many health professionals are likely to be involved. Family physicians are well-suited to this role because of their special training in interpreting, integrating, and implementing care. Yet, despite its benefits, continuity has a potential disadvantage. The physician may become so much a part of the patient's family system as to lose the ability to see problems of management differently from the way the family sees them. The range of options then narrows and the physician becomes increasingly unable to intervene in situations in which family interactions contribute to the chronicity of the illness. Calling in a consultant—a family therapist or a family physician—will add a new perspective in such situations.

There is another aspect in which the relationship is important. When no more new procedures or medications can be helpful, the physician's personal involvement, over and above medical expertise, continues to be an essential ingredient in clinical management. The fact that the relationship with the physician provides encouragement and strengthens emotional resources makes it never true to say that nothing can be done.

Care for the Whole Family

Accurate information and instruction to the patient and the immediate family avoids misunderstanding and "drives out fear" (Maxwell & Gane, 1962). In addition to the general recommendation to provide comprehensible explanations, there are these more specific ones for families of patients of all ages (Anderson, 1981; Harding et al., 1979; Heisler & Friedman, 1981; Maddison & Raphael, 1971; Rose-Williamson, 1981):

1) Ask repeatedly about the family's perceptions of the illness to facilitate discovering and correcting misunderstandings.
2) Schedule a follow-up session with the family soon after the one in which the diagnosis is first given. Such a plan acknowledges that pain and shock have kept the family from understanding fully what was said the first time.
3) In family sessions, set the stage for the expression of feelings of guilt, fear, anger, and resentment that may otherwise be politely suppressed. Assure family members that they are entitled to such feelings. As they put their feelings into words and as they sense understanding from the physician, they begin to experience the emotional support so crucial for coping with chronic illness.
4) Encourage older children and adolescents to ask their own questions. Their concerns may be quite different from their parents'. Include them in sessions and decisions as much as possible.
5) Elicit from families their own ideas about how to shift priorities and reallocate tasks in the household. Asking rather than telling can help family members maintain their sense of mastery. Repeat such sessions periodically to ensure that changes occur as the patient's condition changes.
6) Aid the family to assess realistically the needs of the patient and to balance dependence and autonomy. Patients, especially children, need a great deal of touching and attention but, if at all possible, and even if they are children, they need to do their own feeding, dressing, and bathing.
7) Sometimes family members see their needs as boundless and the physician as inexhaustible. Such perceptions result in constant telephone calls and unnecessary visits. Shorten the time between visits, but insist on regularity and appointments.

8) Help the family modify its health behaviors to help the patient follow treatment regimens. For example, dietary patterns and exercise programs may need to be changed. Such changes by the whole family minimize the patient's sick label and improve the other members' health.
9) Assist the family in mobilizing a strong network of social support, including such resources as extended family members, clergy, colleagues, friends, and community groups.

When the ill member is a child, these are additional suggestions (Cyphert, 1973; Heisler & Friedman, 1981; Isaacs & McElroy, 1980; Kagen-Goodheart, 1977):

10) Give the child written instructions. These not only increase compliance but help reduce feelings of dependence.
11) Prepare teachers for the child's return to the classroom. Communication between medical and school personnel is necessary for the child's successful reentry. Counsel the teacher to relate to the child as normally as possible and to keep expectations at a level sufficient to help the child feel academically accomplished and socially accepted.
12) Coordinate the separate efforts of the significant adults in the child's life. Surveys have revealed that sources of support for the chronically ill child—family, teacher, health care providers—tend to function independently of each other, thereby producing duplication as well as gaps in the care of the child.
13) Especially if the child is nine years old or older, he or she may have fears of and fantasies about death, and these may interfere with cooperation with treatment. Encourage the young patient to talk about these, because the physician may be the only person with whom the child will risk asking questions and telling fears.
14) Whenever possible, include time to deal directly with the child. To communicate with the child always via the parents may convey doubts to the child about his or her own capability and may undermine strivings for autonomy and independence.

Understanding Resistance

So far, our suggestions about clinical management have assumed a relational context in which direct advice and logical explanations on the part of the physician are welcomed and followed by the family. At times, however, the physician may discover that the more she or he pushes in one direction, the more the family pushes in another. Each side responds by increasing its pressure.

Mutually resistive and mutually escalating types of interaction are fairly easy to recognize, once one adopts the viewpoint that resistance is a characteristic of a certain situation, rather than a trait in a certain personality. These interactions are not easy to interrupt, however. We suggest consultation with a family therapist trained in the use of strategic approaches (Weeks & L'Abate, 1982). In these approaches, one or more participants in the situation—including the health care professionals—are induced to use a different (and usually less direct) method for trying to obtain their goal.

Relabeling and Reframing

Earlier in this chapter, we referred to the formative role that labels play in organizing the meaning of symptoms and the reaction to symptoms. To reiterate, patients and families respond to a diagnostic label on the basis of the meaning it has for them. This meaning is not based solely on the information provided by health care professionals but rather includes prior experiences, hearsay, envisioned impact on their lives, societal opinions, religious views, and various other influences. In cases where the response to the label is causing trouble, the physician may find it useful to undertake changing the response through further explanation, correction of error, examination of beliefs, shifting of basic assumptions, and so on. Many times, however, it is more efficient to change the response by changing the label.

Reframing is also a powerful technique for altering a response. Reframing involves putting an event into a new context that gives it a different meaning, thereby evoking a different reaction. One example of reframing was given in the section on coping strategies. Parents who can reframe their child's chronic illness from a senseless tragedy into a plan from God have certain strengths, resources, and options for managing that would otherwise not be available to them.

The use of reframing and relabeling requires close attention to and great respect for the beliefs and values of patients and families and the ways these are expressed. Relabeling and reframing are not tricks; they are ways of pointing to another side of the families' reality (or to another possible reality) than the one currently in focus. Further examples and discussion can be found in Chapter 5 and in *Change* by Watzlawick, Weakland, and Fisch (1974).

Access to Expertise

In an effort to assist patients with chronic illness, physicians often refer them to superspecialists in case any aspect has been overlooked or some new approach has been developed. As our chapter has shown, family life and chronic illness are intertwined in a way that can create complications in the illness and in the family. We therefore suggest that the family physician deserves a family specialist among the other specialists called upon—either a family therapist or a family physician trained in family therapy. The contribution of the family therapist from the early diagnostic period on through the other phases can be invaluable to the physician, the patient, and the family.

REFERENCES

Advanced Data No. 92 (Sept. 14, 1983). In *Vital and health statistics*. National Center for Health Statistics, U.S. Dept. of Health and Human Services, Hyattsville, MD.

Anderson, J.M. (1981). The social construction of illness experience: Families with a chronically-ill child. *Journal of Advanced Nursing, 6*, 427-434.

Apley, J., Barbour, R.F., & Westmacott, I. (1967). Impact of congenital heart disease on the family: Preliminary report. *British Medical Journal, 1*, 103-105.

Balint, M. (1957). *The doctor, his patient and the illness.* New York: International Universities Press.

Binger, C.M.H. (1973). Childhood leukemia—Emotional impact on siblings. In E.J. Anthony & C. Koupernik (Eds.), *The child in his family* (pp. 195-210). New York: John Wiley & Sons.

Blom, B.E. (1968). The reactions of hospitalized children to illness. *Pediatrics, 42*, 590-597.

Boyle, C. (1970). Difference between patients' and doctors' interpretation of some common medical terms. *British Medical Journal, 1*(704), 286-289.

Brantley, H.T., Stabler, B., & Whitt, J.K. (1981). Program considerations in comprehensive care of chronically ill children. *Journal of Pediatric Psychology, 6*, 229-237.

Breslau, N., Haug, M.R., Burns, A.E., McClelland, C.G., Reeb, K.G., & Staples, W.I. (1975). Comprehensive pediatric care: The patient viewpoint. *Medical Care, 13*, 562-569.

Bruhn, J.G. (1977). Effects of chronic illness on the family. *Journal of Family Practice, 4*, 1057-1060.

Commission on Chronic Illness (1956). *Chronic illness in the U.S.* (Vol. 2). Cambridge, MA: Harvard University Press.

Cyphert, F.R. (1973). Back to school for the child with cancer. *Journal of School Health, 43*, 215-217.

Friedrich, W.N. (1977). Ameliorating the psychological impact of chronic physical disease on the child and family. *Journal of Pediatric Psychology, 2*, 26-31.

Geist, R.A. (1979). Onset of chronic illness in children and adolescents: Psychotherapeutic and consultative intervention. *American Journal of Orthopsychiatry, 49*, 4-23.

Harding, R.K., Heller, J.R., & Kesler, R.W. (1979). The chronically ill child in the primary care setting. *Primary Care, 6*, 311-324.

Heisler, A.B., & Friedman, S.B. (1981). Social and psychological considerations in chronic disease: With particular reference to the management of seizure disorders. *Journal of Pediatric Psychology, 6*, 239-250.

Herr, J.J., & Weakland, J.H. (1979). *Counseling elders and their families.* New York: Springer.

Hoffman, L. (1981). *Foundations of family therapy.* New York: Basic Books.

Iles, J.P. (1979). Children with cancer: Healthy siblings' perceptions during the illness experience. *Cancer Nursing, 2*, 371-377.

Isaacs, J., & McElroy, M.R. (1980). Psychosocial aspects of chronic illness in children. *Journal of School Health, 50*, 318-321.

Joyce, C.R.B., Caple, G., Mason, M., Reynolds, E., & Mathews, J.A. (1969). Quantitative study of doctor-patient communication. *Quarterly Journal of Medicine, 38*, 183-194.

Kagen-Goodheart, L. (1977). Reentry: Living with childhood cancer. *American Journal of Orthopsychiatry, 47*, 651-658.

Katz, E.R., Kellerman, J., Rigler, D., Williams, K.O., & Siegel, S.E. (1977). School intervention with pediatric cancer patients. *Journal of Pediatric Psychology, 2*, 72-76.

Klein, S.J.D. (1976). Chronic kidney disease: Impact on the child and family and strategies for coping. *Dissertation Abstracts International, 36*, 5580-A.

Krulik, T. (1980). Successful "normalizing" tactics of parents of chronically-ill children. *Journal of Advanced Nursing, 5*, 573-578.

Lau, R.R., Williams, H.S., Williams, L.C., Ware, J.E., Jr., & Brook, R.H. (1982). Psychosocial problems in chronically ill children: Physician concern, parent satisfaction, and the validity of medical records. *Journal of Community Health, 7*, 250-261.

Ley, P., & Spelman, M.A. (1965). Communications in an outpatient setting. *British Journal of Social Clinical Psychology, 4*, 114-118.

Ley, P., & Spelman, M.S. (1967). *Communicating with the patient.* London: Staples Press.

Livingston, S. (1957). The social management of the epileptic child and his parents. *Journal of Pediatrics, 51*, 137-145.

Lowit, I.M. (1973). Social and psychological consequences of chronic illness in children. *Developmental Medicine & Child Neurology, 15*, 75.

Maddison, D., & Raphael, B. (1971). Social and psychological consequences of chronic disease in childhood. *Medical Journal of Australia, 2*, 1265-1270.

Mahaffy, P.R., Jr. (1965). The effects of hospitalization on children admitted for tonsillectomy and adenoidectomy. *Nursing Research, 14*, 12-19.

Maslach, C. (1978). The burn-out syndrome and patient care. In C. Garfield (Ed.), *Psychosocial care of the dying*. New York: McGraw-Hill.

Mattsson, A. (1972). Long-term physical illness in childhood: A challenge to psychosocial adaptation. *Pediatrics, 50*, 801-811.

Maxwell, G.M., & Gane, S. (1962). The impact of congenital heart disease upon the family. *American Heart Journal, 64*, 449-454.

McAllister, R.J., Butler, E., & Lei, T.J. (1973). Patterns of social interaction among families of behaviorally retarded children. *Journal of Marriage & Family, 35*, 93-100.

McAnarney, E.R., Pless, I.B., Satterwhite, B., & Friedman, S.B. (1974). Psychological problems of children with chronic juvenile arthritis. *Pediatrics, 53*, 523-528.

McCollum, A.T., & Gibson, L.E. (1970). Family adaptation to the child with cystic fibrosis. *Journal of Pediatrics, 77*, 571-578.

Meissner, W.W. (1967). Family dynamics and psychosomatic processes. *Family Process, 5*, 142-161.

Moore, D.C., Holton, C.P., & Martin, G.W. (1969). Psychologic problems in the management of adolescents with malignancy. *Clinical Pediatrics, 8*, 464-473.

Pearlin, L., & Schooler, C. (1978). The structure of coping. *Journal of Health and Social Behavior, 19*, 2-21.

Pearse, M. (1977). The child with cancer: Impact on the family. *Journal of School Health, 47*, 174-179.

Penn, P. (1983). Coalitions and binding interactions in families with chronic illness. *Family Systems Medicine, 1*(2), 16-36.

Pinkerton, P. (1971). Psychosomatic interrelationship in the management of childhood asthma. *Psychotherapy and Psychosomatics, 19*, 257-265.

Pless, I.B., & Pinkerton, P. (1975). *Chronic childhood disorders: Promoting patterns of adjustment*. London: Henry Kimpton.

Pless, I.B., & Roghmann, K.J. (1971). Chronic illness and its consequences: Observations based on three epidemiologic surveys. *Journal of Pediatrics, 79*, 351-359.

Pless, I.B., Roghmann, K.J., & Haggerty, R.J. (1972). Chronic illness, family functioning, and psychological adjustment: A model for the allocation of preventive mental health services. *International Journal of Epidemiology, 1*, 271-277.

Querido, A. (1963). *The efficiency of medical care*. Leiden: Stenfert Kroese.

Reddihough, D.S., Jones, H.S., & Richard, W.S. (1978, October). Asthma: The doctor's failure in communication. *New Zealand Medical Journal, 88*, 322-325.

Rose-Williamson, K. (1981). Counseling parents of seriously ill children. *Journal of Enterostomal Therapy, 8*, 12-13.

Salk, L., Hilgartner, M., & Granich, B. (1972). The psycho-social impact of hemophilia on the patient and his family. *Social Science and Medicine, 6*, 491-505.

Samora, J., Saunders, L., & Lawson, R. (1962). Knowledge about specific diseases in four selected samples. *Journal of Health and Human Behavior, 3*, 176-185.

Schmitt, B.D. (1973). The chronic disease flow sheet in ambulatory pediatrics. *Pediatrics, 51*, 722-730.

Steinhauer, P.D., Mushin, D.N., & Rae-Grant, Q. (1974). Psychological aspects of chronic illness. *Pediatric Clinics of North America, 21*, 825-840.

Tisza, V.B. (1962). Management of the parent in pediatric practice—Workshop, 1960. I. Management of the parents of the chronically ill child. *American Journal of Orthopsychiatry, 32*, 53-59.

Truax, C.B., & Carkhuff, R.R. (1967). *Toward effective counseling & psychotherapy: Training & practice*. Chicago: Aldine Publishers.

Venters, M. (1981). Familial coping with chronic and severe childhood illness: The case of cystic fibrosis. *Social Science and Medicine, 15A*, 289-297.

Voeller, K.K., & Rothenberg, M.B. (1973). Psychosocial aspects of the management of seizures in children. *Pediatrics, 51*, 1072-1082.

Watzlawick, P., & Coyne, J.C. (1980). Depression following stroke: Brief, problem-focused family treatment. *Family Process, 19*, 13-18.

Watzlawick, P., Weakland, J., & Fisch, R. (1974). *Change*. New York: W.W. Norton.

Weeks, G.R., & L'Abate, L. (1982). *Paradoxical psychotherapy: Theory and practice with individuals, couples, and families*. New York: Brunner/Mazel.

16

A DEATH IN THE FAMILY

JAMES G. O'BRIEN, M.D. and ROY J. GERARD, M.D.

Man is in love,
And loves what vanishes;
What more is there to say?

—W.B. Yeats

In this chapter we will tell about a death in a family from the perspective of the four individuals who were intimately involved—three family members and the family physician. Without writing this chapter, we might never have told the story nor identified the unresolved issues. Although the critical incident that prompted this account occurred in May 1979, the story continues through the present time. So what is viewed is a frozen section of time in one family's life. The storytellers are the father, who is also the spouse of the deceased, the third youngest daughter, the youngest son, and the family physician. Instead of sitting down as a group and attempting to develop the story, we wanted each person's uninfluenced opinion rather than a consensus documentation of what happened over this period of time. At times the distinction between family physician and family became blurred and the family physician became enmeshed in the family and family dynamics; therefore, the physician's viewpoint is not necessarily that of an outsider who viewed the death with objectivity, but the perspective of an individual who was intimately involved.

This chapter is not a "how to" manual for physicians who deal with families in which a member is dying. We do, however, talk about death in general and about the impact on individuals and families by using a series of vignettes that seem to offer insights into family dynamics and personal feelings. The story may be confusing in that it is not clear when Patsy was actually considered "dead" by her family. Was it at the time of her cardiac arrest when to all intents and purposes she was removed physically and psychologically from her family? Or did death occur two years later with her physical death and burial? Our suggestion is that in terms of understanding the dynamics, one view the *acute event* as an example of a sudden unexpected death with all its attendant sequelae, and then view her death two years later as the *expected death* of an individual who had a chronic illness. Clearly, this story has gaps for many reasons, but particularly because of the discomfort and pain involved in recalling a time that stretched and strained relationships and caused much pain and anguish. The recalling and discussion of these events, however, have proved to be worthwhile and have helped to begin to resolve many formerly unresolved issues that are discussed at the end of this chapter.

Period Preceding Patsy's Cardiac Arrest

Jim O'Brien

Patsy was 50 years old at the time of her illness. I had known the family for about 11 years, serving as family physician to most of its members. Roy and I were very close friends, and I also felt close to most of the other family members. A complex series of relationships existed: friends, physician-patient, professional colleague, and chairman-faculty member. I was one of the first residents recruited by Roy in 1968, and I had subsequently served as chief resident, associate director, and associate to Roy.

Before this time, the family had been under a lot of stress. Roy and Patsy's relationship seemed to have deteriorated in the previous two years. Some of the contributing factors to the current status of their relationship were of recent origin, although clearly some of the difficulties represented an exacerbation of long-term problems. Although I served as family physician to Roy and most of the family, my involvement with Patsy was as a friend. In the past, marriage counseling had been provided by a physician in another community.

The children in general could be characterized as attractive, bright, outgoing, and friendly. Each child seemed to have a special relationship with the mother. At the time of illness, Roy, Patsy, Celeste, Juliette, Marianne, and R.J. lived at home (Table 1). (The six older children who had already left home were Patrice, Michelle, Tim, Tom, Suzette, and Elise. See Table 2 for whereabouts of the family members at present.)

Although they were experiencing significant difficulties, I felt that the family was still capable of coming together and uniting for holidays. An observation that supports that impression occurred every Christmas when

Table 1

Household Members and Family Physician, 1979

Patsy	50-year-old mother of 10 children, spouse to Roy. Homemaker.
Roy	54-year-old father and Patsy's spouse, a physician, and Chairman, Department of Family Practice.
Celeste	19-year-old quiet "brain" of the family, seemed to be doing well as a freshman at a local university.
Juliette	17-year-old senior in high school, tended to be somewhat rebellious and to associate with friends who caused her family some concern.
Marianne	15-year-old sophomore in high school, characterized as very bright and as being "difficult" at times.
R.J.	12-year-old, attended junior high school. He had a particularly close relationship with both parents and was well adjusted and loved sports.
Jim O'Brien	36-year-old family physician. Associate Chairman, Department of Family Practice.

Table 2

Where Are They Now (1984)?

Roy	Continues as a single parent. He has experienced a major adjustment in lifestyle with much more involvement now with the younger children and he still acts as the major resource person for many of the older children. He has benefited significantly since writing the chapter.
Patrice	Practicing as a clinical psychologist, married and living in Michigan.
Michelle	Is happily married with a new baby daughter and is living in New York.
Tim	Happily married in East Lansing and also has a baby daughter.
Tom	Living in Arizona.
Suzette	Is happily married with a new baby in California.
Elise	Has been promoted recently and is now a regional manager.
Celeste	Has received her master's degree in speech pathology and is married to Dean, now living in Saginaw, Michigan.
Juliette	Has moved to Florida this past year and is managing a pharmacy there.
Marianne	Is a senior at University of Michigan and is applying for medical school.
R.J.	Is a senior in high school. Still active in sports and has made a good adjustment.
Cathy	Continues to work on a part-time basis as the housekeeper.
Jim O'Brien	Is Associate Chairman and recently returned from a year's fellowship.

typically all the Gerards were at home, an event that Patsy always captured on film and revealed on the next year's Christmas card, which was no mean feat considering the number involved. Often the family mood could be very upbeat and happy, but at other times labile and sad. During times of stress some children allied with one or the other parent while others tried to stay uninvolved and neutral. During those times I tried to support Roy, which strained the relationship between Patsy and me.

Roy

It is difficult to talk about Patsy's death without reflecting on the events that preceded her illness. Looking back to 1979, I think the most significant event was the opening of the trout season. I postponed going fishing on the first day because the winter had been quite cold, and then there had been snow on the ground. So we decided to wait until the first Saturday in May to go to our cabin. R.J., then 12, went up with Patsy and me, and we took our dog Andy, a schnauzer. Early morning Saturday was lovely, but as the day progressed it began to get cloudy and rainy, and then it snowed. Patsy had invited some friends to visit us. The snow began to get thicker, so wet and heavy that a large bough broke off from a pine tree next to the cabin. The branch looked like a Christmas tree, so I put it inside a ceramic jug, and we had Christmas in May. That was really significant because Patsy would not be at home for Christmas that year, and I never dreamed that the events of the next two weeks would change my life, her life, and our lives forever.

Celeste

Before mother became ill, she basically ran the whole household. She was the dominant person. Dad was weak in comparison, but together they balanced each other. She was the person you would go to to ask permission about something. She would be the one who kept Dad in line. She would calm him when things went wrong. I can still hear her say, "For God's sake, Roy, calm down!" She always tried to make everyone feel special. She would send cards and presents. She gave all the kids a lot of emotional support, especially my sisters Elise and Michele. She and R.J. were particularly close. She always got all the kids birthday and Christmas presents, and she tried to find "special" gifts that would mean a lot to the person who received them. I would have to say she was the center of the family and everything else rotated around her, even Dad. She was stubborn and made known her wants (which she usually got). But she was kind of the one who kept everything moving smoothly. She was a very good mother, and although she was going through a lot of her own special problems, she loved everyone very much, and you knew this. She was a "fun-loving" and "crazy" type of person. I have to smile when I think of her own personality and the effect it had on every life she touched. She had so much spirit and personality. Even with her own problems and during her own depression, she seemed so alive. There was no one quite like her and never will be.

May 1979: Patsy's Cardiac Arrest

R.J.

The last time I saw her was when she took me to my piano lesson. She made me go back in the house for a raincoat. Then she dropped me off and told me she was going in for a check-up. I never saw her again.

Jim O'Brien

Roy asked me to see Patsy for an illness characterized by a cough, shortness of breath, and orthopnea of a few days' duration. I discovered she had atrial fibrillation and congestive cardiac failure with acute pulmonary edema. I admitted her to the coronary care unit and requested a cardiologist to see her. She was extremely anxious about hospitalization at that time, and I reassured her that I would let nothing happen to her. Within two days, a second cardiology consultation was requested because of her slow response to therapy. At 11:00 P.M., two days after her admission, I received an urgent call from the hospital asking me to come right away. The resident informed me that Patsy had suffered a cardiac arrest and was being resuscitated.

Roy

After leaving the hospital I drove around for a while, and by that time it was around 11:30 P.M. I pulled my car into the driveway only to meet my daughter, Celeste, who was hysterical and said that the hospital had just called, that something terrible had happened to Mother, and that we ought to get over there right away. At the hospital I saw Jim O'Brien and, from the look on his face, it was clear that a terrible thing had happened because he looked like death warmed over, and he said that Patsy had arrested. He said he didn't think she would live through the night. The whole episode I don't remember very well. I never left that place. I don't know how long I was there, but it was awful because she was obtunded and lay there with a tube in her mouth and her head stiff. I was angry at myself, at Patsy, at the hospital, and at the doctors because of what had happened, and I had a hard time talking to people about the whole situation. I remember trying to get in touch with my kids and telling them to come home, particularly Suzette in California. For me the first few days were like being unconscious.

Celeste

Dad was gone. I was in bed sleeping, and I heard the phone ring. Marianne answered it and then came and woke me. The hospital wanted to talk to Dad. When she informed them that Dad wasn't home, they asked her to have Dad call the hospital. When I heard this, I had a sinking feeling that something was really wrong. I tried to call Dr. O'Brien, but when his line was busy, I knew something was really wrong. Dad came home shortly afterward; I told him to call the hospital immediately. Next thing I heard him screaming and sobbing. He said, "Mother's had a heart attack." I threw on some clothes and we raced to the hospital, Dad driving through every red light and sobbing hysterically. I can still see him pounding on the hospital door. At the Cardiac Care Unit, I think we saw Tim, my oldest brother, and Dr. O'Brien; I can't remember. I remember seeing Mother; she looked so sick. She was having some kind of subcortical reaction and her hands were curled and her arms were waving in slow motion. It was so sickening. I thought for sure she was going to die and I almost wanted her to. She looked so terrible. I remember staying at the hospital until about 5:00 A.M., then going home and lying in bed (I didn't sleep). I felt so bad for R.J. and Marianne; they were so young. I don't remember all the details, but all the family got home. I was so glad. I thought Mother would die before Suzette and Michelle got home and I knew that would be terrible for them. The next few days we took turns staying with Mom at all times; we didn't want her to be alone. I just couldn't bear the thought of her dying alone. I remember getting up at 3:00 A.M. and going to the hospital and just holding her hand. I felt so helpless; she had so many tubes and equipment attached. I remember staring at the respirator, watching it go up and down, and being so terrified that it would stop. It was like the only sign of life and movement around her. It was like she was dead but yet alive; it was so sickening.

R.J.

I remember being in bed and hearing Dad crying and getting up with Celeste and everybody being upset. Then I was told to fall asleep and in the morning was told by Patrice that Mom was really sick but that she would probably get better. I didn't know how sick she was until I saw her two days later, and she was in a coma, and I remember she had a baseball in her hand that Dad had gotten autographed by one of her favorite baseball players. I was really scared, and I didn't think she was going to get better, so I talked with Patrice who told me what everything was. I didn't see her again while she was in the coronary care unit.

Jim O'Brien

Patsy was on a respirator, deeply comatose, unresponsive to any stimuli and exhibiting decerebrate rigidity. Gradually, the family trickled in, obviously devastated, exhibiting shock, denial, and asking for explanations that were difficult. This initial phase, during the first few days, was characterized by family members' being extremely sad, present most of the time in the hospital, coping with chaotic schedules, experiencing loss of a sense of time, and despite what appeared to be a very bleak prognosis, attaching great significance to any sign of hope, even if it was no more than "no further deterioration." There was much visible support for the family during this period from friends, neighbors, colleagues, and hospital personnel. There seemed to be a lot of togetherness and cohesion in the family with just some minor flare-ups.

As the physician, it was difficult for me to relate to so many people, so most of my contacts took place in the waiting room or hallway. On one occasion, I invoked the wrath of a family member by not holding out much hope for a better prognosis. This was a particularly difficult time for me, with a great sense of having failed as a physician and friend and now being incapable of meeting the needs created by the new problem. I was totally immersed in what was going on at the hospital. All the minute changes in Patsy's status were reported to me. Roy did not want any other physicians making decisions without my prior approval. I was able to keep up this pace because I believed this would end very soon.

Gradually, over the next weeks, it became apparent that we had all invested ourselves in this problem emotionally and physically as if it were a sprint, only to realize we were in fact running a marathon and were now exhausted. Work, my own family, and my other obligations now needed to be given some attention, but because of the model of family practice Roy and I had always believed in and promoted, I felt that anything less than my present effort would not be appropriate.

Roy

I went through the motions for a while. Patsy was still unconscious and everything seemed blurred. By that time it was Juliette's graduation and I had never been alone like that before. Like most families, we always got together for significant events. We went through the motions and I don't remember ever being so frustratingly lonely. Graduations are joyous events and I was miserable. Then my dog was killed, and that was probably the crushing blow for me. I could talk to the dog and the dog couldn't talk back. I don't know the day now, but it was some time in June when Jim O'Brien said we needed to do a tracheostomy. This is really freaky because one of my biggest fears in medicine is a tracheostomy. When the surgeon told me he was going to do a tracheostomy, I waited for three hours and he never came back to tell me about it. I asked the nurses when my wife was going to be out of the operating room and found she had been out for two hours.

TWO MONTHS LATER: SUMMER 1979

Roy

Patsy gradually improved a bit to the point where, if we asked her to move her toes or eyes, she would make an effort, and I knew that was going on although it was difficult to convince friends, family, physicians, and nurses. Her friend Mary who came to visit her had faith in God that with prayer Patsy would get better, and then Patsy did improve a little.

September was kind of the magic time when either she was going to improve or not. By now the medical reality of her prolonged illness was beginning to sink in and I was being deluged with bills. Medical economics were a major problem for me. The one feeling I remember most was my anger. I was angry at doctors. Here I was working at a medical school teaching future doctors, and I was at a point where I absolutely hated them.

R.J.

I used to come home for lunch from school and I could no longer do that. Also, in the evenings after school I really missed her. Oftentimes she would fry apples for me and do other small things that no one else could do. At first when she was in the C.C.U., I didn't want to see her. When I saw her I thought she looked useless, but then afterwards I always felt good. Celeste helped most at home at that time. She stayed home more and took care of me, also my Dad and other sisters, but nobody could really replace Mom. Gradually, Mom improved a little bit and when they said she could hear and see, I used to talk with her. I also missed her helping me with my schoolwork. She always helped when I had homework.

Celeste

When Mother started to stabilize, everyone went to their own homes and it was just immediate family who lived here in East Lansing. It was like "life goes on" and "everything returns to normal" but it never really did. For the people who weren't here maybe life returned to normal, but not for me. I guess I too got into a routine; it involved daily visits and newhousehold responsibilities. I felt guilty if I didn't go to the hospital every day. On the weekends, I went to Saginaw (65 miles away, to see my boyfriend Dean). I felt terribly guilty and Dad didn't really help. I felt like I was deserting her. I liked going to see Mom every day, but it did get depressing. You can only say so much and talk about so many things. One of the hardest things was just thinking of what to talk to her about. I felt like I would run out of things to say after about five minutes. I just didn't know what to say. I did feel good about seeing her almost every day. It made me feel like I was doing the most I could, but on the other hand, I wanted to do more but didn't know what to do. It was hard going to see her, especially on slow days when she was worse than ever and didn't respond at all. Yet on her good days one smile or wink would make it all really worth it! Things at home were difficult. I felt I was expected to take over and assume the responsibility for the things Mother did, like buying birthday presents, buying R.J. clothes, etc. Marianne and R.J. couldn't stand my telling them what to do, and at the same time Dad expected me to assume this role. Maybe I took too much upon myself but I felt so bad for Dad, and someone had to assume Mother's role. Dad was going crazy between worrying about Mother, Marianne, and R.J.; he was beside himself. I felt like someone had to be the strong one, and at times I felt there was no one there to give me the support I needed.

Five Months Later

Roy

By now Patsy had improved enough that we were sitting her up in a wheelchair and trying to support her. It was difficult for her to hold her head upright when she was in the wheelchair so we would have to put the chair back a little bit. But at least she was out of bed and we were making progress, and there was some hope. In addition to taking her to physical therapy, we were working on transferring her some place. I remember we had a faculty retreat around that time, and I had to leave it because she went into pulmonary edema. I would find myself having a little bit of hope on the one hand and then despair on the other. She was really sick again. Jim kind of indicated to me that this could happen again and again. I remember a woman saying to me at that time, "Well, why doesn't she just die? This isn't fair to anyone." I thought how could anyone say that to me, and then on the other hand, part of me felt that way too.

I think the next most significant event was that my house was chaotic. My kids were trying to hold the household together, but it was a lot of work. I decided I had to have some structure in my home for R.J. and Marianne and take some of the pressure off the older kids, Celeste and Juliette. A family practice resident who was involved in a religious community helped me to find a housekeeper, Cathy, a member of his group. She was a different kind of woman, 26, very kind, a good cook; she looked at the kitchen and figured it would take two weeks to clean it up.

There was nothing we could do except be there, and I felt desperate most of the time. During one of the most difficult periods, I was concerned that R.J. had not said much about his mother. I remember driving home from the hospital with him. He really didn't like to go, and he said that he wished Patsy would die because she wasn't going to be the same again, and then he started to cry. I don't remember much after that.

Winter 1979

Roy

Finally, during the winter Patsy stabilized some and we decided to try and take her home for the day on a Sunday afternoon. I remember that vividly because I was terrified. How could I manage her at home even for a few hours? What if something went wrong? What about her tracheostomy? What if it became congested? I gave all kinds of excuses for not wanting to take her home because I was afraid I couldn't take care of her. I remember we did. Kathy, a medical student, and a licensed practical nurse from the hospital stayed with Patsy most of the time. The visit helped to some extent because I began to think that maybe she could come home and maybe she would get better, although nobody said that. That was just a kind of fantasy that I had.

Jim O'Brien

Gradually, the family began to pick up the pieces and resume some normal activities. Roy began to appear at work, which at least lessened one of my burdens. Patsy was in a private room in the hospital though still quadriplegic, aphasic, with feeding tube, catheter, tracheostomy, IVs, and only able to communicate by expression and eye movements. Not really a chronic phase, this was an intermittent acute-on-chronic phase with multiple medical problems including pneumothorax, pneumonia, anaphylaxis, congestive cardiac failure, urinary tract infections, and renal failure. These events were particularly devastating and disruptive as the family and caregivers tried to develop a comfortable routine. I was really struggling now to see her every day and coordinate her care at Roy's request, which was extremely restrictive and exhausting. Being enmeshed in the family or at least in the family dynamics, I found it difficult to retain my objectivity as physician and function as caregiver, friend, and colleague.

Christmas 1979

Roy

Christmas that year we planned to take her home again, and we were getting kind of brave about it. We had made all the arrangements, and then on Christmas eve morning Patsy almost died. Her fever spiked and she had pneumonia. Christmas evening we were all in her room and her fever was down. We all sang Christmas carols. Even though it was sad, it was kind of beautiful.

Jim O'Brien

Another of the many crises occurred on Christmas eve seven months after Patsy's cardiac arrest, on a day that I had planned to spend shopping with my wife and children. I received a call from the hospital notifying me of Patsy's 104-degree temperature. I directed the nurse to call the doctor who was on call for our group that day. Within minutes, I received another call from Roy requesting me to please come see her as he was really concerned. I responded and solved one family problem but created a major one in my own family. I am not sure to whom I was responding—friend, fellow physician, chairman—and why. Was it because Roy induced guilt feelings if I delegated the responsibility to another physician, or did I need to maintain control over this case to meet some personal needs? I was very angry because I was not allowed to share this responsibility with other physicians, but I had difficulty expressing this anger to Roy because he was so vulnerable at that time.

I could offer little support as a friend and colleague because the only energy left was to perform my medical tasks as a physician. The whole problem was so overwhelming that even my role as a physician to Patsy became automatic and programmed, as I felt this was the only way I could survive, namely by conserving my physical and emotional reserves.

My relationship with Roy became strained because of the excessive expectations he imposed on me as friend, physician, and colleague, and it was difficult for me to deal with that. I thought seriously of leaving but stayed because I felt I was leaving for the wrong reasons; in addition, I felt Roy's excessive demands were prompted not by malice but by helplessness. Roy was my conduit to the family and the person who controlled the flow of information; he was also the "family medical decision-maker." I made many attempts to break out of the web and disengage from the family or at least drop one of my roles, either as physician, colleague, or friend. Somehow this was difficult to negotiate. It was not just Roy's need to keep me involved but also a desire on my part to see this through.

During this time, a person emerged who I think contributed much to the family and to my survival. Kathy, a sophomore medical student, had befriended Patsy and was a frequent visitor to the hospital. I first met her when I arrived at the hospital at 4:00 A.M. to do an emergency cutdown, only to find her holding Patsy's hand and reading to her. She served as an incredibly valuable person by being an informed monitor for Patsy, which I believe contributed greatly to Patsy's quality of care. She became triangled with Roy and me, and subsequently she communicated my plight to the family and communicated their problems and needs to me at a time when my communication with the family was difficult because the family expected Patsy to get better and I expected her to die. This did result in some respite for me. My impression was that the family, despite the horrendous ordeal and struggle, was getting by.

Spring 1980

Jim O'Brien

During this period I saw Roy many times about a variety of medical problems he was having, such as tachycardia, palpitation, and shortness of breath. These were terrifying to him and had definite similarities to his wife's condition. But in contrast, his symptoms were benign. On one occasion I made an emergency house visit to see his 16-year-old daughter, Marianne, who was having chest pain, palpitations, and shortness of breath. This also proved to be an anxiety attack. The similarity of husband and daughter's physical symptoms to Patsy's presentation is interesting. R.J. was having difficulty in school with failing grades and social misbehavior. One time, when he spent an evening at my house, he tore one of my daughter's dolls to shreds. I felt this might represent anger at his mother although it was not well directed. I discussed this with Roy and he received help primarily from open discussion and assistance from Kathy, the medical student, who took great interest in R.J. and served as a substitute figure for his mother in many ways.

I was able to sense Roy's feelings of grief and frustration. Because of my own frustrations, I could express only sympathy for him, which I think he sensed, and this worsened the closed communication between us. My comfort level with the other family members was much greater and there may have been multiple reasons for this, not the least of which had to do with Roy's being the family leader, ambassador, and requester of difficult tasks. I think Roy and I, because of our expertise as physicians, exhibited much in the way of telepathy, but because of feeling overwhelmed and exhausted were unable to offer empathy to each other.

In retrospect, I felt that as long as I was making a contribution at my present level of involvement, the empathy would have to come from another source or from within the family, because physically and emotionally I was drained. There was criticism from many colleagues about my being overinvolved, which I think was correct; yet few colleagues helped to find solutions to the problem. I believe many of my colleagues could identify my degree of involvement as being problematic but perhaps were concerned about being placed in a similar position if they were to join in the management of the problem.

I was concerned about Celeste, whose commitment was unswerving and constant. While others around her were crumbling, she remained steadfast. I still cannot believe the load she carried without complaint while continuing to achieve straight A's at school. Some of the major tasks of holding the family together were carried out by Celeste.

Roy was the one most hopeful of Patsy's recovery, which was not congruent with how the rest were feeling. He continued to work very hard on a rehabilitation program for Patsy which was typical of him as a physician: never give up. Some of the staff members became so attached to Patsy that they would frequently come in on their days off to attend some of our planning sessions with family members and staff or just to visit.

Our assessment at this time was that Patsy exhibited the features of a "locked-in syndrome." A computed tomography, at first resisted by the family, suggested that this diagnosis, brainstem infarction, was accurate. It was difficult to ascertain really how much Patsy understood of any communication, although I think we all believed she did know and seemed to respond appropriately to stimuli. But people varied a great deal in how they communicated with and related to her. The impact of the illness had a disruptive effect on our department, which was in limbo for a while with most of the members afraid to communicate in a direct fashion with Roy about Patsy. The department was like a family experiencing a crisis, lacking direction and guidance from its parent, Roy.

Roy

By February 1980, there was pressure on me to take my wife out of the hospital and place her in some kind of extended care facility. I was desperate and didn't really know what to do. Jim O'Brien said he would help me, so we visited some extended-care facilities. We went to a county facility and had mixed feelings about it. It looked all right, but God, I thought, how can I put my wife in a place like this? What will people think about me as a physician if I put her in a nursing home? About that time two chairmen colleagues suggested I consider taking her to a convent in a rural area. Initially, I felt this was too far from our home—45 miles. But I visited the convent and met Sister Mary and the whole group of nuns. Although they were very kind, it seemed completely unrealistic for me to put Patsy in a convent by herself. They showed me the room she would be in and how they would provide for her. This is not a nursing home; but the sisters said they accept challenges they dedicate to God by caring for people who have no other means of supporting themselves and need special care. In addition, they have a lay ministry which includes some physicians. In terms of receiving the best medical and nursing care and having a group who would be totally devoted to her, we could not ask for more. But I felt I was hiding Patsy away. I knew it was a dead-end street and she wasn't going to get any better. After talking it over with my family and with Jim O'Brien and other colleagues, I finally came to the conclusion that the convent was the place to take her.

The Sunday afternoon we transferred her there I explained to Patsy what we were doing. We got in the ambulance and drove to the convent, got her situated and comfortable, but I really had mixed feelings. I knew the nuns would love her, but she belonged in my home and this was just another phase of distancing myself from her and from her illness. Jim O'Brien had said I needed to do that but it was hard. I felt like I was being programmed for her death and that I had to get used to her being away and to being alone.

Summer 1980

Celeste

The convent was a relief on the one hand with no more daily visits to that damn hospital, but at the same time it brought guilt feelings. I felt terrible just seeing Mother once a week and for one hour, which was all I could handle. The nuns drove me crazy. I hated driving up there, and I felt terrible because I should have gone to see her more. I still do. I should have gone twice a week or more. When I think of her lying in that bed all alone, I still feel terrible. I know I saw her a lot more than some of the other kids, but maybe it still just wasn't enough. I don't know if anything would have been enough. It used to make me really mad when people used to say she would be better off dead. How do people know that? How can you say that one hour a week holding one of the kids' hands and smiling doesn't make life worth living and bearable for her? It used to make me mad that the other kids didn't visit her more, but who am I to say? They have their own conscience.

Jim O'Brien

The family desperately needed a respite from the continuing demands of caring for a terminally ill person for 10 months. Clearly, the problem was all the more difficult because of our inability to estimate her survival time, which could theoretically continue for years; the multiple acute problems superimposed on the chronic problem; and the fact that Patsy could not really communicate with her family made it incredibly difficult for them to receive thanks, anger, advice, and love in a way that could be appreciated. So many of the family members were concerned by the fact that perhaps this input and commitment to her were unrecognized, especially by Patsy. Did her memory remain intact? This last factor imposed a huge burden on the family. If only she had been able to communicate, she could have lessened their physical and emotional burden by applying limits to their involvement and by sharing their grief and by showing acceptance and appreciation.

FALL 1980

Roy

Patsy's going to the convent gave me a little peace from the standpoint that I began to get more of a routine in my life. I was trying to do my job as chairman and trying to be a father to my kids, which I found difficult. I would usually visit her once during the week, sometimes twice, but I would always go there on Saturday and Sunday. I hated to go there, but I felt I should. One incident stands out. I drove to the convent with Dr. O'Brien who had not visited Patsy since her transfer two months before. She was asphyxiating as we entered her room and, without thinking whether we should or should not, we intervened, and she was transferred to the local hospital for emergency treatment. This was significant because at that point I was out of synchrony with the nuns and her new physician in terms of her potential for recovery. I believed that there was no hope, and they believed God was going to make her better and functional again. Despite my disbelief in their prognostications, I tried to make my visits more meaningful, reading to her more and playing music that she enjoyed.

A new difficulty for me at this time stemmed from the nuns' feeling that I could help Patsy, myself, and my family more if I were to join their lay physician order. Because this was contrary to my beliefs, I had to resolve the dilemma of not offending a group who was vital to me and my family and yet participating in my wife's care in the best way possible and the only way I was capable of at this time.

Jim O'Brien

After Patsy's transfer to the convent, my life was much less complex. I had been relieved of one major obligation, and I think I was able to support the rest of the family in a more direct way—both as physician-adviser and as a friend who cared. When Patsy became part of a new committed and enthusiastic group who really believed her full recovery was possible, this was in conflict with most of the family who felt she was in a definite decline which would terminate in death. This was a dilemma.

Christmas 1980

Roy

Christmas 1980 was one of the most beautiful I have had in my life. Christmas had always been a special time since our marriage when I was a medical student. You planned for Christmas for two or three weeks and this was something that Patsy had always impressed on our kids. It was extremely rare not to have the whole family together for Christmas. Probably the two things we loved most in our lives were Christmas and football, so Christmas of 1980 was my gift to her. To get her home was a great undertaking as she was not very well at the time. I had to get a hospital bed, oxygen and suction equipment, and 24-hour nursing care. All of that and decorate the house. We went to the convent to pick her up and somehow the trip was okay. I was always a nervous wreck worrying that her tracheostomy tube would plug up and so on, but it never did. I put her in the living room and she seemed really happy. I never told her our dog had died. She was at home for almost a week. I was scared about it but I had the nurses, and Kathy, the medical student, helped greatly during that time. On Christmas day we carried Patsy to the couch in the family room, and all the children opened their gifts in front of her. She seemed to enjoy it and smiled, and we had a beautiful Mass with Father Mac, our local priest, whom she loved. It was a beautiful Christmas that my children and I will always remember. It was Patsy's last time at home and, taking her from the house to the ambulance, I think she knew she would never be home again. It was as though a little bit of her died at that time. I believe that all the children felt she was going to die and in their own way prepared for the inevitable.

Celeste

It was great when she came home for Christmas. She seemed so happy to be home. Yet it was terrible to send her back there. It just broke my heart when she cried as she left. I wanted her home, but I knew it was impossible. It was so sad to send her back up there to be alone in terms of not having her family all the time, although she had the nuns.

Spring 1981

Jim O'Brien

Patsy had the undivided attention of the nuns who accepted her as one of their own. She became their challenge. This approach was worthwhile, and the cohesion between nuns and family increased when the nuns, too, became convinced Patsy was not going to get better but was going to die. The problems were not having her family close by and her inability to determine the type and extent of her care.

Patsy was deteriorating rapidly. I had not seen her for months. I drove to the convent one morning about a week before she died and chatted with her while two nuns were in the room. I wondered if she really understood what I was saying as there was little response from her that day. When I told her I wanted to say goodbye, she cried. I embraced her and left. She really did know.

Celeste

I was with her the afternoon she died. She was really out of it. I wished she would have been more alert. I wanted to tell her goodbye and that it was okay for her to go, but I never had a chance. I really wish I could have said that to her. I know she knew that I loved her, but it just would have made me feel better to say those things. I needed to say goodbye. I was alone at home the night she died; Dad was with Mom. I kept waiting for him to call. All the kids were calling wanting to know how Mom was. We all knew she was going to die. It was one of the worst nights of my life. When Dad got home at 3:00 A.M. and told me she had died, a part of me died. It wasn't true, I thought, but I knew it was. I think everyone was kind of relieved that she had died, but I wasn't. I wanted her back sick or healthy. I just wanted her to be there. It made me feel so terrible to think she was gone forever.

Roy

The drive to the convent, as always, was boring. The noises of my VW convertible drowned out the car radio as I drove on U.S. 23 toward the small town to visit my wife. At least the inconveniences and noises of the car were a distraction and kept me from thinking of Patsy and what I was to do from now on. I knew the end was near, but how could I talk to her about it? Even though I am a doctor and have faced death and dying many, many times before with others, I found I could not do it now with my wife. I kept thinking if she could only talk, say something, at least I could have some feedback. Over the past two years the most she could give me was an occasional wink, a smile, and maybe if I was lucky, a nod. I fantasized that this was all a dream; Patsy hadn't really had a cardiac arrest with massive brain damage. She wasn't really paralyzed, unable to speak, swallow, or even brush a strand of hair from her cheek.

I saw the "infernal" flame of the oil refinery near the convent and was brought back to reality. Patsy *is* paralyzed, lives with the sisters, and I am on my way to visit her, a trip I had made so many times during the past months. As I got closer to the convent, I could smell the refinery; no wonder there were never any birds in the feeder outside Patsy's window. I had put a finch feeder near her window more than a year ago. At home we had many feeders and at times it seemed as though I was feeding the whole bird population of Michigan. Not so here. There had not been a single bird on that feeder in a year. Often I would see Patsy looking wistfully through the window at the feeder only to find it empty. I thought of the time I read *Jonathan Livingston Seagull* to her and about the episode where Jonathan says that one can be free if one truly wants it badly enough. Suddenly, I knew what I could say to Patsy.

Sister Stephanie met me at the door and said, "Patsy is fine; I have talked to her about dying, now it is your turn." She said her temperature was down and that she was looking forward to seeing me. I entered her room and she looked great. That was one of the ironies—she never looked sick. She was always in a fresh nightgown; her sheets fresh and clean; her hair neatly combed and, in spite of her 51 years, she had only one or two gray hairs. She smiled ever so slightly as I walked in. It was a small room and looked like a photographer's studio because of the pictures of our 10 children all over the walls. We could have had a bigger room, but I chose this one because it was next to Sister Stephanie's.

I told Patsy of the events of the day, how the kids were, about the budget crisis where I work, and that the Easter candy had been taken care of. Endless trivia that make our day. Finally, I looked through the window at the finch feeder swinging in the wind and said, "Patsy, I realize now that you will never see a finch again while you are alive, but after you've gone, whenever I see a goldfinch, I will feel your presence near me." She smiled with understanding, gave me a twitch of a wink, and that was the end of our discussion about death.

The next day she became feverish, septic, unresponsive, and lapsed into a terminal coma. This was Easter week and on Good Friday I felt she was near death. Again I drove to be with her at the convent. When I arrived, I was told that she was indeed near the end. I sat with her Friday night, held her, prayed for her, and at 1:30 A.M. she was free like the gull in *Jonathan Livingston Seagull.* The next morning, Holy Saturday, the finch feeder outside Patsy's window at the convent was alive with goldfinches. A coincidence? Maybe, but I like to believe not.

R.J.

For a while everything seemed so drawn out that I wanted her to die. I knew she was going to die. I remember Suzette being called and asked to come home. I cried when I found out she was dead; it was different than after the heart arrest. Now there was no hope. Death is final. At times I felt particularly fine, but then I felt sad and it came on in waves. It was scary. I hated the atmosphere; it was a gloomy day. Seems like when someone dies it's gloomy. She looked so different—not like Mother. Everyone was so upset. I remember there was a gardenia on the casket. I said "Goodbye, I miss you." I didn't think until we left the casket that I would never see her body again, although I knew she was up there. I'm doing a lot better now and can talk about it. The death brought the whole family together. Even though there were 10 kids, she treated each kid as unique and now each one can cherish their own relationship with her.

Celeste

One of the worst experiences was viewing her body at the funeral home. She looked so shitty! So dead! I'll never forget how terrible she looked. Life goes on though. I still think of her, although some days more than others. I miss her and think it is so unfair I don't have a mother. I feel terrible for R.J. growing up without a mother. Mother would be so excited about my sister Michele's baby. It's just not fair. There are so many things I have never said that I should have and so many things I never should have said. So many things I would do over but I'll never have a chance. It's just so unfair. I guess I just accepted her death. I know that my life has to go on, but I don't want it to in a sense. I don't want to lose the good memories of her when she was healthy, but they seem like such a long time ago and they grow dimmer. I just want to remember the happy and positive experiences and not the negative ones, but I remember some of both. I guess I am at least glad that I remember something. I hope R.J. remembers her as a healthy, beautiful mother—he was so young. I want him to remember how very much she loved him. It is so important.

Roy

It has been eight weeks since Patsy's freedom and the weeks have been harder for me than I had ever dreamed they could be. The loneliness is suffocating, but the finches help me to hold on. At our home the finches continue to come and at the convent they are frequent visitors. The story could end here but it doesn't.

Recently, I was at a medical meeting in Kansas City and stayed at the Crown Center, a place where Patsy and I had stayed many times before. My sadness, grief, and loss became overwhelming. Before leaving the room for the airport and the journey home, I knelt down to say a prayer. The words were difficult to find. Finally, I just blurted out, "Patsy, I hope you are happy. How can I know you are?" Sorting through the mail when I arrived home that day, I opened a letter from Patsy's niece, Susan, with whom I had shared the goldfinch story. Susan commented that she was touched by the story and was sending me the cover of *The New Yorker* magazine for the week of April 13th, the week that Patsy died. I was awe-struck. It showed an old Victorian home with a bird bath and a tree full of goldfinches. Tears came to my eyes. Patsy really did hear me—but that's not all. My son came into the room and turned on a preview of a program on HBO which traces the history of radio. In one scene the narrator turns to a young boy and says, "What are the kinds of finches native to North

America?" The young boy answers, "The goldfinch and the purple finch." My hair almost stood on end and my flesh was cold and covered with goosebumps. I shivered, but my heart was full. She heard me, and I can hear her!

Discussion

It is within the family that individuals first develop the feeling of belonging, a sense of self-worth, the ability to trust others, and a capacity for intimate relationships (Arndt & Gruber, 1977). Stress experienced by one family member clearly has an impact on all other members and affects relationships and communication within the family unit. It is also within the family that an individual first experiences frustration and the pain and agony of losing a loved member. Thus, the family is the primary group that provides preparation for life as well as for death (Arndt & Gruber, 1977).

The loss of a family member may be the single most traumatic and upsetting event in a person's life and losing a spouse is the most significant life change in terms of the amount of stress produced (Geer, 1965). It is possible, however, that the falling birth rate, the emotional investment families have in their children, and the expectancy that children will live to be adults make the death of a child the most traumatic loss of all, especially when one considers a child's vulnerability and the seeming meaninglessness of his or her death.

Factors that Influence Grief Response

The effects of the dying process on family members vary with the nature of the terminal illness, the personalities of involved family members, the history of family relationships, the importance of the dying person to each family member, the ability of all concerned to establish the kind of communication that is most satisfying to everyone, and the rapidity with which death occurs (Arndt & Gruber, 1977). To create a great sense of loss in other members, the deceased family member does not necessarily have to be the breadwinner but can be an individual who, for example, influences the mood or the togetherness feeling in a family (Bowen, 1978).

Among deaths that cause the most serious effects on the family are deaths of either parent, especially when the children are young (Kalish & Reynolds, 1976). This not only disturbs the family's emotional equilibrium but also removes the function of the parent, breadwinner, or mother at the time when these functions are most needed. In contrast, there are family members who may have been a burden in their final illness and whose deaths are a relief to the family. Even this type of person, although dysfunctional, may have played a valuable role in maintaining family equilibrium.

When death is sudden, unexpected, and occurs in a younger individual, the family has no time to prepare and deal with it, no time to process what is happening, no time to reminisce and no opportunity to work out unfinished business. Such a death seems to cause a great deal of denial among survivors.

Statistical evidence shows convincingly that the death of a family member provokes serious effects, including death of other family members. Young (1963), in his study of the effect of widowhood on survival, found that the widows' mortality rate increased by 40% during the first six months of bereavement. In a controlled case study of the impact of death on surviving family members, Rees and Lutkins (1967) found a significant increase in mortality of bereaved relatives, the greatest number of deaths occurring during the first year but continuing to be high for three to four years after the family member's death. This study also indicated a higher risk of death for male than for female relatives. Mortality among widowers increased by 19.6% in contrast to a 5% increase among widows.

Another interesting finding from the Rees and Lutkin study was that the place of death of the relative had subsequent effects on the mortality of the bereaved. If the first-to-die relative died in the hospital, in contrast with dying at home, the risk of mortality to the bereaved was doubled. Further, the risks of subsequent death were increased fivefold if the first relative died at a place other than the home. This finding might be influenced by the fact that many of these deaths were accidental and more likely to have been sudden and traumatic.

A family's past response to losses will influence its current response. Grief may be greater for the surviving family members who perhaps had a more dependent relationship with the deceased, or in situations in which the loss is unexpected and sudden with no anticipatory grief. Parkes (1964) noted that high stress during the last two years preceding the death and losing a parent during childhood are other factors that accentuate and intensify grief reactions.

Grief in the Individual

The shock and numbness of the first phase of grief resemble a physical illness. Grief has, in fact, been identified by Parkes (1964) as a disease state and a legitimate cause of death. Bereavement often means multiple losses: loss of a partner, a lover, supporter, audience, disciplinarian, social facilitator, and income provider.

Lindemann (1944) defined grief as a definite syndrome with somatic and psychological symptoms. Although in the strict medical sense it may not be accepted as such, weeping, sighing, respiration, decreased strength, physical exhaustion, guilt, sense of unreality, anger, agitation, insomnia, and depression are usually present. Many of the somatic complaints are secondary to a sympathetic overactivity, as was perhaps exhibited by Roy after Patsy's death and by Marianne before her mother died. This overactivity generally peaks during the first month. Parkes (1972) discovered in his study of London widows that the more pronounced these somatic symptoms were, the greater was the potential for anger and for poor health subsequently.

Although many people believe that the most characteristic feature of grief is prolonged depression, this is not so. Brief, frequent episodes of grief accompanied by acute anxiety and extreme psychological pain are much more common. Family members experience these during the first few weeks, and the episodes often peak between the fifth and fourteenth day (Parkes, 1964). Stimuli like a photo or a familiar sound may trigger this response. Bowlby (1961) has referred to this as "yearning and protest." When it is accompanied by sympathetic overactivity, it is obvious why the newly bereaved person suffers palpitations, insomnia, difficulty concentrating, and aimless activity.

Pining is a persistent and obtrusive wish for the person who is gone. This is often accompanied by the "searching phenomenon or an attempt to recover the lost object," perhaps an example of which is Roy's goldfinch story. The searching phenomenon may also explain the high incidence of hallucinations experienced at this time. Bowlby (1961) identified the need for empathy during this period as being critical for the bereaved person's ability to move through this stage. If this is absent, the bereaved person may become fixed at any one of these stages.

Bowlby defined mourning as the psychological process set in motion by the loss of a loved object and which, when completed, is associated with the relinquishing of that object.

Grief in the Family

As Hill (1958) described it, the family response to crisis occurs in several phases: an initial period of stunned denial; confusion, anxiety, and frequent resentment toward the dead or dying person; a period of recovery and reorganization with a gradual move toward a new homeostasis, which may be equal, lower, or higher than the previous level of functioning. Often the family's stages of grief parallel those of the individual as described above; but they may be asynchronous in the family, and not all members go through all stages (Kalish, 1977). Mourning tends to unite family members in a common purpose and goal, but often there are intense feelings of pain and grief about the loss and a sense of abandonment. Pain and fear arising from the loss of a loved one are eased by mutual grief and expression of feelings, but guilt is often projected by blaming others, and sometimes a family scapegoat emerges to bear the brunt of the anger.

There are many unknowns and many new tasks. The loss of someone who died essentially before her natural life span was over will provoke a much greater response in family members than the death of an older person who was chronically disabled, was no longer a breadwinner, and whose family achieved independence. The younger person who died still had roles to play, was still productive, and often had young children who are now deprived of a source of emotional stability and love and have lost a model for developing sex-role behavior. Often the family will change when children take on an adult role and attempt to act as a substitute parent (Kalish, 1977).

Guilt

Because no relationship is perfect, guilt may be a very powerful feeling at this time, especially when one reflects on how things might have been and on how one might have contributed more. Now the stark reality that nothing can be done and nothing made up in a way that matters strikes home. Mild death wishes are common, especially in children. Since death has occurred, the survivors may now feel that they contributed to it in some way. Obviously, most adults are able to deal with these thoughts intellectually and know that this way of thinking has no validity. Lacking the same intellectual capacity, a child may continue to struggle with this feeling of guilt. Anger and guilt may alternate in a vicious cycle (Kalish, 1977). Family members may be angry with the dead person for having abandoned them, but they may repress the anger, knowing intellectually that the dead person did not choose to die. They may reason that for most people death is a tragedy, and that compared to the dead person's loss, their one loss is small. Yet, these thoughts often provoke feelings of guilt, which in turn intensify the anger, and so the cycle continues.

Anger

According to Bowlby (1961), anger is a normal component of grief, particularly early on, but it may alternate with apathy and depression. For the family, death may be personalized and viewed as harm done to the bereaved. Sometimes the blame is directed at physicians, the hospital, other family members, and God (Kalish, 1977), because anger is an emotion often misdirected. Quarrels with those closest to the bereaved may result in alienation and social isolation when the need for support is greatest. Occasionally these feelings are expressed by family members who had an ambivalent relationship with the dead person.

Equilibrium

Family responsibilities need to be reassigned, and later the family must establish new relationships (Kalish, 1977). A family that has demonstrated its ability to adapt and to cope effectively with crises is more likely to mourn in a way that ends with satisfactory resolution. The more open the communication among family members, the better the chances for a reasonable outcome. Barriers to communication tend to grow out of a need to protect family members from hurt or sadness or out of accumulated feelings of bitterness. The family system experiencing the death of one of its members is in a state of disequilibrium, and relationships will show evidence of strain. Readjustments, new roles, and new responsibilities tend to create an emotional overload when compounded with relational conflicts and dysfunctional communication in a family system.

Fatal Illness

The person who is chronically and terminally ill needs to make changes to allow the family to compensate for losing him or her. If this person is the main breadwinner and major decision-maker, responsibility for tasks like managing finances needs to be relinquished to another or several other family members. The family member then has to accept the task. Such transitions may have a major disruptive effect on the family because, as power changes hands and new roles and responsibilities must be assumed, there may be a domino-like effect on all those within the family system.

Each family has its own set of rules and regulations for family behavior. If the system is to continue to function effectively, the rules may have to be changed. They may now be challenged because their major enforcer is ill and incapacitated. A new system of functioning needs to evolve and new roles and responsibilities need to be negotiated.

Usually spouses, most often wives, bear the brunt of care for each other, and most of the responsibility for support and sustenance rests with the nuclear family.

Chronic illness changes the ways in which family members relate to each other, often with disintegrative rather than integrative effects (Bruhn, 1977). As the responsibilities for direct care often fall to a few family members, others may offer assistance in a more peripheral manner, perhaps by financial help or moral-emotional support. But the primary caregivers' stresses are great. In addition to suffering through the demands of caring for the patient, they may be subjected to criticism and unhelpful suggestions by less involved family members. The primary caregivers' greater control over the situation, their ability to limit access to the patient and control information flow, and their closer contact with the physician and greater influence on treatment are a natural source of conflict with other family members.

After the patient dies, the primary caretaker may have the greatest difficulty at first because of the tremendous void in his or her life, but may probably have the least feeling of guilt (Bruhn, 1977). The impact of chronic illness on the individual is poignantly described by Kathleen Lewis (1983), a nurse who has systemic lupus erythematosus: "I have come to believe that dying is the easy part, the breathing out of spirit, requiring no effort. The real challenge is to grieve one's losses, let go of the past and face living complicated by chronic illness, rejoicing in the gift of life."

Anticipatory Grief

Many close family members go through anticipatory grieving, a psychological rehearsal for the death that will come soon (Kutscher, 1973). In this fashion, they work through a part of the distress and are presumably better able to handle the death when it happens. Feelings of anxiety about separation or the dread of being abandoned may induce anticipatory grief and mourning. Detachment begins to occur with acceptance but, it is hoped, not to a degree that leads to isolation or abandonment. In our situation, with Patsy located a significant distance from her family, the visits of family members decreased, Roy and Celeste being the most frequent and consistent visitors. Roy recalls vividly the pain of visiting once or twice a week and the temptation to withdraw and have the nuns assume more responsibility for Patsy's care. If this phase is drawn out, it can cause feelings of impatience and frustration in the family members. We do not know, in our case, whether or not the classic sequence described by Kubler-Ross (1969) occurred. Certainly, the anger, depression, and gradual withdrawal were part of our experience.

Families struggling with the anticipation of death need to realize that it is important that children, in particular, be prepared and not shielded from the dying person or death. In our culture children tend to be protected from this stark reality (Hollingsworth & Pasnau, 1977). This in itself is a tragedy, as mourning is a way of emphasizing the difference between life and death, the separation of the dead from the living. This difference is glossed over and minimized when death and dying are spoken of in euphemisms.

Some people believe that an important stage for the dying patient, between the stages of acceptance and detachment that Kubler-Ross described, may be in "saying goodbye." This often will be initiated by the dying person, usually not overtly but perhaps by expressing appreciation for what close family members have done (Meares, 1981). The dying person attempts to let family members know they have been loved and valued. Contrast this with suicide in which the dead person has deliberately refused to say farewell. This may cause guilt feelings and depression in the survivors, especially when the suicide has been particularly vindictive. The dying person saying goodbye must receive reciprocity; it is the last opportunity to complete unfinished business.

Like the patient, the family may not go through all the stages outlined by Kubler-Ross (1969) of denial, anger, depression, acceptance, separation but may pass through many of them (Kutscher, 1973). As is true for the dying patient, the family members may not be synchronous with each other. A family that accepts death as being inevitable one day may bargain the next for some new drug or treatment. Physicians should remember that acceptance of death by patient and family does not necessarily mean that one does not have to deal with the same issue again.

Probably the most difficult phase for the family is the final stage, when a dying person begins to detach from life. Family members need to understand that this is not rejection and does not mean the dying person resents them in any way. To state this may be superfluous, but most experts seem to encourage the retention of some hope for all dying patients.

When is the best time to tell the dying patient, "You are dying"? Most able clinicians allow the patient to initiate such a conversation by asking skillful and probing questions. Some patients don't want to know, which creates a particularly difficult situation because of the incredible burden it imposes on the family and on the patient. How can the patients participate in decisions about their management or how they will live the rest of their lives? Another strain comes from trying to create a script that is untrue at a time when most dying patients suspect or know they are dying. This is a time for reconciliation. The game of mutual pretense seems to serve an important function: It protects the patient's and family member's psychological self. But one consequence is a form of social isolation when the patient and family member is in greatest need of human contact (Orcutt, 1977). How this difficult issue is handled will influence not only how the person will live, but also how he or she will die.

The opportunity to have a humane and dignified death may well depend on how effectively the individual can negotiate active participation with the family in what is possibly her or his most significant personal transition (Benoliel, 1974).

Family members of different ages need help in dispelling any myths that might hinder their involvement and participation in the death. According to Kutscher (1973),

> the presence of grief in anticipation of the loss in both subtle and pronounced ways alters the trauma of the aftermath. When death has been prepared for by those who will survive, those bereaved may more readily find their way back to normal functioning. There is a kind of symmetry and replication of effects. The more the anticipatory grief reaction before the loss, the less the bereavement effects following it. Conversely, the less the anticipatory grief before a loss, the greater the bereavement effects afterwards, such as in sudden death.

The goal in the patient's final days should be a time of sharing, loving, planning, and anticipatory grief. If this does happen, the possibility that family survivors will have a foundation on which to rebuild their lives will be much greater.

Role of Physicians

Family physicians have a unique opportunity to participate in the care of their dying patients. The demands on physicians who care for dying patients and their families are high. The physicians' role may change often, depending on the needs of patients and families and the stage of the illness, but they will often alternate between being diagnostician, coordinator, facilitator of communication, counselor, and family supporter.

To contribute successfully in this whole process, physicians need to know themselves, their reaction to and comfort with death and dying. They need to know the dying patient and that person's coping strategies, uniqueness, and role in the family. Knowing a family's attitude toward death and dying and how the family characteristically deals with stress and crisis is of great importance. Most families have no experience in dealing with death and often need to be coached and advised on how to deal with their dying member.

The physician needs more than common sense in this situation. There is a whole body of knowledge that he or she should be acquainted with. Frequently episodes of anger and discouragement need to be dealt with; without understanding how common and normal this response is, physicians may personalize it and further withdraw from their patients.

Some insight can be gained from the perspective of a dying individual and his response to hospitalization. In the book *A Private Battle* (Ryan & Ryan,

1979), Cornelius Ryan described his hospital experience vividly: "You take off your clothes and you're in their hands, unable to decide when you come or go or to plan the next day yourself. You aren't a person any longer, you're a patient without dignity or sense of self" (p. 10). An awareness of the sense of helplessness and inability to be involved in decisions that many dying patients experience should dictate to physicians to give their dying patients the opportunity to participate to the fullest extent possible in determining the type and extent of their care. Helping the family to ventilate and work through unresolved conflicts is beneficial at this time.

Cassata (1979) noted:

> Stigma is the invisible shield that surrounds terminally ill individuals and grief-stricken survivors and which mediates the communication process. All social interaction is greatly affected by the stigma surrounding death and, to a large extent, such interaction depends on the meaning that the death holds for each participant. When one is intimately or emotionally involved with the dying person, one can be restricted by a sense of loss and grief; when one is responsible for the care of that individual, vulnerabilities as a helping professional must be faced as well. This is clearly aggravated in a hospital setting. (p. 1)

The family physician can help the family decide whether or not children are to be involved in the ritual of death and dying, the funerals, and other ceremonies that serve to separate life from death and allow expression of grief and termination of relationships. Features predictive of increased risk of unresolved grief include excessive clinging, those who have reacted poorly to separation in the past, and ambivalent relationships. These factors should prompt follow-up of family members, especially when the death has been unexpected.

There are personal costs for those who undertake the undeniably stressful task of caring for the bereaved. Burnout is a risk and only knowing one's limits will prevent overcommitment. Hospice and other community support services can complement medical care and the family physician's role.

Telling our story identified unresolved problems for the participants and prompted a number of counseling sessions in which the family members and the family physician discussed and relived their experiences. Without writing this chapter, we would not have dealt with these issues, which, for some of us, clearly represent unresolved grief and anger with all the negative sequelae these can entail. Writing the chapter elicited different feelings from all of the authors. Particularly for both of us (Roy and Jim), reading the other's report of various events elicited further and perhaps more intense feelings. On one occasion, when both of us were meeting with a counselor, it quickly became apparent that Jim had a much greater need to express previously unexpressed feelings about Patsy—grief for her as a friend, anger toward Roy for keeping him involved. This response, which was unexpected then, put Roy in touch with feelings that slowly emerged in the subsequent months, and resulted in gradually increasing comfort in discussing all aspects of this experience. The process continues through today and we suspect will in the future.

A quote attributed to Cecily Saunders seems to have much relevance to us at this time: "Hopefully when the time is over, that we would be able, all of us, patient and family and us the professionals, to look back on the good hours in that period as some of the best we ever had and at least look back on the bad hours with pride."

REFERENCES

Arndt, C.M., & Gruber, M. (1977). Helping families cope with acute and anticipatory grief. In E.R. Prichard & J. Collard, et al. (Eds.), *Social work with the dying patient and the family*. New York: Columbia University Press.

Benoliel, J.Q. (1974). The dying patient and the family. In S.B. Troup & W. Greene (Eds.), *Death and the family*. New York: Scribner.

Bowen, M. (1978). *Family therapy in clinical practice*. New York: Jason Aronson.

Bowlby, J. (1961). Processes of mourning. *International Journal of Psychoanalysis*, *42*, 317-340.

Bruhn, J.G. (1977). Effects of chronic illness on the family. *Journal of Family Practice*, *4*(6), 1057-1060.

Cassata, D.M. (1979). Death and dying: Communication parameters and perspectives. Paper presented to the Annual Conference of Speech Communications Association, San Antonio, Texas.

Geer J.H. (1965). The development of a scale to measure fear. *Behaviour Research and Therapy*, *3*, 45-53.

Hill, R. (1958). Social stresses on the family. *Social Casework*, *39*, 139-158.

Hollingsworth, C.E., & Pasnau, R.O. (1977). *Response of children to death in the family in mourning: A guide to health professionals*. New York: Grune & Stratton.

Kalish, R.A. (1977). The family and death. In H. Feifel (Ed.), *New meanings of death*. New York: McGraw-Hill.

Kalish, R.A., & Reynolds, D.K. (1976). *Death and ethnicity: A psychocultural investigation*. Los Angeles: University of Southern California Press.

Kubler-Ross, E. (1969). *On death and dying*. New York: Macmillan.

Kutscher, A.H. (1973). Anticipatory grief, death and bereavement: A continuum in caring for the dying patient and his family. In A.H. Kutscher & M.R. Goldberg (Eds.), *Conference on caring for the dying patient and his family*. New York: Health Sciences Publishing Corp.

Lewis, K. (1983). Living with chronic illness. *Postgraduate Medicine*, *74*(3), 179-183.

Lindemann, E. (1944). Symptomatology and management of acute grief. *American Journal of Acute Grief*, *101*, 141-148.

Meares, R.A. (1981). On saying good-bye before death. *Journal of the American Medical Association*, *246*(11), 1227-1229.

Orcutt, B.A. (1977). Stress in family interaction when a member is dying: A special case for family interviews. In E.R. Prichard & J. Collard, et al. (Eds.), *Social work with the dying patient and the family*. New York: Columbia University Press.

Parkes, C.M. (1964). Recent bereavement as a cause of mental illness. *British Journal of Psychiatry, 110*, 198-204.

Parkes, C.M. (1972). *Bereavement studies of grief in adult life*. New York: International Universities Press.

Rees, W.D., & Lutkins, S.G. (1967). Mortality and bereavement. *British Medical Journal, 4*, 13-16.

Ryan, C., & Ryan, K.M. (1979). *A private battle*. New York: Simon & Schuster.

Young, M. (1963). Mortality of widows. *Lancet, 2*, 454-456.

17

EVALUATING THE FAMILY IN CRISIS

FRANK S. PITTMAN, III, M.D.

Crisis Theory

Crisis is a useful concept for problem-solvers. All people have problems, of course, but some have the luxury of devoting a season or a lifetime to solving or not solving some cherished problem. Others of us either have too many problems of our own, are responsible to too many people who have problems, or solve problems for a living or a hobby, so we must get efficient at problem-solving. We must get on with it. For us, the concept of crisis can be extremely helpful.

A crisis is the state of things at a time of impending change. It is the turning point at which things will either get better or worse, the intersection of events at which change is possible. Crisis and change are related concepts. It is possible to have a crisis that does not result in change, although that would require that everyone remain very still and in place, and that no one do or say anything new. But, as a matter of definition, it is not possible to have change without crisis.

When a stress bears upon a system, the system is thrown into a state of crisis, which can be resolved by change in the system or by removal of the stress. To define four words: A *stress* is a force that tends to distort; a *system* is a set of interacting parts; a *crisis* is a state of impending change; a *change* is a new or unaccustomed action outside one's usual repertoire.

Systems in general—families, individuals (each person is a system, too, of course), or other groups—have certain qualities that affect their crisis response. One characteristic of a system is that anything that affects one part of the system will affect the other parts, too. If one member of the family is in trouble, changes his or her functioning, or is concealing a secret, the shock waves will be felt throughout the family, and someone else may develop symptoms.

Another characteristic of a system is its inherent resistance to change. Families may even overlook or misinterpret stresses to avoid responding, because response might mean change. These two qualities of systems make family members exquisitely sensitive to changes in one another, yet highly resistant to outside forces. The family may grow tighter and closer the harder the world tries to change it. Our attention was first drawn to crisis theory by Erich Lindemann (1944/1965) in his classic study of the acute grief reactions of survivors of the Coconut Grove Fire. From his psychoanalytic viewpoint, the crisis was seen as surviving childhood conflicts. Since then, we have assumed that a characteristic process follows stress; whatever the stress, a crisis follows a predictable pattern.

A few years later, Gerald Caplan began publishing his extensive investigations of crisis and he identified the typical phases of crisis resolution (1956). After a stress, according to Caplan, a system will attempt its traditional problem-solving mechanisms. If these don't resolve the stress, the crisis will become more intense. Thus, the system will be mobilized to do something outside its usual range and repertoire. The mobilization either works and resolves the stress, or fails and leads to disruption of the system or such intense pressure on one person to change that that individual becomes symptomatic and serves as a new stress. Caplan observed that if some resolution does not take place within six weeks, the disequilibrium will become a way of life. Caplan also expanded the concept of crisis from an individual phenomenon to a family situation (1964).

David Kaplan, who had worked with Gerald Caplan, studied such specific stresses as the premature birth of a child (Kaplan & Mason, 1960), and he described acute emotional upsets (1962). Kaplan, Reuben Hill (1958/1965), and others expanded the family focus, moving from a psychoanalytic framework to one of systems. They described crisis behavior as more related to the specific nature of the stress or hazard rather than only to the premorbid personality.

Kaplan joined psychiatrist Donald Langsley in Colorado to organize a study of crisis-oriented family therapy as an alternative to psychiatric hospitalization. In 1964, at the University of Colorado Medical Center, Langsley and Kaplan recruited a clinical team of social worker Kalman Flomenhaft, psychiatric nurse Carol DeYoung, and myself. Psychologist Pavel Machotka supervised the research. The theoretical framework of the project was the assumption that the request for psychiatric hospitalization of a family member represented an effort to solve a family crisis. On one level, the project tested the effectiveness of family therapy as an alternative to psychiatric hospitalization. On a second level, the project developed techniques of crisis therapy.

On still another level, the project tried to explore the relationship between family crisis and serious mental illness. In its simplest form the theory was that a stress comes to bear upon a family system, throwing it into a state of crisis, which the family may attempt to resolve by hospitalizing one of its members (Langsley, Kaplan, Pittman, Machotka, Flomenhaft, & DeYoung, 1968).

The project's clinical team took a random sample of patients who had been evaluated by the emergency room psychiatrist and were determined to require immediate psychiatric hospitalization. Each of the 150 patients lived with some adult relative within an hour's drive of the Denver hospital. One-third of the patients were suffering from acute psychoses, another third were suicidally depressed or had made suicide attempts, and the rest were in manic states, had organic brain conditions, were in alcohol withdrawal, were adolescent runaways, or had school phobias or other disorders. The clinical team prevented the hospitalization, offering crisis-oriented family therapy and appropriate medication, visiting the home, making collateral contacts, and arranging appropriate outpatient follow-ups. The group was compared to a matched group of hospitalized controls and followed for several years.

The results revealed that essentially all patients with families could be treated outside the hospital, with less disruption of functioning, less family disruption, and no increase of suicides or other ill effects. In addition, family crisis therapy cost about one-sixth as much as the average 28-day hospital stay. All experimental patients were kept out of the hospital initially and only about 15% went on to subsequent hospitalizations, while 40% of those hospitalized initially had subsequent hospitalizations. Most strikingly, later hospitalizations of the experimental patients were not only far less frequent, but also much briefer than those of the controls.

The widely reported data from the Denver Project had considerable influence on the community mental health movement. The destructiveness of psychiatric hospitalization—its tendency to encourage chronicity—may result from removing the problem from the family. This removal of one member prevents the family from learning how to solve its own problems and makes mental illness seem more mysterious and difficult than it needs to be. One retrospective conclusion from the study might be that in general, it may not help psychotic people to remove them from a hospital, but it does hurt them to remove them from their family in a time of crisis. The family's involvement is an important part of the treatment of serious mental illness. If there is no family, the prognosis is worse. If the family is not involved in treatment, the treatment will be more costly, less efficient, and more likely to lead to chronicity or disruptive recurrence. The Denver Project's conclusion was that any treatment that does not involve the family bypasses the core of the problem. No family and no patient are too crazy for family therapy. Since family therapy is the treatment of choice for acute psychosis, the presence of a psychotic member, acute or chronic, hospitalized or at home, is certainly no contraindication to family therapy for family crisis.

Freeman and Simmons, in *The Mental Patient Comes Home* (1963), found that patients did better if the family was tolerant of symptoms but intolerant of nonfunctioning. By contrast, society in general and the medical profession in particular have tended to regard cessation of functioning as an appropriate response to symptoms. Anxious or depressed people are seen as suffering from excessive functional stress and encouraged to take it easy, take time off from work, give up productive activity, tranquilize themselves, get out of conflictual relationships, or even, horror of horrors, go on disability. This may be appropriate for a day or even a week, but not for long. People's lives cannot be protected by sacrificing their functioning. There are rare exceptions to this but, generally, a stressful, even a stark raving mad, family should not be avoided. A misguided effort by family members undercuts the therapy more if they are uninvolved than if they are involved in the treatment. The more mysterious and isolated the treatment process, the more likely the family will be to misunderstand what is therapeutic about it and thus to sabotage it quite inadvertently. We cannot protect families from their patients without damaging the patients, and we cannot protect patients from their families. The best protection we can offer comes from requiring them to live with the results of their effects on one another and to take responsibility for driving one another crazy or sane.

When we are presented with a symptomatic individual, we must assume that he or she represents a family in crisis, even if the family crisis may be no more than a helpless reaction to the symptomatic member. As often as not, our first contact with a family is with a relative who is concerned about another family member's behavior. It is insufficient to focus our evaluation solely on the person with symptoms or only the one concerned about the person with symptoms. We must evaluate the system, the context in which the problematic behavior occurs.

Evaluating the Family System

However simple the crisis, there are elements we need to consider about each family. Each family system has certain characteristics that influence its crisis proneness and crisis response. These characteristics determine how families differ from one another even while facing the same stress or undergoing a similar crisis.

Boundaries

Each family has a set of members. Some belong to the immediate family, others to the extended family, and some are merely relatives. The degree to which they are included in the family functioning, family activities, and, perhaps most importantly, in family decision-making varies. The relatives are included in ceremonial occasions, may have the right to visit informally, may exchange appropriate favors, and may be privy to family business. Aunts, uncles, and cousins are sometimes treated like siblings or parents, sometimes like friends, sometimes like duties. Siblings, and even parents, are sometimes treated like duties and seen only on ceremonial occasions or not at all. Most families, however, have some extended family members who are involved in essentially all decisions and many activities. Families with close functional ties to many extended family members are more resistant to sudden change and are cushioned through life's crises. On the other hand, families with close functional ties to only one extended family member may be somewhat immobile and dependent. Loose-boundaried families, in which the members have close relationships to outsiders but little closeness to one another, may lack the mechanisms for subtle changes in functioning, and tend to drift apart rather than change in response to crisis. By contrast, families with tight boundaries may intensify internal conflict and pressure on one another more easily than call for help from outside.

In evaluating a family in crisis, we must know whether someone else—another family member or someone outside the family—needs to be consulted for change to take place. The appropriate questions here are: How do the others react to the problem? Who can help with this? Whom do we need to talk to about doing things differently? Who else sees it as a problem? Whom do you talk to about it?

It is not unusual for the family to have undergone boundary changes before the request for professional help. Some family members may have moved out or been sent away. Members of the extended family may have moved in for a time. Close friends, even casual ones, may have been brought in, too. We must know who is included as stabilizers for the family during the crisis and who is part of the usual family structure. We cannot assume that the members of the household and the members of the functional family are the same.

Some people, even when they marry, maintain strong boundaries between themselves and their spouses, treating a wife or husband much as an adolescent treats parents—as a functional necessity but a threat to individuality. Bigamists, male chauvinists, people who are having affairs, or those who are in psychoanalysis may similarly leave a spouse out of decision-making. Somewhat more common are marriages that are too tightly bound to admit any third person, even a child. Some couples have children but keep their life secret from them. The parents may even divorce and remarry without considering the children or even explaining the situation to them.

At the opposite end of the spectrum are those couples who use their children as marriage counselors and referees in marital battles. Occasionally a parent will go so far as to let one of the children know the details of an affair that is being kept secret from the other parent. It is probably healthier for parents to air their differences around the children than to pretend the children do not or should not notice. But for one parent to conspire with a child to keep secrets from the other parent can only be destructive; it gives far too much power and responsibility to the child, who needs to know that the parents are more or less together as security and stability for the family. Subgrouping across generations is a major cause for crisis-proneness.

Subgrouping occurs also when one spouse conspires with a parent, a sibling, a friend, a lover, or a therapist to keep problems secret from the other spouse. In family decisions, such alliances may outvote or overpower the other spouse, and they can certainly outmaneuver the left-out spouse, who is then trapped behind enemy lines. The domestic devastation produced by a secret affair is well known, as are the more insidious effects of a conspiring in-law.

Anyone, even the family doctor, who crosses family boundaries to champion one party of a domestic dispute can be just as destructive. This is true even if the championed party appears to the outsider to be an abused child, a battered husband or wife, or the misunderstood mate of a paranoid person. It is characteristic of families in crisis to loosen their boundaries and cry for outside help. The police officer, the divorce lawyer, the mother-in-law, the hairdresser, and the family physician may all cross the boundary at the same time and all may be equally destructive if they see their function as protecting one family member from another one.

Clearly, a parent who abuses a child must be reported to the legal authorities. Yet clinical experience has shown that when the physician sides with the child against the parent, or if the emphasis is mainly on protecting the child, the child is endangered even more. The physician must recognize the child's guilt-producing effects and convey to the parent the message that he or she will also be protected from the child. The function of the intruder in the family crisis—the physician—is to respect and protect power alignments sufficiently to help stabilize the family.

Roles

Each family assigns roles to its members. Some roles are functional (breadwinner, cook, banker, dumper of the kitty litter); others are emotional (jester, family doctor, etiquette advisor, family problem). Functional role assignments are generally quite clear and obvious, though they may be conflictual. Rigidity in roles is a frequent source of crisis-proneness. Well-functioning families provide some degree of backup for a member whose role is not being performed. Some families, though, assign roles on gender, which prevents the flexibility necessary to adapt to change. As repugnant as it is to most of us, the "me Tarzan, you Jane; me hunt, you cook" arrangement is as workable as any other if both parties agree. But if Tarzan can't cook and Jane can't hunt, either would starve if the other one ceased to function. The male need to be served can get bizarre. One man inspected the faucets each evening to be sure his wife had polished them as his mother would have. Another man could be sexually aroused only by the sight of his wife on her knees scrubbing the floor. By contrast, there are women who actually believe that they should never have to hold a paying job outside the home and therefore never prepared themselves for a career. Such people, when called upon to perform roles they consider inappropriate for their gender, may feel quite oppressed. It seems difficult to maintain a family that contains a prince or princess who feels too special to do the work that needs to be done. And when such a person also usurps a full-time emotional role, such as family critic or family patient, without also becoming "the family problem" and therefore the one to be changed, the family's range becomes greatly limited and crisis-prone.

Crisis-proneness is not just the result of functional or emotional rigidity. It can also result from functional looseness. Some families prefer to ignore certain roles, as if they are not really necessary. There are families in which no one cleans up, pays the bills, oversees the schedule, or determines the appropriateness of other people's behavior. Thus, when the power is cut off, or the garbage blocks access to the kitchen, or various members drift away, a crisis occurs. The situation is treated as unique, and the member who expressed dissatisfaction is seen as the problem.

Families can become crisis-prone, too, when the more emotional roles go unperformed. Not only must the family members be loved and encouraged and comforted, they must also be criticized. It must be someone's job to comment on the appropriateness of behavior. When that job is not done, behavior may become bizarre and offensive. Politeness is not necessarily helpful in family living. Someone treating a family in which someone behaves inappropriately should realize that no one may ever have noticed or complained before.

In some families, one person, perhaps an adult, perhaps one of the children, is defined as vulnerable—as one who can't help it but must always be obeyed and catered to. Asthmatic children who could stop breathing if upset, alcoholic parents who could start drinking if angered, or those defined as mentally ill are prime candidates for this role. If anyone questions the vulnerability of the family patient, it is the questioner who becomes the family problem—the one whose behavior must be changed. The family gives its highest priority to protecting the family patient from becoming self-sufficient.

It takes at least two people to produce a family patient, but they also produce a crisis-prone family. Other emotional roles may stifle families. If the father must always know best, if the second child must always be at fault, if the child marked for success must always be blameless in his failures, if mother's actions must always be seen as love, if anyone must always be anything, then nothing can ever be understood, and no change can take place.

Family Rules

Just as family roles determine who does what, family rules determine who can't do what. Family rules are even more ubiquitous than family roles, and often just as bizarre. Crisis-proneness results when rules prohibit the family from functioning, or from having friends outside the family, when the rules interfere with normal socialization and development of the children, or prevent awareness and discussion of problems that require change. The possibilities for stifling growth are limitless, but they seem proportional to the degree with which the family fears the world around them. Some families protect themselves from adolescent sexuality by prohibiting normal adolescent socialization. A rule commonly taught young girls is that any man who wants sex with a girl does not respect or love her, which means she must marry a man who is not attracted to her. Men may fear their wives' adultery or rape to such a degree that they keep them in a virtual chastity belt, preventing them from working, driving at night, or going out with friends. Other families have rules against any alcohol use because they fear alcoholism. Rules against language are not uncommon. One old woman had a large sign over the mantle spelling out the four letter words that could not be spoken in her house.

Rules for protecting the home can become imcompatible with comfortable living. Joan Crawford's rule against wire hangers is well-known. Some families have rooms tended like museums, which no one may enter, and yards too well kempt to permit children to play in.

Few rules are more explosive than those involving infidelities. Although most people agree at marriage to remain faithful, and a majority actually do, occasionally adultery is common and continual adultery not at all rare. A few couples negotiate the conditions under which extramarital sex will be permitted or even encouraged, and therefore the adultery is open and shared and seen as not quite an infidelity, at least in theory. In practice, it may be surprisingly stimulating, or it may be unsettling. More often, people move around furtively and compound their infidelities with lies or even efforts to blame the cuckolded spouse for some deficiency that drove the other spouse to do it. Such an infidelity tears at the heart of the marriage by the insult, desertion, rivalry, insecurity, and sudden loss of trust; the results may be devastating. Yet, people who want to have affairs and intend to do so may find it hard to negotiate openly about their intentions, because they would prefer that their partner follow the rule of fidelity. Some couples permit extramarital sex while physically separated or on a trip. Affairs may be more permissible with prostitutes, with members of the same sex, or with strangers. One man, an artist, insisted that he had never been unfaithful "except with ex-wives and models and they didn't count." His wife saw it otherwise and left him. The rules on such an emotionally charged issue must be clear. Many women assume all men are adulterous, and some men assume it of all women. If a marriage is conducted under the assumption of infidelity, a faithful spouse may be kept at a distance with little opportunity for intimacy to develop.

Rules against open communication stifle problem-solving. Early family researchers spent years analyzing fragments of family conversations to delineate the rules about who speaks after whom. These rules, about who can say what to whom, and about what and when, are usually subtle and uncodified and may not even be apparent to the family members. Many family fights ignore content entirely and focus exclusively on whether people are speaking respectfully or have a right to say what is being said. The most basic job of a family problem-solver is to cut through this and let the family members deliver the necessary messages and opinions.

Communication rules may always be in conflict. When a man from a diplomatic, silent family marries a woman from a noisy, conflict-loving family, both spouses may be continuously uncomfortable. When a liberated child decides to open communication with a closed family, or a cautious, sneaky child enters a stormy family, the child's style may trigger a crisis.

Goals and Values

Some people never question their reasons for believing as they believe. Those who aren't very bright remember only the first thing they learn about any subject and reject any subsequent information that doesn't seem compatible with it. As a result, their belief and value system may be strongly held, yet never examined. It has been said that no one is fit for life until they realize that their parents were stark raving mad and everything they've been taught is dangerously suspect and must be continuously reexamined until they are sure it is a belief of their own choosing and therefore changeable in the face of new data. Families that constantly reexamine their goals and values become more interesting and more flexible. Of course, families with no long-range view of themselves and their place in the world have little ability to inspire their children. The result could only be children who are either as nonconflictually complacent as their parents or who show unexpected, but unprotested, talents and ambitions.

Crisis-proneness results from unachievable goals and values; some goals and values are innately at odds with one another. We know, for instance, that popularity of junior high school students results from social comfort—the unquestioned assumption that people will like them. Parents' anxious efforts to keep children constantly alert to rejection or to potentially offensive aspects of their behavior or appearance can only result in the social anxiety antithetical to such popularity. Some goals and values are simply incompatible with the nature of the human animal or with that of the individual family member. Any effort to rid oneself of normal or even abnormal feelings only increases those feelings. Still, parents may set for their children the goal of not feeling certain things. I still see mothers who spank small children for crying in grocery stores, which invariable causes the child to cry harder. When anxious, some people attempt to appear calm, which surely increases their anxiety. Similarly, guilt over sexual attraction can remove the pleasure of the attraction while turning it into an obsession, which then takes on far more importance than it deserves.

Some families try to avoid certain experiences. Their goal is to get through life without any member's having a divorce, abortion, affair, imprisonment, psychiatric hospitalization, or even a failing grade or any overt acknowledgment that all has not gone ideally well. Occasionally one sees in the newspaper the story of a couple who have lived through 50 years of marriage without an unkind word or of a child who had not missed Sunday school in 15 years. Most of us realize that life is a comedy, not a tragedy, and no one gets through it without an occasional pie in the face. Yet families who must have only ideal experiences may believe that there is no recovery from a bad one. The failing grade, the abortion, or the adultery marks the individual and the family for life, an ineradicable blot on the family that makes further efforts pointless since the primary goal of avoiding these unpleasant but common experiences is unachievable. Some families feel little will to continue after a child becomes illegitimately pregnant, fails in school, or goes to jail or a hospital. Divorce is common after a rape or the death of a child, even when there is no blame or distrust—just a sense of unachievable perfection. Less traumatic experiences, even minor slights, have also sufficiently dispelled the magical perfection to bring a particular family to grief.

Issues from the Past

Every family has certain unresolved issues that are kept in storage for an uproar whenever needed. These past conflicts fall into two categories: those that are secret or lied about, and those that are open, symbolic, and past. Obviously, any real issue has to be handled in some way as it occurs, with some people taking action and others at least accepting or tolerating that action. But secret issues can't be resolved to anyone's satisfaction, and symbolic issues exist for the primary purpose of remaining unsolved.

Secrets usually involve past rule-breaking. Someone has an affair, lies about it, and offers no explanation for his or her changed behavior, leaving everyone vaguely confused. The mystery may continue to disorient the family for years, postponing solution of the problems. Much energy may go into protecting a secret item of past history—a degree not earned, a debt not reported, a child given up, a marriage not acknowledged, a dread secret from the family of origin. The secret may affect behavior and decisions only slightly most of the time but, like a lightly mined field, may make a few areas hazardous. Suspicious people may know there is a secret and become increasingly uncomfortable around the person who holds the secret, but do a terrible job of guessing what the secret is.

Tension

Tension is the family members' awareness of one another; it may be seen as a measure of the members' fears of displeasing one another or of the degree to which they experience one another's pain. Tension may be so low that no one feels involved in anyone else's life. One 14-year-old girl lived at home through a nine-month pregnancy without her parents noticing she was pregnant. Adolescents may develop severe drug habits, young adults may have affairs, or older ones deteriorate as a result of Alzheimer's disease, before anyone is aware of anything unusual.

A more visible problem is a family with a high level of tension, in which everyone bounces off everyone else and it is unclear where each emotion begins or who owns any problem. There are enmeshed families—smothering mothers, folies à deux, "gruesome twosomes," and other relationships in which the emotional tension is so intense that one person's feelings are felt instantly by other family members and seem owned by the reactor rather than the originator. Some people even experience others' physical sensations or think they can do so. One theory concerning anorexia nervosa suggests that the anorexic person may be reacting to parental efforts to feed her when the parents experience hunger, a process that goes on so long that she never learns to experience hunger on her own. Likewise, obesity has been seen as a result of the child's learning to eat when the parent is anxious. By contrast, paranoid people seem more aware of other people's anger than of their own, failing to notice their attacks on others but being acutely aware of the other person's response to their unrecognized attack. This leaves them, inexplicably, feeling attacked. When tension is high, symptoms and emotions are transmitted rapidly.

Some years ago in Colorado, John McDonald (1968) set aside a ward of the hospital for patients who had threatened to kill others. Since there were too few people who had made such threats, the ward was not filled and other patients were housed there. The anxious staff knew it was the "Threat To Kill Ward" and lived with acute sensitivity to the possibility of violence. Soon, even the depressed little old women were threatening murder in order to use the telephone or get their PRN medication.

Stress

A stress is a force that tends to distort. What is stressful for one family may not be stressful for another; stresses are specific to the system in question. Efforts to quantify stress have not been impressively successful. The death of a spouse or bankruptcy might be considered more stressful than a fistfight with neighbors or Christmas, but there are families in which a bankruptcy or the pregnancy of an unmarried daughter would be routine, while a family gathering would constitute a crisis. In many marriages a husband's death is far less stressful than his retirement. The degree of stress depends on the family's values and expectations and on the nature of its relationships.

Stresses might be categorized according to whether a stress is overt or covert, whether it is unique or habitual, permanent or temporary, real or imagined, and whether it is seen as structural or situational.

Overt-covert. In general, overt stresses create fewer problems. In a misguided effort to avoid embarrassment, pain, blame, or change, many people keep secrets, compounding the confusion created by an event that affects one family member for reasons not understood by the others. If a stress is overt (the house burns down), then the family can band together and outsiders can offer help. If it is covert (a secret affair or loss of money), then no one knows how to help.

Habitual-unique. Response to habitual or recurrent behavior is different from response to unique behavior. One episode of drunkenness is quite different from chronic alcoholism. One lost job is different from recurrent job instability. Many family battles occur over the question of whether a stress is unique or habitual, and the distinction is significant. The sixth failed grade, affair, arrest, suicide attempt, or episode of violence becomes obnoxious rather than alarming to the family. A person called in to help may be shocked by the irritated complacency of families who have been through such an episode many times. The same helper, on the other hand, may be surprised later when the family reacts to the next episode in the series as if it had never occurred before. Determination of habitual versus unique requires accuracy by all concerned.

Temporary-permanent. Families may also battle over whether a certain stress is temporary or permanent. The family member pushing for change may concentrate on the permanent effects and stigmas of an abortion, an arrest, a failing grade, or an affair, even if a more permanent baby, imprisonment, expulsion, or divorce did not occur. Likewise, people who resist change may see only the temporary impact and downplay long-range consequences. The mother who didn't want her son to wear an earring treated the pierced ear as if it were permanent like a tattoo, rather than temporary like a hairdo. Many adolescents, dropping out of college, insist that they'll return to school in the fall. One young man, marrying for the seventh time, had nothing more permanent in mind than the dental work his prospective father-in-law could perform.

Real-imagined. Sometimes it is not clear whether or not a stress is real. Incest may be reported by a child when it did not actually occur, or it may have happened and been denied by the accused parent. The same thing is true of infidelities. Sometimes people destroy their children to prevent incest from becoming known, and they often convince everyone of a spouse's insanity to keep an affair secret. Yet, from the standpoint of a therapist, whether or not the act occurred may not matter as much as the reality of the disturbed relationships and high tensions. It is not uncommon for a child to report an act of incest by a new stepparent who is actually intrusive in nonsexual ways. An imagined affair may not yet be sexual but may accurately identify the direction of someone's attentions. Emotional reality may take priority over physical reality. Emotional accuracy is enormously important, even if the physical details are fuzzy.

Situational-structural. Stresses may arise from within the structure of the family, or a family may find itself in a stressful situation brought on by outside forces. In facing an enemy, it helps to know, as Pogo did, whether or not it is us. Families in whom the blame is always externalized may feel no need to change the behavior that is causing the stresses. Parents of failing children may blame the school system, addicts blame doctors or Vietnam, blacks blame whites, men blame women, and everyone blames parents, while nobody takes the responsibility for change. On the other hand, it is equally unhelpful to internalize each stress and blame a favorite defect in the family structure for whatever comes up. Children of divorcing families may blame their poor school grades or messy rooms for the marriage problems. Battling couples may blame everything that happens on an ancient affair, an unpleasant in-law, or some old offense. Depressed people may blame any crisis on some internal defect, constantly asking, "How have I failed?" By doing that, they miss the opportunity to appropriately assign responsibility within the family or to escape or understand difficult realities.

If these parameters can be properly evaluated and defined, the stress, its characteristics, effects, and sources, can be understood clearly enough to point the way to change. When the stress is clearly understood, the crisis can be minimized. When the stress is confusing, the crisis extends unnecessarily and amplifies uncontrollably.

Crisis

A crisis results when a stress bears upon a system and requires change outside the system's usual repertoire. The state of crisis is marked by nonspecific changes in the system. The boundaries are loosened, which enables a therapist or anyone else to enter and influence the way the system operates. Rules and roles become confused. Both expectations and prohibitions become relaxed. Goals and values lose importance and may even be lost altogether. Unresolved conflicts are revived and become the focus of much attention; tension between family members rises. A physician observing a family in crisis may find the family disorganized, nonfunctional, directionless, battling over long-dead issues. The doctor may assume the family is far sicker than it is, may assume the revived conflicts to be the real issues, and may overlook the stress entirely. By this time, the family may want to dump its stress in some way that will reduce tension without solving the problem. Members may decide to dissolve the family, ship someone off, get a divorce, have an affair (the loosened boundaries permit this), or put someone in a hospital. On a vulnerable family member, the pressure may reach a level sufficient to bring forth symptoms, even psychosis. The scapegoating of one member may become the focus of everyone's attention and that person may be isolated or punished or treated. To an observer who doesn't understand the stress, this may appear perfectly appropriate.

Perhaps each crisis is unique, but most crises fall roughly into four categories. The first, simplest, and least common is the *"bolt from the blue."* The stress here is overt, unique, real, and situational. Someone may die, the house may burn down, the economy may collapse, the plumbing may overflow just before the guests arrive, the sweepstakes ticket may win, the expressway may come through the front yard, or the child may be kidnapped. If everyone can pull together to define the stress and the changes required, the crisis may not destroy the family; functional changes will vary with the duration of the stress. Bolts from the blue are obvious, clearly arising from forces outside the family. The stress is real, it could not have been anticipated, it hasn't happened before, and it is unlikely to happen again. Neither soul-searching nor blame are appropriate or helpful, though they occur. Anticipating a recurrence would be a mistake, though such anxiety is almost universal. Most of the family's attention can be directed to the regrouping necessary to keep the family going.

Obviously, bolts from the blue are as likely to occur in well-functioning families as in families with all manner of problems, but old problems and the new crisis may become confused. One example is a house burning down around a family in which there was incest, drug abuse, alcoholism, and a matriarchal, intruding grandmother. The fire, however, caused the family to focus on a young child's hyperactivity, which had been ignored in the large house, but became intolerable in the motel where the family lived temporarily.

The danger of bolts from the blue lies in the search for blame—the effort to find something someone could have done to prevent the disaster. This attempt will undoubtedly uncover all sorts of personal and structural deficiencies to which responsibility for the crisis becomes attached. As a result, the real task of pulling together and adapting to the situation is bypassed in favor of attack and defense.

Developmental crises are expectable. They are overt but may have a few covert features. Instead of temporary phases, they represent permanent changes in status and function that clearly arise from the nature of biology or society, not the family structure. They are real, even as they provoke fantasies and expectations that may not be real. There is nothing unique about developmental crises, and above all they cannot be prevented. The usual developmental crises include: marriage; birth of children; children starting school, going through puberty, becoming independent and leaving home; and parents growing older, retiring, and dying. Teenage sexual activity and pregnancy, drug use, or school deficiencies are not true developmental crises, but they are so prevalent that they might as well be. Infidelities, midlife crises, and divorce seem to be on the verge of becoming expectable crises in our society. Children born to unmarried mothers, jail terms, unemployment, and addiction may be almost as common, but these remain aberrations that are preventable if the people involved are aware of choices as they make them. Preventable crises are characteristic at each stage of development; knowing they are expectable may help to keep them from being inevitable.

More subtle developmental crises occur in marriage. One is the cooling of romantic love that occurs during the first year or so as mates see each other more clearly. When the honeymoon is over, it is usually replaced by a far more mature partnership. Another marital crisis is the cooling of sexual intensity in the thirties as the sexual drive becomes less hormonally urgent and more dependent on the relationship. During the forties, awareness of patterns of career success or failure emerges and a rethinking of goals takes place.

Subtle developmental stages occur also in child-raising. Two-year-old children learn to say no, six year olds work to please, 12 year olds become aware of their parents' deficiencies. Fourteen-year-old adolescents ignore their parents' values in search of the assurance of popularity from their cruel peers and find manifold deficiencies in themselves. Sixteen year olds want freedom; eighteen year olds are afraid of it.

At each developmental stage a crisis of some sort is inevitable. Problems arise when one part of the family tries to prevent the crisis rather than define and adapt to it. A common developmental crisis centers on adolescent sexuality. Parents may go to amazing extremes to prevent their children, especially their daughters, from being actively sexual. One mother cut off her 16-year-old daughter's hair to make her less sexually attractive; another mother tried to have breast reduction surgery performed on her 14-year-old daughter. A parent's intervention into a child's sexuality may go as far as incest or voyeurism. Someone must tell frightened parents what is normal, and they certainly won't take the adolescent's word for this.

Adolescent sexuality cannot be dictated. One pair of parents who were proud of their liberality, allowed their 15-year-old daughter to acquire birth control devices, required her to drink and smoke marijuana with them, and encouraged her to have "experiences." They objected only to cigarettes as bad for asthma. She refused "experiences" and sat in her room sullenly smoking. The parents had overlooked the cardinal rules of developmental crises: They cannot be stopped, they cannot be produced prematurely; they can only be understood and thereby dampened and coordinated with all the other forces that operate in the family.

Caretaker crises occur when a family has an inherent defect that makes them dependent unilaterally on some power outside the family. While the family's structure may be faulty, the stresses arise from forces outside its control. The structural defect may be permanent; the stress may be overt or covert, but it is often habitual and represents a situation of chronic dependency. Families subject to caretaker crises include those dependent on outsiders for financial support, like families supported by welfare payments, trust funds, alimony, or the kindness of strangers.

Similarly, families with a chronically ill member are unable to control their destiny, as the treatments, orders, and restrictions leave everyone helplessly dependent upon the physicians—who may be caring, sensitive, and communicative, but are still outside the give-and-take of equal relationships. Families dependent on a psychotherapist are in the same situation, with the added mistrust created by a vague air of mystery and a definite air of secrecy.

Another situation of dependence arises when a single parent has an affair with a married person. No matter how much a married man or woman may love the other person, he or she spends all holidays with the spouse, and that is not negotiable.

Some chronic psychiatric illnesses also create conditions outside a family's influence. Manic depression seems to be a predominantly chemical, genetic disease the patient and family cannot control. The family's efforts are unlikely to influence its course and are usually destructive, encouraging the manic-depressive patient to control his or her emotions. Schizophrenia, which probably is at least partially chemical in origin, often becomes recurrent or chronic and is incompletely influenced by the individual's or family's efforts. The family's attempts to find a once-and-for-all "cure" may prevent acceptance of the chronic or recurrent nature of these conditions. Schizophrenia is often managed and stabilized without invalidism, but it may well require long-term medication and therapy. The family's resistance to continuing treatment frequently results in the patient's relapse.

In all caretaker situations, the family must assess the need for continuing dependence on the caretaker. If dependence cannot be avoided, the family must establish a relationship with the caretaker in which the family is being considered. Equally important may be the family's understanding of the nature of the dependence, the purpose of the caretaker, and the rules of the relationship. If the modus operandi of the caretaker is mysterious to the family, the relationship loses any semblance of predictability. Caretaker crises occur when the caretaker's rules change and don't seem negotiable, or when the caretaker makes decisions without explaining them.

Structural crises are those that exacerbate struggles within the family. They may occur without any perceptible external stress but seem like an earthquake that arises periodically from underground forces. Unless the first crisis in the series is handled well enough to resolve the internal problem, structural crises are likely to recur, caused perhaps by an overt, but more likely by a covert, stress. And if a real stress doesn't trigger the next structural crisis, then an imaginary one will. These crises have nothing to do with stress, and are not an effort to avoid, understand, or change anything. They are the most difficult crises to treat because they represent an effort to prevent the change. Families with an alcoholic member, violent families, and adulterous families all fall into this category. So do families in which a member intermittently uses divorce, suicide attempts, job changes, running away, or creating an uproar as reactions to ordinary stresses. Because of the excessive, nonspecific quality of the typical structural family crisis, the family may never deal effectively with the stresses it encounters, putting all its energy into avoiding the usual crisis. Therefore, nothing ever changes.

Alcoholic families are especially difficult. Nothing should be easier to resolve than alcoholism: Don't drink. But an alcoholic may be a joyless, difficult person without alcohol, so the family may not require or even tolerate his or her sobriety. Of course, even if the family objected, the alcoholic might not completely control the drinking, but the family does not have to tolerate it if it chooses not to. Nor do people have to tolerate violence with its guilt-producing remorse, adultery with its disorienting lies, or suicide attempts with their threat of eternal guilt. Yet families do choose to retain such members. The crisis pattern itself seems to be its own reward, keeping reality from being considered and deficiencies from being dealt with rationally.

In treating families of this kind, the practitioner must shift the focus from the current crisis and isolate the problem from the surrounding chaos. I am always astounded to see people take responsibility for having caused someone else's recurrent outlandish behavior. One must find out how anyone got the idea someone else is not responsible for his or her own behavior. What is so frightening about rationality? Families who tolerate bullies (and suicide attempters are no less bullies than alcoholics, adulterers, and husband- or wife-beaters) are not victims but accomplices. If the bully unilaterally stops the chaos, he or she may destroy the raison d'être of the family.

One common pattern of structural crisis occurs in marriages in which one partner recurrently threatens divorce. He or she may believe the marriage is unworthy of him or her, that the marriage belongs to the other spouse who uses it tyranically. Taking little responsibility for making the marriage work, such a person does not leave but from time to time precipitates a crisis in which the other spouse must prove commitment to the marriage by some tolerance or sacrifice.

Treating Families in Crisis

The treatment of families in crisis is conceptually quite simple. In psychoanalytically oriented psychotherapy of either individuals or families, the definition of the problem is made increasingly subtle and complex. Crisis therapists—whether they are psychiatrists, family physicians, family counselors, or family therapists—above all, simplify.

The format developed by the Denver group is easy to follow and provides sufficient structure to keep us oriented in even the most chaotic family or the wildest array of intersecting crises. The format has a simplicity and logic unusual in psychiatry, and it seems especially suited to the more practical, less esoteric activities of the family physician or counselor. There are seven steps. The physician should enter the situation with an air of calmness but urgency, convey a clear sense of how things work, be impatient but not unkind with people who seem to prefer chaos to change, and be optimistic that obstacles can be hurdles if one knows what's going on. Sympathy is out of place, as is a passive interest in understanding people's feelings better, disapproval of behavior on moral rather than practical grounds, or a protective willingness to join in conspiracies. The physician's central posture is that of the friendly, impartial, sensible expert.

Emergency Response

This means we must respond right away, within days certainly, preferably within hours. Perhaps our being there, calm and interested, is enough to prevent the family from doing something drastic to relieve the tension. The first therapeutic person on the scene is admitted into the loosened boundaries of the family and granted great power and influence. He or she may have more power to bring about the second step than any therapist subsequently. He or she can take over some of the family's administrative functions during the crisis, an action that would have been resisted a few days before and will be resisted a few weeks later. The physician has to arrive quickly and work fast. A few minutes when all hell is breaking loose are worth more than hours of work later on.

Focus on the Family System

This second step is usually easy for us to bring about, especially after the other family members have been made aware of the crisis. We bring together whomever needs to be involved in understanding and solving the problem. If the member crying for help is not involving the others, we may have to call them.

Ordinarily in a crisis, the family will choose an individual to be changed so that the rest of the family won't have to do so. If family members are sufficiently concerned, they will be willing to be involved. But the therapist must be willing to start with whomever shows up. As Anderson and Stewart (1983) said, someone who treats families is in the position of the salesman who "must be willing to agree to anything that will get his foot in the door" (p. 46). Once started we involve the others as quickly as possible by whatever means we can. A telephone call to the missing members may be sufficient, but sometimes a home visit is required. The guiltier people feel about their involvement, the more frightened they are of seeking help. A friendly, competent voice on the telephone may seem sufficiently tolerant to offer some protection. Even on those rare occasions when a family member refuses to come in or talk, he or she can be included in the formulations. He or she can be sent a specific message explaining the situation and suggesting actions. The absent member must, however, be protected from blame.

Small children need not be included, but all other family members must be involved, particularly those who have the power to sanction or prohibit change.

Defining the Problem

This step is crucial and complex; it involves finding out why the crisis is happening now. The past needs to be explored only far enough to identify the points of crisis, when things went so wrong that the family felt the need to call for help. The step is complex because the family may already have defined the problem so unhelpfully that their efforts were futile or destructive. Every family has collected a lifetime of extraneous information and many unresolved problems that are being connected to the current crisis. When we treat families in crisis, we must wade through all that and focus everyone's attention on the current problem.

In the midst of the chaos, as everyone blames everyone else and digs for the roots of the problem in the past, in the stars, in the society, the doctor's small voice keeps repeating, "Why now?" The information the doctor is given is not incorrect or irrelevant, and it will be helpful later on. But without the understanding of why the crisis has happened now, the other information can be misleading.

If this crisis is a bolt from the blue, the doctor may be told quickly, but the information may not apply to the family's functioning before the crisis. In a caretaker crisis, the information also surfaces rapidly. In a developmental crisis, the information may be distorted, most likely being the story of one person's troublesome or psychopathic behavior, although the person described may not be the one forcing the change from one developmental stage to another. The individual identified may be the one opposing the development or contributing to its distortion. With persistence and patience, the practitioner should be able to figure out who is changing.

Structural crises are the misleading ones. No matter how often the same crisis has occurred, a family member will describe it as unique and brought on by external circumstances, or as a caretaker crisis, in which one person has a chronic defect outside his or her control and the world has not been supportive enough. The blame may be put on another member's development.

If the focus is sharply on the question, Why now?, and it turns out the crisis is one of a series, it has been caused by a structural problem no matter how much the current episode may be related to other stresses. So, in addition to asking, Why now?, the doctor must ask if this has happened before and explore the past deeply enough to find out when the family was last functioning well enough not to need help. There are pitfalls in getting the story, because people tell the history according to the way their family looks at things.

A classic example is: "The whole problem is me. I've never been good at anything. Just ask my parents. They'll tell you." Or, "Everything was OK until she started dating. That was when my husband began to drink. So I helped her sneak out of the house. When he found out about it he beat me up and that was when I took all those pills."

If the information is put together in such a way as to explain the interaction and everyone's part in it, then the symptomatic behavior seems to be an understandable, if not necessarily a reasonable, reaction to the situation. Until it makes sense, the doctor must keep on probing and act as though he or she doesn't understand the situation yet. The "one-down" position outlined by Fisch, Weakland, and Segal (1982) is a powerful one; it requires patients to come up with coherent explanations rather than resisting the diagnosis.

General Prescription

As soon as the crisis is defined, efforts can be made to calm everyone in preparation for some sensible action. Someone or everyone may need to take sedative medicine for a day or so, or the doctor's reassurance that he or she now understands the situation and knows what to do about it may be tranquilizing enough. If someone's hospitalization cannot be avoided, this should be done now or later never before the family situation is clear. Simplistic as it may sound, I have found that chamber music, refreshments, and an air of confidence calm everyone as much as putting someone in the hospital. Yet calming the situation should not interfere with the therapeutic effort of solving the problem. The family may have to remain upset until the problem is clearer.

Specific Prescription

This fifth step flows directly from step three and, in its simplest form, is an act of logical, practical reality-testing. We tell the family to do something sensible that will either solve the problem or symbolize a change that will solve it eventually.

The physician must describe the situation without blaming anyone, but with the unshakable conviction that everyone wants to do something sensible and is perfectly capable of doing so. Family members may object to the formulation, but they are less likely to reject it if the physician is supportive. With some families, vagueness about some aspects of the problem is permissible, but vagueness about the solution is not. The doctor tells them what sensible people would do under the same circumstances. This step can't be faked; it marks the difference between helpful helpers and unhelpful ones.

The prescription may be quite simple: "Stop drinking. If you're not an alcoholic, it should be easy. If you are, Antabuse will help." "Stop the affair, at least for now. You can call him from here. I'll call if you're embarrassed to." "Don't commit suicide tonight. We'll find other alternatives tomorrow." "Go on to school/work, they'll help you if you need it." "Stay home tonight. The family needs to be together."

The prescription should also be directed towards the symptom in question. When such simple directions are given, they are usually joined with instructions to the other family members to either talk or not talk about the issue, and to help in various ways to perform the prescribed task.

If there is conflict about who is to do what, separate prescriptions can be given to each member of the "You go ahead and hunt, and you go ahead and cook" variety. For example, "You job hunt tomorrow, and she'll write the letter to your mother." Each person's task performance must be independent of the others', so that one person cannot avoid the task because someone else did: "You are to hunt, whether or not he cooks."

In bolts from the blue, simple structure is usually sufficient—returning to normal functioning in most areas and doing the special tasks produced by the crisis. In caretaker crises, the doctor has already done the job by becoming the new caretaker, but he or she must now assign an end to the dependence or an acceptance of it. The doctor tells the unemployed to look for a job and work, the manic-depressive patient to resume taking lithium. In developmental crises, if the crisis-producing change is in a child, the doctor supports the parents' authority, but then allies himself/herself with the developmental phase, asking the parents to accept it while they maintain control and the child demonstrates responsibility in going through it. In adult developmental changes, the doctor must support the family's authority as the adult adapts his new goals and patterns to the family. In structural crises, the bully is defined as responsible for his or her behavior, and the tasks involve a cessation of bullying and encouragement of the family to protect itself from it, while the issues are negotiated from positions of greater equality. If the doctor has been skillful in defining the crisis as one in which all are players, then this should not be difficult. Everyone is given a task, even if it is only to oversee someone else's task. Then the meeting ends, perhaps with the admonition that the doctor knows that perhaps not everyone will do their work—and that's OK because, if they don't, the real problem will surface. The tasks are not only realistically useful, but they have symbolic value and are tests of cooperation.

Negotiating the Resistance to Change

The family has been gathered quickly, the chaos reduced, the problem defined as a solvable one, and everyone told some simple things they can do to help solve it. Sometimes they will do those things. When they do not, we must explore their reasons for not doing the things that would solve the problem. This may take time and require further explorations into the innate peculiarities of the family, but if we keep everyone's attention on the solution of the presenting crisis, the process has a focus.

In this sixth step, which usually takes place at the second session with the family, the physician will learn much more about the family than during the first meeting. Most likely, the person protecting the family from change is not the initially identified patient.

New tasks, new explorations, and even revisions of the original definition are in order. Bolts from the blue will be resolved quickly. Caretaker crises will return rapidly to the point at which the last caretaker ran away, so that the doctor may discover that the previous caretaker misjudged the problem and the doctor can now solve it. Developmental crises always require some negotiation but usually not many sessions before the family will accept objective wisdom from an outsider.

Families in structural crises often resist change. They may drop out of the treatment process early, try to send only one member, or play a touch-and-go game. It is these families who often need to be referred to family therapists and psychiatrists, but they are most resistant to therapy. It is these families about whom the family therapy books are written.

Do not expect them to change quickly, because when one member improves, another may sabotage the improvement. The family members are accustomed to doing the opposite of what they are told, so one technique may be for the doctor to admit helplessness and defeat, at which point the family may change to keep the doctor involved. But if the doctor can persuade just one person that change is possible, that the bully is competent, that the victims are free to escape the pattern, the impasse will be broken and change will become possible. The question at this stage is: "What, above all, do you not want to change?" The answers are often amazing.

Termination

This seventh step is the last, although not all problems will be solved. Appropriate referrals are made, and they may be accepted or not. Either way the family has a resource available for the subsequent crises that are inevitable in all families.

The people who need psychotherapy least want it most, and those who need it most resist it most stubbornly. The biggest crises are the fastest to treat. In treatment of family crises, change, if it occurs, is achieved quickly and, whether the change occurs or not, the crisis is over in a few weeks.

Let families experiencing bolts from the blue go gracefully and they will be back when they need a doctor. If these families don't terminate quickly enough, and if the physician gets lost in the situation, then the families should be encouraged to try getting along on their own, and check in later.

In certain caretaker crises, especially those involving schizophrenic and manic-depressive patients, someone may have to manage the patient's medication indefinitely. If the patient has a good working relationship with the family, then the medication management can be done efficiently by one individual. These situations involve important family work. The family of a manic-depressive patient taking lithium must learn that the danger is over and there is no need to protect the patient from emotions. With schizophrenic persons, the converse is true, in that a low level of emotionality seems helpful, as are firm expectations of functioning. Schizophrenics, once past the acutely psychotic episode, benefit from associations with groups and other opportunities for learning to be normal. Family protectiveness from normality should be stopped, even if the schizophrenic must leave home to accomplish this.

Structural crises often end quickly and return in time, the second round of treatment often being more helpful. Eventually, families who have recurrent structural crises may become amenable to serious family psychotherapy to prevent the crises, rather than use the crises to prevent therapy.

There is a limit to how much saving any of us can offer to families who don't want to be saved from their problems. But each family crisis is an opportunity for the family and the physician to learn more about how people can get through life without driving one another crazy.

REFERENCES

Anderson, C., & Stewart, S. (1983). *Mastering resistance*. New York: Guilford Press.

Caplan, G. (1956). An approach to the study of family mental health. *U.S. Public Health Reports, 71*(10). Washington. D.C.: U.S. Government Printing Office.

Caplan, G. (1964). *Principles of preventive psychiatry*. New York: Basic Books.

Fisch, R., Weakland, J.H., & Segal, L. (1982). *The tactics of change: Doing therapy briefly*. San Francisco: Jossey-Bass.

Freeman, H., & Simmons, O. (1963). *The mental patient comes home*. New York: Wiley.

Hill, R. (1965). Generic features of families under stress. In H.J. Parad (Ed.), *Crisis intervention: Selected readings* (pp. 32-52). New York: Family Service Association of America. (Original work published 1958)

Kaplan, D. (1962, April). A concept of acute situational disorder. *Social Casework*, 7, 15-23.

Kaplan, D., & Mason, E. (1960). Maternal reactions to premature birth viewed as an acute emotional disorder. *American Journal of Orthopsychiatry, 30*(3).

Langsley, D., Kaplan, D., Pittman, F., Machotka, P., Flomenhaft, K., & DeYoung, C. (1968). *The treatment of families in crisis*. New York: Grune & Stratton

Lindemann, E. (1965). Symptomatology and management of acute grief. In H.J. Parad (Ed.), *Crisis intervention: Selected readings* (pp. 7-21). New York: Family Service Association of America. (Original work published 1944)

McDonald, J. (1968). *Homicidal threats*. Springfield, IL: Charles C Thomas.

18

FAMILY ASSESSMENT TOOLS

GABRIEL SMILKSTEIN, M.D.

Knowing how family members interact has long been appreciated by family physicians as important in understanding a patient's health status. Yet, systematic application of this knowledge has not been the rule in clinical practice. Much of the explanation for the incongruity between what is known intuitively and what is practiced actively by family physicians may be found in the failure to integrate existing psychosocial knowledge into the clinical training of medical students, and the failure of physicians to employ in practice useful techniques that will facilitate the identification and management of family problems. This chapter deals primarily with the rationale for the use of family function assessment in clinical medicine. Instruments helpful to physicians for evaluating family function will be identified.

Health and Family Function

Although a caring attitude and sensitivity to family problems have served family physicians well, doctors can render greater service if they know how a family in trouble contributes to its members' disequilibrium and altered health status. The literature that yields this knowledge is primarily a product of the second half of the 20th century. Credit belongs to Richardson (1945) for documenting the negative impact on health of conflictual interaction among family members. Other pioneers were members of the psychosomatic movement (Alexander, 1950; Dunbar, 1947), as well as family-oriented social scientists (Ackerman, 1958, 1966; Hill, 1949; Kluckholn, 1958; Koos, 1946). In recent years Engel (1980) has been the champion of the biopsychosocial model in clinical practice.

The tie-in between psychosocial family issues and health has been clarified by those who have studied the illness-inducing effect of stress. The basic literature deals with the relationship between stress and illness (Antonovsky,

1979; Coelho, Hamburg, & Adams, 1974; Dohrenwend & Dohrenwend, 1974; Gunderson & Rahe, 1974; Hinkle et al., 1958; Hinkle & Wolff, 1958; Holmes & Rahe, 1967). Analyses of the stress-illness phenomenon have demonstrated that a variable of considerable influence is the family's role as both a source of stress and a resource to buffer stress (Cassel, 1974; Chen & Cobb, 1960; Cobb, 1976; Masuda & Holmes, 1978; Pratt, 1976).

Evidence has mounted to support the concept that the functional relationship between patient and family members is a major factor in the outcome of illness. Berkman and Syme (1979) found it to be true in age- and sex-specific studies, while morbidity studies have related family function to outcomes of such illnesses as streptococcal infection (Meyer & Haggerty, 1962), angina pectoris (Medalie & Goldbourt, 1976), myocardial infarction (Theorell & Rahe, 1971), and asthma (DeAraujo, Dudley, & Van Arsdale, 1972; Lask & Matthew, 1979). Many studies also suggest strongly that outcome of pregnancy not only is related to biomedical risk, but is also a function of psychosocial risk (e.g., family dysfunction) (Laukaran & van den Berg, 1980; McDonald, Gynther, & Christakos, 1963; Nuckolls, Cassel, & Kaplan, 1972; Smilkstein, Helsper-Lucas, Ashworth, Montano, & Pagel, 1984).

Family as a Resource

An understanding of the family as a resource requires a definition of the family in health. A healthy family is one whose members perceive it as cohesive and offering the emotional and physical nurturance and resources that are necessary for personal growth and sustenance in the face of life's challenges.

The family is, in general, the most important social support available to patients. However, in considering the social support available to patients, physicians should also recognize the resource strength of friends and other support groups (Berkman & Syme, 1979; Brandt & Weinert, 1981; Pratt, 1976). A nurturing family uses its available resources on a day-to-day basis to meet the routine needs of its members. Stressful life events, however, which require special coping responses, challenge the adequacy of family resources. Physicians who wish to study family in depth will find that resource analysis facilitates family assessment. One approach, which uses the acronym SCREEEM, lists family resources as social, cultural, religious, economic, educational, environmental, and medical (Smilkstein, 1980).

These resources are considered effective when they meet all or most of the following conditions:

1) Social interaction and open communication are evident among family members. Family members also have well-balanced lines of communi-

cation to such extrafamilial groups as friends, social groups, and other community organizations.

2) Cultural pride or satisfaction can be identified, especially in distinct ethnic groups.
3) Religion offers satisfying spiritual experiences as well as contacts with a like-minded extrafamilial support group.
4) Economic stability is sufficient to provide both reasonable satisfaction with financial status and an ability to meet the economic demands of usual life events.
5) Education of family members is adequate to allow members to solve or comprehend most of the problems that arise within the format of their lifestyle.
6) Environmental conditions are such that the family is favored by clean air and water, and space to satisfy its needs for work, play, and home life.
7) Medical resources are available through channels that are easily established and have previously been experienced as satisfactory.

Family Resources for Buffering Stress

Formulating the role of family as a resource in buffering the illness potential of a stressful life is as simple as ABC. Hill's (1965) ABCX conceptual framework clarified the factors that participate in the stress-illness-resource interaction. As he stated: "A, stressful life event, interacting with B, the family's crisis-meeting resources, interacting with C, the definition the family makes of the event, produces X, the crisis." It should be recognized that the interaction of A, B, and C may also produce resolution of the disequilibrium associated with the stressful life event if the family's resources and coping style are appropriate.

Family crisis is a function of the interaction of stressful life events and resources. That is, if the family experiences life events that are perceived as being of great magnitude, and the family is resource-poor, the usual outcome is failure to cope and its ensuing anxiety state. At these times of crisis, the physician may be consulted as the extrafamilial resource to relieve the anxiety of the crisis or to recommend intervention that will resolve the family problems associated with the crisis.

The Double ABCX Model described by Patterson and McCubbin (1983) extends Hill's work by emphasizing the need to view a given stressful life event in the context of a family's history of a "pile-up" of life events, as well as the availability of resources.

The study of family stress in the context of the family's social community (Oliveri & Reiss, 1981) is a natural extension of assessing internal family dynamics. The family may be the primary psychosocial influence in the patient's life, but the full spectrum of study is not established until the family's community stresses and resources are examined.

The physician who wishes to understand the family's crisis must investigate all factors (A, B, and C) that contribute to family crisis. Analysis of the stressful life event(s) and resources alone will not adequately facilitate resolution of the crisis. Information must also be obtained on the family's orientation to the life event(s) that induced the crisis (Kluckholn, 1958). Elucidation of a family's orientation to a crisis is important to the family physician, for it will help clarify the family's explanatory model or sociocultural view of an illness or psychosocial crisis (Kleinman, Eisenberg, & Good, 1978). Knowing the patient's explanatory model is also valuable because it establishes the congruence of the patient's view with that of the physician. Lack of congruence may lead the family physician to attempt to resolve a family crisis with resources that the patient may consider inappropriate. The consequences are usually noncompliance and prolongation of the crisis state (Becker & Maiman, 1975; Gillum & Barsky, 1974; Gordis, Markowitz, & Lilienfeld, 1969).

Indicators for Initiating Family Function Assessment

In general, there are four situations in the doctor-patient encounter in which knowledge of family function may facilitate assessment and management of health problems: 1) when a new patient enters a practice; 2) when family members are called upon to assist in patient care, especially when the problem will result in a role change (e.g., pregnancy and chronic illness); 3) when a negative life event of major consequence (e.g., death, cancer) occurs in a family; and 4) when a patient's history overtly or covertly suggests family dysfunction as the cause of a health problem.

1) The physician who obtains knowledge of a new patient's family structure and function will be in a position to anticipate illness behavior (Kleinman & Smilkstein, 1980) and in some instances start preventive measures. One example is educating parents to enhance family nurturing. To facilitate data gathering, Bauman and Grace (1974) recommended a home visit when new patients enter a practice, but because of time and financial constraints, few physicians are able to do this and not all families require it. In general, physicians assign priorities to assessment procedures. McWhinney (1981) noted basic indications for home visits, listing management of certain health problems, and assessment of home conditions and family function. McWhinney emphasized that "this kind of assessment (home conditions and

family function) may be the by-product of visits for other purposes." The physician who is sensitive to the impact of family conditions on the health of members will always be attuned to receiving family information.

2) When family members must help with patient care, the physician's knowledge of patient-family member interaction can be beneficial in anticipating compliance. Studies have shown that family members' motivation to care for the sick is influenced by family function (Davis, 1963; Kearnes, 1979; Litman, 1974). Physicians should recognize also that a possible response to the stress of caring for a family member who is ill will be an increase in the appearance of health problems in those who do the caring (Bruhn, 1977; Klein, Dean, & Bogdonoff, 1967; Meissner, 1974; Widmer, Cadoret, & North, 1980).

3) The impact on family members of a major life event has been documented quantitatively. Holmes and Rahe (1967) showed that in diverse community and cross-cultural studies, divorce, death of a family member, and marital separation scored highest among all life-event items surveyed. These major life-changing episodes represent times when a physician should consider convening a family to facilitate resolution of the family members' worries, fears, anger, and guilt.

The management and outcome of other life events, such as pregnancy and chronic illness, may be enhanced by patient and family education (Schmidt, 1983). At these times, biomedical information should be augmented by psychosocial evaluation and, when needed, counseling. This recommendation is especially applicable in resource-poor families (Charles, Norr, Block, Meyering, & Meyers, 1978; Cobb, 1976; Thomas & Wyatt, 1951).

The worth of documenting life events was highlighted in a longitudinal study of more than 1,000 children one to four years old (Beautrais, Fergusson, & Shannon, 1982). Family life events were associated with increased risk of office visits by and hospitalization of the children for such health problems as lower-respiratory infection, gastroenteritis, accidents, scalds, and poisoning. Furthermore, children from families experiencing a large number of life events had an increased risk of hospitalization for improper or inadequate care (family function was not evaluated in this study). Even when these data were subjected to multivariate analyses to take into account differences in the mothers' age, ethnic status, and education, as well as differences in family size, the child's place in the family, and family living standards, the correlation between life events and child health was the same.

Not all families require the same degree of support. Resource assessment, primarily of the quality of social support from family and friends, will guide physicians in estimating how deeply they should be involved in families whose members have experienced a major stressful life event. The rationale for this is the knowledge that families who are resource-rich, particularly in social support, usually resolve their own problems (Pratt, 1976). The physician can play a major role, however, as an educator or support person in helping resource-poor families resolve life crises.

The physician may also use family assessment in deciding on nonintervention. Study of the family may reveal that it is appropriate for family members to work through their difficulties by themselves. Those who argue for the physician's involvement whenever a family experiences a traumatic life event fail to recognize the growth that may occur when family members resolve their own problems.

4) The physician should intervene when the patient overtly or covertly declares family dysfunction to be the critical problem. Overt and easily identifiable manifestations of family dysfunction are impending divorce or separation, excessive arguing, fighting, poor communication, incest, child abuse, juvenile delinquency, runaway children, school behavior problems, and school failure.

Family members will frequently not admit the presence of psychological problems. Instead they may focus on the health problem of a family member or the behavior of the member. This commonly occurs when a child is truant from school. Only careful assessment of the child and family will reveal whether the truancy is a manifestation of family problems or not. The child's truancy may be related to a conflict at school or perhaps even delinquency with peers. In any event, the family physician should be cautious in addressing family problems when the family prefers to identify only one of its members as the patient. Parents may react defensively to any suggestions that they may be the problem. If the physician is willing to accept the parents' limited definition of the problem, it may be possible later to redefine the problem as a family problem, or as a marital problem, if this is appropriate, without alienating the family and perhaps losing the patient.

In practice, however, many physicians err by dealing with the symptom, school truancy for example, as the primary problem and will not even consider the possibility that the symptom is a reflection of a more general family dysfunction that requires proper assessment and treatment.

Studies suggest, moreover, that most family dysfunction problems brought to the physician are hidden under a facade of physical symptoms — psychosomatic illness, vague symptoms of organic disease, long lists of physical problems, and visits to multiple physicians (Rosen, Kleinman, & Katon, 1982). It is in patient problem areas such as somatization, high medical utilization, multiple complaints, and chronic pain that assessment of family function will be most rewarding. Recognition of the dysfunctional family should aid the physician in understanding patient behavior and in planning treatment.

Family Function Assessment

It may seem simplistic to say that family function assessment techniques should meet the needs of those who teach, study, and serve under the rubric of family medicine. Yet this statement reflects a valid concern, for in general, physicians have resisted family assessment and management schemes that do not harmonize with their total practice responsibilities (Cowan & Sbarbaro, 1972; Marinka, 1976; Merkel, 1983). The following section deals with issues of family structure and function data that should be considered when the physician recognizes that information on family may contribute to the resolution of a patient's problem.

Family Structure Data

The physician's biomedical assessment of patient problems requires that the time-honored data base on family structure be part of the patient's record. The format that best displays information on the age, sex, and health status of a patient's family members is the family tree or genogram (Jolly, Froom, & Rosen, 1980). The family tree has the advantage of giving the physician a rapid view of family membership (nuclear and extended), relationships (e.g., marriage, divorce, adoption), and genetic implications of family members' illnesses (e.g., death from heart disease or cancer) (Medalie, 1978). Although use of the family tree encourages and facilitates family study, it is not an instrument of inquiry into family function.

Family Function Data

What information does the family physician require to assess the quality of family member interaction? The basic question most physicians will want answered is the degree to which a family is a resource for the patient or a source of stress. There is no dearth in the quantity and variety of tests available to assess family function. Straus and Brown (1978) reported almost 100 instruments designed to assess family function alone. Many more were available to assess relationships between spouses, parents and children, and siblings. Miller, Rollins, and Thomas (1982) also wrote an excellent review of methods for studying marriages and families. When an attempt is made to adapt these instruments to family practice, however, methodological problems become apparent. The length and complexity of the instruments, as well as their sociocultural specificity, are major impediments to their use by most family physicians.

To be responsive to the family physician's needs, the ideal family function assessment instrument should be completed by the patient, understood by the patient with limited education, brief, useful for patients from different socioeconomic or cultural groups, and capable of supplying data that will indicate the integrity of important components of family function.

Probably no instrument now available meets all of these qualifications, but a number of them have pragmatic worth and deserve review.

Family Function Assessment Instruments

Family physicians vary considerably in their interest in family function. For those who wish to obtain a rapid view of relationships in a household or family, one of the most effective strategies is the use of the Family Circle Method. As Thrower, Bruce, and Walton (1982) described the technique:

> Family circles may be collected from an individual, a family subsystem (marital, sibling or parent, child) or individually from all the members of a family group in the presence of one another. The clinician draws a large circle on a piece of paper, blackboard, or flipchart. The persons interviewed are instructed as follows:
>
> "As a family physician, I am interested in you, your family, and people who are important to you. Let this circle stand for your family as it is now. Draw in some smaller circles to represent yourself and all people important to you—family and others. Remember, people can be inside or outside, touching or far apart. They can be large or small depending on their significance or influence. If there are other people important enough in your life to be in the circle, put them in. Initial each circle for identification. There are no right or wrong circles."

Examples of family circles are shown in Figures 1 and 2. Although the family circle does not permit in-depth interpretations of family function, the use of the method announces to the patient the physician's interest in family and frequently establishes an entree for discussion about family issues.

Another instrument that is playing a growing part in clinical and research studies of family function is the family APGAR (Smilkstein, 1978; Smilkstein, Ashworth, & Montano, 1982). The family APGAR (Figure 3) was introduced

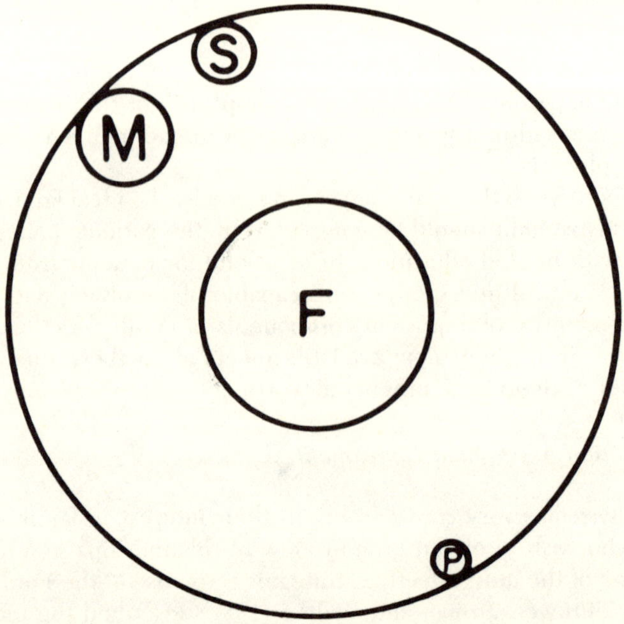

Figure 1. P is a 43-year-old, white, single patient whose father dominated the family. The patient has a low self-image and rarely used the family as a resource. F = father, M = mother, S = sister, P = patient.

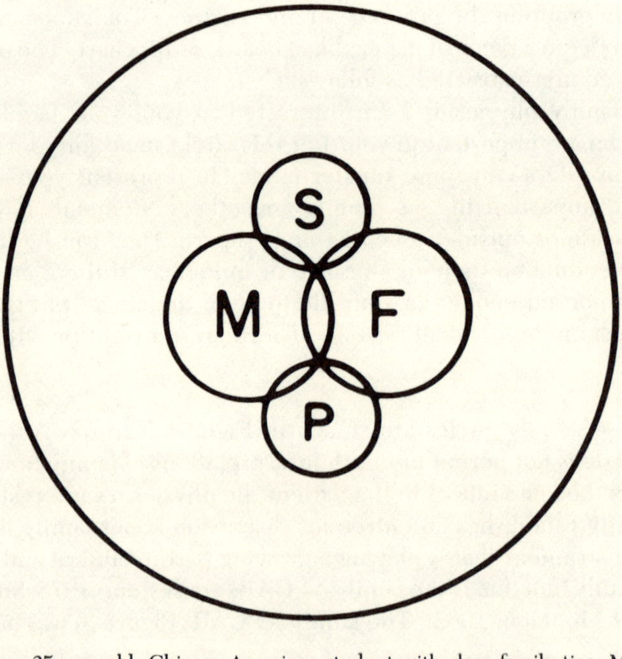

Figure 2. P is a 25-year-old, Chinese-American student with close family ties. M = mother, F = father, S = sibling, P = patient.

The following questions have been designed to help us better understand you and your family. You should feel free to ask questions about any item in the questionnaire.

Comment space should be used if you wish to give additional information or if you wish to discusss the way the question applies to your family. Please try to answer all questions.

"Family" is the individual(s) with whom you usually live. If you live alone, consider family as those with whom you now have the strongest emotional ties.

	For each question, check only one box		
	Almost always	Some of the time	Hardly ever
I am satisfied that I can turn to my family for help when something is troubling me. Comments:	☐	☐	☐
I am satisfied with the way my family talks over things with me and shares problems with me. Comments:	☐	☐	☐
I am satisfied that my family accepts and supports my wishes to take on new activities or directions. Comments:	☐	☐	☐
I am satisifed with the way my family expresses affection, and responds to my emotions, such as anger, sorrow or love. Comments:	☐	☐	☐
I am satisifed with the way my family and I share time together. Comments:	☐	☐	☐

Family APGAR

Figure 3. Family APGAR.

as a utilitarian screening instrument for family function. The five-item questionnaire was developed on the premise that a family member's perception of family function could be assessed by scoring that member's report of satisfaction with five parameters of family function: adaptation, partnership, growth, affection, and resolve (commitment) (Smilkstein, 1978; Smilkstein et al., 1982).

In clinical studies the family APGAR has shown positive correlations with school performance and behavior (Chen, Hsu, Hsu, & Lin, 1980), compliance with use of medication for hypertension (Pian, 1983), motivation to comply with physicians' postoperative instructions to ostomy patients (Kearnes, 1979), and adaptation to parenthood (Lobo, 1982). Negative correlations have been found with depression (McNabb, 1983) and the frequency of birth and postpartum complications (Smilkstein et al., 1984). The instrument's limitations are those of a brief screening instrument that restricts specificity.

Five other examples of self-report questionnaires on family function that deserve review by family physicians are the Family Function Index (FFI), 15 items (Pless & Satterwhite, 1973, 1975); Family Environment Scale, Form R, 90 items (Moos, 1974); Faces II, Family Adaptability and Cohesion Scales, 30 items (Olson, Sprenkle, & Russell, 1979); McMaster Family Assessment Device (FAD), 53 items (Epstein, Bishop, & Levin, 1978); and Feetham Family Functioning Survey (FFFS), 21 items (Roberts & Feetham, 1982).

The first of these, the FFI, has the advantage of being a "simple, easily administered test to reflect the dynamics of family interaction" (Pless & Satterwhite, 1973). The instrument estimates family function by evaluating areas of nuclear family interaction such as marital satisfaction, frequency of disagreement, communication, problem-solving, and feelings of happiness and closeness. The validity of the FFI was established by comparing index scores with ratings of the same families by experienced case workers. The FFI has been used to study the nuclear families of children with chronic physical disorders. Its authors say it can accurately identify chronically ill children who are likely to experience secondary psychological difficulties. Sociocultural biases of certain questions should be considered by those planning to use the FFI.

In the proper socioeconomic setting, the Family Environment Scale has proved to be effective for family function research. For use in a family physician's office, however, the Family Environment Scale suffers from both the large number of questions asked and the middle-class orientation of the questions.

Faces II is one of several family inventories developed by Olson and associates. The authors provide information for each inventory on conceptual development, construct validity, internal consistency (alpha reliability), test-retest reliability, scoring procedures, cutting points, and national norms. The time patients require to complete the 30-item questionnaire is reasonable for office practice.

The FAD is a self-reporting screening for family function assessment. It is made up of seven scales, six from the McMaster Model of Family Functioning (MMFF) and a "general functioning" scale to assess the overall health and pathology of the family (Epstein et al., 1978). MMFF scale items are problem-solving, communication, roles, affective responsiveness, affective involvement, and behavior controls. The general functioning scale items address such issues as the family as a resource, the rights of individuals to be different, handling of emotions, and the family's ability to work together. Four alternative responses are allowed for the 53-item questionnaire.

The validity of the FAD was established by comparing the questionnaire responses of clinical and nonclinical samples. All seven scales showed significant differences between the two samples. The FAD was also an effective predictor of spouse morale when used in parallel analysis with the Wallace Marital Satisfaction Scale (Locke & Wallace, 1959).

The integration of a 53-item FAD questionnaire into a patient's self-reported health history does not seem feasible. The FAD's authors also indicated their concern that the scales are highly intercorrelated. Therefore, although seven subscales are scored, the FAD seems to measure one construct, which suggests that a shortened questionnaire might yield similar results.

In the FAD validation study, the general functioning scale discriminated best between the two test groups, clinical and nonclinical subjects. Items in the general functioning scale address the family as a resource, rights of individuals to be different, how emotions are handled, and working together. These items have been treated as central to the study of family function in a number of instruments such as Glueck and Glueck's (1934; 1970) family questionaire, the family APGAR, and the Coping Health Inventory for Parents (CHIP) (McCubbin et al., 1983).

CHIP is an 80-item checklist providing self-report information about how parents perceived their overall response to the management of family life with a (chronically ill) child. Because of its length, the instrument has limited use for routine assessment of family function by the practicing physician.

The FFFS, the fifth example of family function assessment, is a well-validated and reliable instrument that measures relationship between family and individual, relationship between family and subsystem, and relationship between family and broader social units. Its strength is in measuring satisfaction with marriage. Its primary weaknesses are that it cannot be applied to single-parent families and its measurement of relationship "with broader social units" is rather limited.

Family Function Testing: Patient or Family?

From whom should family function data be collected? Under what circumstances should the respondent(s) be the patient, selected individuals, or the whole family? The literature does not offer a clear answer to these questions. Confusion exists because investigators have, in general, used the perception of individual members to judge the functional status of the family. In fact, most early sociological data on how families function was based on wives' responses (Ball, McKenny, & Price-Bonham, 1983). White and Brinkerhoff (1977) have commented on the fallacy of assuming that "statements true of individuals are also applicable to the collectives of which they are members."

Can meaningful data be obtained when only the patient completes a family function instrument? The answer is a qualified yes. The qualification is related to the purpose to be served when the family function data are obtained. Numerous studies have shown significant correlations between an individual's perception of his or her family or marital function and that individual's health status (McNabb, 1983; Medalie & Goldbourt, 1976; Smilkstein et al., 1984; Vaillant, 1977). How well an individual copes with life is related also to the individual's perception of his or her family function. In the pediatric age group, parents' perception of family function has been shown to be related to health problems in their children. For example, parents who report their families to be dysfunctional are more likely to have emotional problems in their chronically ill children (Pless & Satterwhite, 1975). Also, children with recurrent throat infections are more likely to come from families perceived by parents as dysfunctional (Meyer & Haggerty, 1962).

These studies suggest there is a place for assessing the patient's view of family function (or, in the pediatric age group, assessing the parents' perception of family function). Thus, when the patient is the focus of care, the patient's perception of family function will, in general, alert the family physician to possible health-outcome problems.

There are circumstances, however, when the problem presented by the patient requires an understanding of the functional relationship of the "collectives" who make up the family. When the family is the unit of care or research (family therapy or family systems research), a "within-family" design should apply to the strategy for obtaining data. "Within-family" information may be obtained "when a family is repeatedly observed by observing more than one of its members" (Ball et al., 1983).

Oliveri's and Reiss's Card Sort procedure, for example, involves all family members in a problem-solving exercise that delineates the family dimensions of configuration, coordination, and closure. Their studies show that these family characteristics have value in predicting response to treatment in family-oriented psychiatric treatment programs.

The problem of family-function testing: patient or family? cannot be resolved by the family physician according to an all-or-nothing principle. Obtaining information on family function from all members of the family would offer the family physician the most data, but volume of data is not necessarily related to optimal strategy in clinical problem-solving. For the present, the issue between "within-family" or patient perception family function testing is not which is better but which is more appropriate for the problem being studied by the family physician. Future research will have to address issues of family-functioning instrument specificity and utility. Family physicians will begin to use family functions instruments more actively when they have clear knowledge of the purpose for which the data are being collected, and when the process of data collection fits their temporal and economic resources.

Summary

Various studies, especially over the last 50 years, have established that the integrity of the family system is a factor in the health status of family members. Family physicians have known this intuitively but, in general, the medical education of physicians has not included guidelines for when or how to study family function, nor what to do when family dysfunction is identified. In this chapter I have recommended the following:

1) The biomedical data base that reveals family structure and genetic patterns should be displayed in the patient's chart by use of the family tree or genogram.
2) Information on family function should be obtained when a new patient enters a practice, when family members are called upon to assist in patient care (especially when the problem will be chronic), when a negative life event of major consequence occurs in the family (e.g., death or cancer), and when a patient's history overtly or covertly suggests family dysfunction as the etiology of a health problem.
3) Family physicians will continue to use the interview as their major source of information on family function. No instrument can pick up the nuances of emotional import that are evident when a patient changes body position or facial expression, or when the patient responds hesitantly to a physician's question. Because of the time constraints under which most physicians work, however, utilitarian instruments designed to give introductory

or supplemental information on family function will be of great benefit to the busy physician.

4) The family should be recognized as a resource and as a source of stress. Furthermore, the family is only one component of the patient's social support system. To understand a patient's social support network fully, inquiry should be made of the quality of the patient's relationship with family, friends, and groups.
5) The issue of how family function data should be collected requires further study. For the present, it appears that the patient's perception of family function is appropriate for most patient-oriented studies. When the family is the unit of care, as in family therapy, "within-family" studies are needed.

REFERENCES

Ackerman, N.W. (1958). *The psychodynamics of family life: Diagnosis and treatment of family relationships*. New York: Basic Books.

Ackerman, N.W. (1966). *Treating the troubled family*. New York: Basic Books.

Alexander, F. (1950). *Psychosomatic medicine: Its principles and applications*. New York: W.W. Norton.

Antonovsky, A. (1979). *Health, stress and coping*. San Francisco: Jossey-Bass.

Ball, D., McKenny, P.C., & Price-Bonham, S. (1983). Use of repeated-measures designs in family research. *Journal of Marriage and the Family, 45*, 885-896.

Bauman, M.H., & Grace, N.T. (1974). Family process and family practice. *Journal of Family Practice, 1*, 24-26.

Beautrais, A.L., Fergusson, D.M., & Shannon, F.T. (1982). Life events and childhood morbidity: A prospective study. *Pediatrics, 70*, 935-940.

Becker, M.H., & Maiman, L.A. (1975). Sociobehavioral determinants of compliance with health care recommendations. *Medical Care, 13*, 10-14.

Berkman L.F., & Syme, S.L. (1979). Social networks, host resistance, and mortality: A nine-year follow-up study of Alameda County residents. *American Journal of Epidemiology, 109*, 186-204.

Brandt, P.A., & Weinert, C. (1981). The PRQ-A social support measure. *Nursing Research, 30*, 277-280.

Bruhn, J.G. (1977). Self-concept and the control of diabetes. *American Family Physician, 15*, 93-97.

Cassel, J.C. (1974). An epidemiological perspective of psychosocial factors in disease etiology. *American Journal of Public Health, 64*, 1040-1043.

Charles, A.G., Norr, K.L., Block, C.R., Meyering, S., & Meyers, E. (1978). Obstetric and psychological effects of psychoprophylactic preparation for childbirth. *American Journal of Obstetrics and Gynecology, 131*, 44-52.

Chen, E., & Cobb, S. (1960). Family structure in relation to health and disease. *Journal of Chronic Diseases, 12*, 544-567.

Chen, Y.C., Hsu, C.C., Hsu, S.H., & Lin, C.C. (1980). A preliminary study of family APGAR index. *Acta Paediatrica Sinica, 21*, 210-217.

Cobb, S. (1976). Social support as a moderator of life stress. *Psychosomatic Medicine, 38*, 300-314.

Coelho, G.V., Hamburg, D.A., & Adams, J.E. (Eds.). (1974). *Coping and adaptation: A behavioral sciences bibliography*. New York: Basic Books.

Cowan, D.L., & Sbarbaro, J.A. (1972). Family-centered health care: A viable reality? *Medical Care, 10,* 164.

Davis, F. (1963). *Passage through crisis: Polio victims and their families*. Indianapolis: Bobbs-Merrill.

DeAraujo, G., Dudley, D.L., & Van Arsdale P.P. (1972). Psychosocial assets and severity of chronic asthma. *Journal of Allergy and Clinical Immunology, 50,* 157-263.

Dohrenwend, B.S., & Dohrenwend, B.P. (Eds.). (1974). *Stressful life events: Their nature and effects*. New York: Wiley.

Dunbar, F. (1947). *Mind and body: Psychosomatic medicine*. New York: Random House.

Engel, G.L. (1980). The clinical application of the bio-psychosocial model. *American Journal of Psychology, 137,* 535-544.

Epstein, N.B., Bishop, D.S., & Levin, S. (1978). The McMaster model of family functioning. *Journal of Marriage and Family Counseling, 4,* 19-31.

Gillum, R.F., & Barsky, A.J. (1974). Diagnosis and management of patient noncompliance. *Journal of the American Medical Association, 228,* 1563-1567.

Glueck, S., & Glueck, E. (1934). *One thousand juvenile delinquents: Their treatment by court and clinic*. Cambridge, MA: Harvard University Press.

Glueck, S., & Glueck, E. (1970). *Toward a typology of juvenile offenders: Implications for therapy and prevention*. New York: Grune & Stratton.

Gordis, L., Markowitz, M., & Lilienfeld, A.M. (1969). Why patients don't follow medical advice: A study of children on long term antistreptococcal prophylaxis. *Journal of Pediatrics, 75,* 957-963.

Gunderson, E.K.E., & Rahe, R.H. (Eds.). (1974). *Life stresses and illness*. Springfield, IL: Charles C Thomas.

Hill, R. (1949). *Families under stress*. New York: Harper.

Hill, R. (1965). Generic features of families under stress. In H.J. Parad (Ed.), *Crisis intervention*. New York: Family Service Association of America.

Hinkle, L.E., Christenson, W.N., Kane, F.D., Ostfeld, A., Thetford, W.N., & Wolff, H.G. (1958). An investigation of the relation between life experience, personality characteristics, and general susceptibility to illness. *Psychosomatic Medicine, 20,* 278-295.

Hinkle, L.E., & Wolff, H.G. (1958). Ecologic investigations of the relationship between illness, life experiences and the social environment. *Annals of Internal Medicine, 49,* 1373-1388.

Holmes, T.H., & Rahe, R.H. (1967). The social readjustment rating scale. *Journal of Psychosomatic Research, 11,* 213-218.

Jolly, W., Froom. J., & Rosen, M.G. (1980). The genogram. *Journal of Family Practice, 10,* 251-255.

Kearnes, D.R. (1979). *Compliance in a home after surgery: Influences of family functioning and individual motivation*. Master of Nursing Thesis, University of Washington School of Nursing.

Klein, R., Dean, A., & Bogdonoff, M. (1967). The impact of illness on the spouse. *Journal of Chronic Diseases, 20,* 241-248.

Kleinman, A.K., Eisenberg, L., & Good, B. (1978). Clinical lessons from anthropologic and cross-cultural research. *Annals of Internal Medicine, 88,* 251-258.

Kleinman, A., & Smilkstein, G. (1980). Psychosocial issues in assessment. In G.M. Rosen, J.P. Geyman, & R.H. Layton (Eds.), *Behavioral science in family practice*. New York: Appleton-Century-Crofts.

Kluckholn, F.R. (1958). Variations in the basic values of family systems. *Social Casework, 39,* 63-72.

Koos, E.L. (1946). *Families in trouble*. New York: King's Crown Press.

Lask B., & Matthew, D. (1979). Childhood asthma. A controlled trial of family psychotherapy. *Archives of Diseases of Children, 54*(2), 116-119.

Laukaran, V.H., & van den Berg, B.J. (1980). The relationship of maternal attitude to pregnancy outcomes and obstetric complications. *American Journal of Obstetrics and Gynecology, 136,* 374-379.

Litman, T.J. (1974). The family as a basic unit in health and medical care: A social behavioral overview. *Social Science and Medicine*, *8*, 495-519.

Lobo, M.L. (1982). *Mother's and father's perceptions of family resources and marital adjustment and their adaptation to parenthood*. Doctor of Philosophy Dissertation, University of Washington, School of Nursing.

Locke, H.J., & Wallace, K.M. (1959). Short marital adjustment and prediction tests: Their reliability and validity. *Journal of Marriage and Family Living*, *21*, 251-255.

Marinka, M. (1976). The family in medicine. *Proceedings of the Royal Society of Medicine*, *69*, 115.

Masuda, M., & Holmes, T.H. (1978). Life events: Perceptions and frequencies. *Psychosomatic Medicine*, *40*, 236-261.

McCubbin, H.I., McCubbin, M.A., Patterson, J.M., Cauble, A.E., Wilson, L.R., & Warwick, W. (1983). CHIP—Coping health inventory for parents: An assessment of parental coping in the care of the chronically ill child. *Journal of Marriage and Family*, *45*, 359-370.

McDonald, R.L., Gynther, M.D., & Christakos, A.C. (1963). Relations between maternal anxiety and obstetric complications. *Psychosomatic Medicine*, *25*, 357-363.

McNabb, R. (1983). Family function and depression. *Journal of Family Practice*, *16*, 169-170.

McWhinney, I.R. (1981). *An introduction to family medicine*. New York: Oxford University Press.

Medalie, J.H. (1978). Family history, data base, family tree, and family diagnosis. In J.H. Medalie, *Family medicine—Principles and applications*. Baltimore: Williams & Wilkins.

Medalie, J.H., & Goldbourt, U. (1976). Angina pectoris among 10,000 men: II. Psychosocial and other risk factors as evidenced by a multivariate analysis of a five-year incidence study. *American Journal of Medicine*, *60*, 910-921.

Meissner, W.W. (1974). Family process and psychosomatic disease. *International Journal of Psychiatric Medicine*, *5*, 411-430.

Merkel, W.T. (1983). The family and family medicine: Should this marriage be saved? *Journal of Family Practice*, *17*, 857-862.

Meyer, R.J., & Haggerty, R.J. (1962). Streptococcal infections in families, factors altering individual susceptibility. *Pediatrics*, *29*, 539-549.

Miller, B.C., Rollins, B.C., & Thomas, D.L. (1982). On methods of studying marriages and families. *Journal of Marriage and Family*, *44*, 851-873.

Moos, R.H. (1974). *The social climate scales: An overview*. Palo Alto: Consulting Psychologists Press.

Nuckolls, C.H., Cassel, J., & Kaplan, B.H. (1972). Psychosocial assets, life crises, and the prognosis of pregnancy. *American Journal of Epidemiology*, *95*, 431-441.

Oliveri, M.C., & Reiss, D. (1981). A theory-based empirical classification of family problem-solving behavior. *Family Process*, *20*, 409-418.

Olson, D.H., Sprenkle, D.H., & Russell, C.S. (1979). Circumplex model of marital and family systems I: Cohesion and adaptability dimensions, family types, and clinical applications. *Family Process*, *18*, 3-28.

Patterson, J.M., & McCubbin, H.I. (1983). The impact of family life events and changes on the health of a chronically ill child. *Family Relations*, *32*, 255-264.

Pian, C. (1983). *Satisfaction with family support and adherence behavior with antihypertensive medical regimens*. Thesis for Masters in Nursing, University of California Los Angeles, School of Nursing.

Pless, I.B., & Satterwhite, B. (1973). A measure of family functioning and its application. *Social Science and Medicine*, *7*, 613-621.

Pless, I.B., & Satterwhite, B. (1975). Family function and family problems. In R.J. Haggerty, K.J. Roughman, & I.B. Pless (Eds.), *Child health and the community*. New York: John Wiley and Sons.

Pratt, L. (1976). *Family structure and effective health behavior: The energized family*. Boston: Houghton Mifflin.

Richardson, H.B. (1945). *Patients have families*. New York: Commonwealth Fund.

Roberts, C.S., & Feetham, S.L. (1982). Assessing family functioning across three areas of relationships. *Nursing Research, 31*, 231-235.

Rosen, G., Kleinman, A., & Katon, W. (1982). Somatization in family practice: A biopsychosocial approach. *Journal of Family Practice, 14*, 493-502.

Schmidt, D.D. (1983). When is it helpful to convene the family? *Journal of Family Practice, 16*, 967-973.

Smilkstein, G. (1978). The family APGAR: A proposal for a family function test and its use by physicians. *Journal of Family Practice, 6*, 1231-1239.

Smilkstein, G. (1980). The cycle of family function: A conceptual model for family medicine. *Journal of Family Practice, 11*, 223-232.

Smilkstein, G, Helsper-Lucas, A., Ashworth, C., Montano, D., & Pagel, M. (1984). Prediction of pregnancy complications: An application of the biopsychosocial model. *Social Science and Medicine, 18*, 315-321.

Smilkstein, G., Ashworth, C., & Montano, D. (1982). Validity and reliability of the family APGAR as a test of family function. *Journal of Family Practice, 15*, 303-311.

Smilkstein, G., Kleinman, A., Chrisman, N., Rosen, G., & Katon, W. (1981). The clinical social science conference in biopsychosocial teaching. *Journal of Family Practice, 12*, 347-353.

Straus, M.A., & Brown, B.W. (1978). *Family measurement techniques, abstracts of published instruments, 1935-1974*. Minneapolis: University of Minnesota Press.

Theorell, T., & Rahe, R.H. (1971). Psychosocial factors and myocardial infarction—1. An inpatient study in Sweden. *Journal of Psychosocial Research, 15*, 25-31.

Thomas, H., & Wyatt, R.H. (1951). One thousand consecutive deliveries under a training for childbirth program. *American Journal of Obstetrics and Gynecology, 61*, 205-209.

Thrower, S.M., Bruce, W.E., & Walton, R.F. (1982). The family circle method for integrating family systems concepts in family medicine. *Journal of Family Practice, 15*, 451-457.

Vaillant, G.E. (1977). *Adaptation to life*. Boston: Little Brown.

White, L.K., & Brinkerhoff, D.B. (1977). Measurement problems in family research: A critical note on units of analysis. *International Journal of Sociology of the Family, 7*, 171-179.

Widmer, R.B., Cadoret, R.S., & North, C.S. (1980). Depression in family practice: Some effects on spouses and children. *Journal of Family Practice, 10*, 45-51.

19

LEGAL ISSUES IN FAMILY PRACTICE

J. RAY HAYS, Ph.D., J.D. and LEONORA MONTGOMERY, M.A.

Medical practice is increasingly recognized as having a moral, ethical, legal, as well as a medical context. Although we shall limit the scope of this chapter to legal issues, it is appropriate first to define the differences between morals, ethics, and the law. Physicians who understand the relationships and differences between them are better equipped to help patients resolve conflicts and identify priorities.

Legal codes are derived from the broad ethical consensus of a community. Legal standards are the formal rules—legislative, administrative, or derived from judicial decisions—that reflect a society's consensus on the conduct of relationships.

Morals may refer to the code of conduct adopted by an individual. Morals are also the rules that the community has adopted so that its members have a clear idea of specific duties and obligations.

Ethics, on the other hand, are the standards by which we judge actions as right or wrong. As we use the terms here, morals are a statement of one's value system; ethics are the values that underlie statements of morals (Frankena, 1963; Hare, 1967).

Common Legal Issues in Medicine

Because laws and regulations reach into medical decision-making, the practitioner has a growing need to know more of the legal vocabulary and the legal procedures and requirements of medical practice. Advances in medical technology have created unfamiliar situations, and patients have been encouraged to ask more questions about their treatment. Thus physicians are increasingly challenged to account not only for their medical practices, but also for the basis in law of these practices.

The following case example illustrates how today's doctor has to meet various requirements to satisfy the demands of different constituents.

An established patient in a private family practice presents with symptoms that suggest venereal disease. With a presumptive diagnosis based on history and clinical findings and before confirmation by laboratory cultures, the physician begins the indicated treatment. Medical treatment of the problem is, however, only one aspect of the treatment the patient deserves and society demands. The social context includes the interest we all have in preventing the spread of communicable disease. The physician's obligation, which stems from this social interest, is to find the individuals who have had contact with the carrier and to let them know that they have been exposed, should be alert for symptoms and, if infected, seek treatment.

This concern has been subsumed in the legal requirement of mandatory reporting by the physician of certain communicable diseases. The social obligation to search out the exposed individuals has been acknowledged by society by providing public health services to do the fieldwork of locating individuals at risk. The law's requirements, however, might well come into conflict with a physician's belief that such disclosure might damage a marriage or jeopardize a person's employment, and that reporting will do little social good. At this point values seem to be in conflict. A doctor who views the practice of medicine from a systems perspective is in a better position to integrate medical with social and legal concerns, ultimately serving both the patient and society better.

The law that is applicable in a specific setting depends on the law of the state in which the practice occurs. No attempt will be made here to illustrate comprehensively the law of specific jurisdictions. Not only may it differ from one jurisdiction to another, but the law on any issue is dynamic and may change any time a legislature meets or a case is decided in court. Issues that underlie the current expression of the law do not, however, change so rapidly.

Individual Rights Versus Group Rights

The system of justice in Western society is based on the individual, who is the unit of measure for the creation of duties, obligations, responsibilities, and rights. This is not true throughout the world. In some Eastern cultures, for example, the welfare of society is held above that of the individual.

Family practitioners who deal with family systems must be aware that they are on the forward edge of a new relationship between professionals and the unit of analysis and treatment. This is not to say that for the family physician the *patient* is the *family*. It *is* to say that the client who is injured or ill is to be viewed more holistically—as a member of his or her group, not as an isolated individual. That is, the doctor is not merely treating this knee; the doctor is treating this knee of this woman, in this particular family group, in this specific community. Such practice is, in a sense, an update of the approach of the family doctor before so much specialization occurred. For this broader concern the legal system will be playing "catch-up" and will develop as a result of the interactions of professionals and consumers of service. This has, of course, always been true; new remedies are found in the law to cope with new situations. It is the dynamic nature of progress in the law to respond to the needs of society.

When developing new remedies, the law may for a period of time create inequities. Because dealing with a family system as an extension of the treatment of an individual patient is new, the physician may run into issues not considered in the legislation, which was developed with emphasis on rights of the individual patient. Inequities may result that may harm both the practitioner and the consumer. That is true of any new enterprise, and it is part of the price of change and growth that comes from a new orientation.

Duty to Care

One guiding principle of all ethical codes of the helping professions has been the concern for the client's welfare. In the Oath of Hippocrates, physicians swear to follow regimens that will benefit the patient and to abstain from whatever is mischievous or deleterious. The principle is best embodied in the proscription, *primum non nocere*—first, do no harm. The ethical code of psychologists tells them to "respect the dignity and worth of the individual and strive for the preservation and protection of fundamental human rights" (American Psychological Association, 1981, p. 633). A family systems approach intends to expand this focus of concern from individual patients to the system in which they function. Yet problems occur when we deal not with separate persons, but with persons in the interactive groups we call systems. The ethics code of the American Medical Association provides an excellent guide for the physician (American Medical Association, 1973). We address some of these problems below.

Informed Consent

Case example. The mother of a 14-year-old adolescent calls you to request that a chemical screen for drugs be done for her son. She believes he is abusing several drugs and wants to get the "goods" on him. She wants the screen done without his knowledge.

The physician knows that several drug screens are available to detect the presence of drugs of abuse or their metabolites. The physician also believes that he should try to maintain the adolescent's trust in order to continue to treat him. Conducting a drug screen without the boy's knowledge would almost certainly alienate him and perhaps eliminate the physician as a source of help. Discussing the issue of trust with the boy's mother is one way of showing her that she might need to be more open with her son, but it is time-consuming. There may be many other patients who could benefit from the time the physician would spend on this matter.

In a systems-oriented practice there is the assumption that any procedures may have an impact well beyond the identified patient. The results of the physician's work affect not only the patient but also, to some extent, the individuals in contact with the patient. The legal requirement of obtaining informed consent before beginning diagnosis and treatment applies, however, only to the persons who have direct contact with the physician. But the physician with a systems orientation knows that intervention in the life of the identified patient with the consent of the patient is but one element of the whole. Although physicians have a moral obligation to be sensitive to the ramifications of treatment throughout the family system, their responsibility is limited by the extent and distance of the impact and the power to predict the consequences of treatment.

Failure to gain the "legally adequate consent" of those in direct contact with the physician, however, results in the risk that the medical procedure may be considered a battery or unconsented noxious touching of another (*Natanson* v. *Kline*). "Legally adequate consent" has been defined as consent by a person who has the following characteristics: legal capacity, comprehension of information, and voluntary agreement. Legal capacity means that the person giving consent is of minimum legal age and has not been adjudicated as incompetent to manage his or her affairs. Informed consent has four elements. The person giving consent must have been given information relating to 1) the risks and 2) the benefits of the procedure, 3) the risks of forgoing the procedure, and 4) the procedures available as an alternative to the proposed treatment.

Standards for Disclosure

According to *Natanson*, "the duty of the physician to disclose, however, is limited to those disclosures which a reasonable medical practitioner would make under the same or similar circumstances." This relative standard has been gradually replaced by an absolute standard that requires the physician to disclose all "material" information. In *Canterbury* v. *Spence*, the court defined material information as relating to "the inherent and potential hazards of the proposed treatment, the alternatives to that treatment, if any, and the results likely if the patient remains untreated" (*Canterbury* at 877).

In *Cobbs* v. *Grant*, the California Supreme Court contrasted the relative standard found in *Natanson* with the absolute standard required by *Canterbury*. The court concluded that requiring a physician to disclose those risks that only other physicians disclose is "irreconcilable with the basic right of the patient to make the ultimate informed decision regarding the course of treatment to which he knowledgeably consents to be subjected" (*Cobbs* at 243).

In the legal context, consent is required before proceeding with treatment. The systems-oriented physician should tell the prospective patient that the physician believes in looking beyond treatment of a specific, diagnosed problem to a broader view of the patient's health. The patient's consent involves some awareness and understanding of the physician's orientation. Exceptions to the informed consent rule occur under emergency circumstances and with minor children and incompetent persons.

The law on informed consent relates to individuals rather than systems, and it developed as a branch of the general law of torts or the law of personal wrongs. The general rule of case law is that a person must be given enough information for a reasonable and prudent person to decide whether or not to undergo the proposed procedure.

In the case of the mother who wants the drug screen of her son, the physician may or may not wish to perform diagnostic tests on a teenage child even though the child is not old enough to consent to the procedure the mother has requested. The age of legal capacity to consent varies among states and among presenting problems. Most states, for example, allow young adolescents to consent to treatment for venereal disease without requiring parental permission or parental knowledge, but many states will not allow them to consent to other procedures until they are adults.

Consent by Whom?

Most of the case law on informed consent has developed in surgical cases and the examples, although applicable to systems-oriented practitioners, do not always fit. Who, for example, consents when family therapy is proposed as an adjunct to medical treatment of a child's asthma? Obviously, each parent can consent to the procedure, and the child can assent to it. Assent is defined as the affirmative agreement of one who lacks the legal capacity to provide consent. It is obvious that no one member can consent for the family; each member is responsible for his or her own decision about pursuing treatment. Several authors have dealt with the ethical issues in dealing with family systems which confront physicians and therapists (Hays, 1975; Hines & Hare-Mustin, 1978; L'Abate, 1982; Margolin, 1982).

For certain purposes, a couple is treated as a legal unit so that an action by one member of a couple is binding on the other. When a husband enters into debt by purchasing a car, for example, both husband and wife are liable for the debt. For most medical treatment, however, a spouse may not consent for the other. As such treatment is personal and relates to the individual's bodily integrity, consent may be given solely by the individual directly affected.

Children do not generally have the right to consent to medical treatment, although many states give minors the right to seek contraceptive information and devices and to have abortions, treatment for venereal disease, and psychiatric treatment without parental consent. These laws arose from the belief that requirement for parental consent might inhibit minors from seeking such treatments, which are in the individual's and society's best interest. In general, consent by either parent is effective for providing treatment for children. The assent of the child should be obtained because the child's cooperation with any procedure aids both treatment and its outcome (Shectman, Hays, Schuham, & Smith, 1982).

Incompetence

Unless adjudicated as incompetent, adults are considered competent to consent to medical treatment. Even persons diagnosed as mentally ill have the capacity to consent when they have the "mental ability to make a rational decision, which includes the ability to perceive, appreciate all relevant facts and reach a rational judgment upon such facts" (*State Department of Human Services* v. *Northern*). If the physician believes that the proposed patient does not have the ability to understand the suggested treatment or is incompetent, a guardianship proceeding must be initiated. The guardian can provide consent for the patient. Most states' laws provide for guardians of persons, of the estate, and guardianship for limited purposes.

Consent by the spouse or next of kin may be sufficient in some states to treat incompetent persons. The more cautious approach is to seek a guardianship, especially before initiating hazardous or experimental procedures.

Emergencies

When a patient is presented in an unconscious state because of illness or trauma, a physician may treat the patient without his or her consent. Consent to the application of life-saving measures when the patient cannot communicate is implied, on the theory that a reasonable, ordinary, and prudent person would consent to the procedures.

Privileged Communication and Confidentiality

Confidentiality and privilege are frequently confused (Everstine et al., 1980; Hays, 1981). Confidentiality refers to information obtained that is not to be revealed outside of a relationship, like that between a physician and patient. Revealing such information without the patient's permission is a breach of confidentiality. Privilege is a narrower concept and concerns the admissibility of information in a court of law. The terms may be distinguished by their scope: Confidentiality covers any information obtained in confidence, while privilege relates only to courtroom testimony. Bersoff and Jain (1980) have written an excellent guide on privileged communication.

The confidential relationship between physicians and their patients is a medical tradition at least as old as the Hippocratic Oath. Like lawyers, physicians and other members of learned professions do not reveal information about their clients to others who have no need or right to know. Physicians may be held liable for revealing such information without the permission of the patient. A physician's duty not to provide testimony exists, if it exists at all, as a result of statutes or case law. It should also be noted that the right not to have such testimony presented belongs to the patient; it is the physician's obligation to preserve and assert this right of the patient. Information becomes admissible in court when the patient or client desires it to be admitted. Once the client wants the information revealed, the professional must provide the testimony.

Two California cases illustrate this point. *In re Lifschutz* involved a psychiatrist found in contempt of court and jailed after he repeatedly refused the court's order to answer questions concerning a former patient. His patient was suing someone, claiming that person had caused him severe mental and emotional distress. Clearly, information about previous treatment could be relevant to such a suit. The psychiatrist believed that there was an ethical obligation not to reveal the information and that the information was irrelevant because of the time that had elapsed between treatment and the suit. The court ordered the psychiatrist to testify.

In *Caesar* v. *Mountanos*, the psychiatrist was held in contempt and sentenced to jail for refusing to disclose information about a patient who had sought financial damages as a result of an automobile accident. The patient was seeking therapy for emotional problems which she believed resulted from the accident. Caesar, a psychiatrist, refused to answer questions about his treatment of the patient, claiming that such revelations would be harmful to her psychological well-being. The court concluded that the competing interests to be weighed were the patient's interest in privacy and the state's compelling interest in ascertaining the truth. Since the plaintiff, Caesar's patient, was attempting to recover damages for a psychic injury, and information about her treatment was therefore relevant and material to the decision, the court required Caesar to provide the information. Professional interests in the client's well-being thus must give way in the presence of the compelling interest the state has in a full and fair disclosure in court. In this case the interest of the group overrode the interest of the individual.

The duty to warn. The matter of privileged communication between a professional and a client has one major exception, and that is the duty to warn an intended third-party victim. The doctrine came to dramatic public attention in *Tarasoff* v. *Board of Regents of the University of California.* A student at the university had revealed to a counselor that he intended to kill a woman who had rejected him. The therapist called campus police who held the student briefly, then released him. Two months later, after the woman returned from a vacation, the student killed her. Her family sued the therapist and the university for failure to warn their daughter or them of the threat. The California Supreme Court ruled that a confidential relationship must yield when disclosure is essential to avert danger to others; the confidential relationship ends where public peril begins. The duty to warn occurs when a therapist has reason to believe that a third party is in imminent danger.

Although considered in a number of jurisdictions, at legislative and judicial levels, California is still the only state which holds that there is a clear duty to warn an intended third-party victim. Other states have either rejected the notion or taken a neutral approach. Physicians should seek local consultation to find out the status of the duty to warn.

Malpractice

Malpractice, a civil legal action, refers to the professional's civil liability when providing services. An aggrieved person has several avenues for obtaining retribution for a perceived transgression by a professional (Hare-Mustin, Maracek, Kaplan, & Liss-Levinson, 1979; Sinnett & Thetford, 1975). Four factors must be present and proved before the injured party may "recover," which refers to the award of money or compensation for the wrong he or she has suffered. The first element in a malpractice action is to define the *standard of care.* It must measure up to the quality of care a reasonable and prudent practitioner would have provided under the same or similar circumstances. This should be a generally accepted or standard professional practice. Second, the practitioner must have *breached* or failed to meet that standard of care in some way; such a failure may include breach of a fiduciary or trust relationship, as when a doctor violates a confidence (Hays, 1980). The breach of care must be the *proximate cause* of *damages* suffered by the patient, which are the third and fourth elements of a malpractice action. Simple negligence or malpractice suits outnumber all other actions against professionals, comprising about two-thirds of all cases (Hogan, 1979). One appropriate statement about malpractice is that there is not so much malpractice in medicine as there is bad psychology when a physician is sued by a patient. The better the relationship between doctor and patient, the less likely is a malpractice action, regardless of the treatment outcome for the patient.

Avoiding malpractice. The best way to avoid a malpractice action by a patient is to be honest and straightforward in explaining treatment, its course and rationale. The systems-oriented physician should state that, from time to time, what is done may not be understood by everyone involved and that the course of the disease and its treatment outcome cannot be completely predicted. A flexible approach is one of the characteristics of a family-systems-oriented practice. If the system members recognize this as the approach taken by their physician, the likelihood of misunderstanding of untoward events, with subsequent displeasure and law suits, will be reduced.

Some individuals believe they have a professional obligation to resist any law that is inconsistent with a principle held by their profession. The laws formulated by the U.S. Congress and the state legislatures are the consensus of how relationships in society are to operate. If professional opinion and scientific evidence run counter to this consensus, the remedy is to work within the system to move society in a more enlightened direction.

Clinical Issues with Legal Implications

Child Abuse and Neglect

Case example. A mother brings her child to a physician's office for treatment of several cuts. The child has bruises in varying degrees of healing and scars from other cuts in various places on her body. The physician treats the cuts and inquires about the other evidence of trauma suffered by the child. The child's mother tells a vague story. The physician does not obtain any further information nor does he tell the mother that he is worried about child abuse. The physician believes the child may have been abused and reports this to the local child welfare authorities. The parents then sue the physician for violation of their right to privacy, interference in the parent-child relationship, and intentional infliction of mental suffering. Should the physician have reported the case? Are there any penalties for a failure to report?

Child-abuse reporting laws are another general exception to the rules on confidentiality and privilege. Most states require any person who has knowledge of or observes child abuse or neglect to report it to the community agency responsible for children's protective services. Abuse or neglect includes the psychological as well as physical health of children. Failure to report child abuse is generally a misdemeanor crime. The responsible agency will investigate the complaint and determine whether or not to initiate termination of parental rights. These agencies have the right to intervene rapidly to protect children from life-threatening situations. Most statutes provide immunity to individuals who report in good faith under such laws. Thus the reporting person should have no fear of libel, or slander, or other suits by accused parents. In the case mentioned, the physician would not have to worry about an adverse judgment if the report of potential child abuse was made in good faith.

Obviously, if the child-abusing family has been in treatment, such reporting, even if done anonymously, may result in the family's termination of treatment. The physician must balance the risk of discouraging the family from treatment against the welfare of the child.

The prudent practitioner must inform parents of the limits of confidentiality afforded to the professional. One of these limits is that, in life-threatening situations, the professional has a duty to protect family members who cannot protect themselves.

Spouse Abuse

The family doctor and emergency room physician may frequently see the results of spouse abuse, most of it of women. Some of the characteristics associated with spouse abuse are "low socio-economic level, frequent verbal arguments, background of family violence, alcohol abuse, and the . . . tendency to adhere to rigid sex role stereotypes. . . . These form a complex picture of the eruption of violence" (Coleman & Weinman, 1981, p.240). Current views of spousal violence are that such violence is interactional, that is, is part of the nature of the relationship between the spouses rather than simply being the responsiblity of one spouse. Most professionals are reluctant to question a patient directly when they suspect spouse abuse. It is sometimes easier to stitch the wound or treat the bruises than deal with the source of the difficulty. Intervention at some level other than treating the outcome could prove lifesaving. In the long run, such intervention might reduce the incidence of the behavior, because violence in adulthood tends to be associated with being raised in a violent family (Gelles, 1974). The statement that "violence breeds violence" is quite true, particularly in the case of family violence.

There are two basic areas of treatment the physician might explore in spouse-abuse situations: One is alcohol abuse; the other is teaching the couple some control over impulsive verbal behavior. Neither of these problems is easily treated, but helping the couple examine events that trigger violent episodes can sometimes be the first step in resolving the problem. Should the family physician not want to or not have the time to deal with such problems at a level other than treating the outcome of the violence, that is, stitching up the wounds, the physician should be aware of local agencies that deal with family violence.

Rape and Sexual Abuse

Rape is a crime of violence in which the act of sexual contact is used to play out the violence of one person toward another. This is the current view of this crime. For the purpose of this chapter, rape is defined as heterosexual intercourse without the female's consent. We define sexual abuse as any other type of forcible attempt at sexual gratification, including sexual abuse of a child, homosexual contact, deviant sexual intercourse, and other forms of abnormal sexual activity.

Whenever the physician is confronted with evidence of rape, he or she should be concerned with at least two issues: proper medical treatment of the victim including counseling; and the legal preservation of evidence. Most frequently, rape victims are seen by emergency room personnel, who should be sensitive to the perceptions of the crime victim. Special training programs are available for medical staffs to aid them in working with rape victims. Rape evidence kits should be stocked in hospital emergency rooms and staff members trained in the use of these kits. Many physicians dislike working with rape victims because of the possibility that they might be called to testify in court. Participation in a trial is a reality for physicians in such cases. As part of the decision to treat such patients, the physician should recognize its broader implications.

Counseling of a rape victim should be started by the first persons from whom treatment is sought. Because of the nature of the act, long-term consequences of the rape should be anticipated. Physical healing may take only a short time, but the psychic wounds may last much longer. Because the long-term consequences of rape are now well-known, the treating physician has a duty to recommend long-term counseling. Obviously, this cannot be forced upon an unwilling patient, but good medical practice calls for offering treatment for problems we believe exist.

Many physicians will see patients whose sexual lifestyles are not the norm. These lifestyles have certain implications. For example, the incidence of acquired immune deficiency syndrome (AIDS) is relatively higher in promiscuous homosexual men. The physician should be aware of patients' sexual orientation and advise them on how to reduce the possibility of exposure to sexually transmitted diseases.

So-called deviant sexual habits also have legal implications because they are frequently proscribed by law. The physician must be careful about information concerning these habits which is written into the patient's record of treatment. The best method for handling sensitive information is to regard the patient's medical record as a legal document. As I (Hays) was told in my training, "Every chart goes to court." Keeping that in mind may help guide the physician in record keeping. Records should be accurate and complete but should not contain speculation, conjecture, and unfounded hypotheses. This is true not only for sex-related cases but also for all others.

When sexual abuse of a child seems to have occurred, the physician is obliged to report this to child protective services or the police. From the standpoint of the reporting requirement, there is no difference between physical abuse and sexual abuse of a child. But there is a difference in the support and counseling that may be required. Children who have been abused, whether physically or sexually, are generally secretive about it. They are afraid that they have done something wrong and that their life will be worse if they tell what has happened to them. Sometimes the adult involved makes overt threats to the child. The child should be helped to understand that he or she will be supported in coping with the problems that have been revealed; physicians should know available resources and how to use them.

Marriage, Divorce, and Child Custody

Marriage is a legal union of two persons who stand in a unique relationship to each other. One spouse can incur debts which must be paid by the other but, in general, one spouse may not consent to medical treatment for the other. Because of the unique legal relationship of married persons, the family practitioner should be aware of some legal aspects of this relationship.

The original purpose of marriage was to provide the social unit for producing, protecting, and educating children. It remains so in most societies. Marriages may be either ceremonial, civil, or common law. A ceremonial marriage is one sanctioned by a religious group and recognized in that church as valid. A civil marriage is conducted in a formal ceremony but without the religious sanctions of a church. Common-law marriages are valid in many jurisdictions and occur without religious or formal civil endorsement.

A common-law marriage generally must have three attributes: an intent by the parties to be married; holding themselves out publicly as husband and wife; and cohabitation. In jurisdictions that accept them, common-law marriages are as valid as other marriages. If a couple is married in one jurisdiction under a common-law statute, they remain married, even though they may move to a jurisdiction which has no such provision. There is, however, no common-law divorce.

Divorce—the family doctor's role. When family physicians are approached by a couple in the process of getting a divorce, they will find themselves at the crossroads of the health care system, the legal system, and perhaps the religious system. The health care system, in this case, specifically addresses the psychological well-being of the couple and the children, if there are any. The legal system, on the other hand, deals with the protection of the legal rights of all parties involved.

The underlying assumptions and operating procedures of the two systems differ. The legal system is an adversarial system and the health care system is not. Lawyers make every possible effort to win their client's case and to discredit the other's side concerning property, visiting rights, and/or custody of the children. Marital counselors and family therapists, in contrast, will attempt to support each person as members of one family.

Similarly, the issue of confidentiality is handled differently. The adversary method of the legal system promotes distrust, guardedness, and competition. Family counseling promotes trust, opening of communication, and cooperation. This is not to say that one system is better than the other. They simply have different methods and purposes. Because they are so radically different, family physicians must know whether or not their patients are already involved with the legal system. What is their purpose in coming for counseling? Is it because their lawyer suggested it or because they wanted to work things out? Does the patient intend to call the physician to testify in his or her behalf and against the spouse? In child custody cases, for instance, are they prepared to accept the physician's opinion of what might be in the best interests of the child, or are they trying to buy the physician's or counselor's expertise and authority to support their claims in court? These goals are all perfectly valid.

Such complex problems and issues are probably best handled by mental health professionals, but we mention them here to alert family doctors that they should help their patients clarify their expectations before becoming involved in family counseling. When the legal system is potentially or actually involved, the family doctor or counselor may have one set of goals and the patients another, based on totally different assumptions.

Divorce-legal issues. Each state provides for the legal dissolution of marriage, but grounds for divorce vary among the states. Drawing most attention in any divorce are property matters and the custody of children.

In general, there are two legal approaches to the division of property acquired during a marriage. The older is that all property belongs to the husband and any division of the fruits of the marriage uses that as its starting place. This approach is followed by more of the eastern states of the United States than the western. The other position is that the fruits of the marriage are the product of joint efforts by husband and wife, and the division of property acquired during marriage takes that premise. This latter community property law generally leads, at divorce, to an equal distribution of property between husband and wife.

Where husband and wife are treated on an essentially equal footing, alimony or support paid by one partner to the other after divorce is generally not a part of the statutory scheme of divorce. Some notable exceptions to this general principle exist, as in California, a community property state in which alimony is awarded.

Many state divorce laws are written so that counseling of couples filing divorce petitions may be required. While such counseling may not reduce the divorce rate, it may have a salutary effect upon the feelings generated by the couple. Many of the issues resulting from divorce are not aired with attorneys or in the court. Mediation and counseling can help work out these problems before they become major. The family physician should know whether or not such services exist and how to refer clients.

Child custody. No single issue has created as much emotion and debate as child custody. In general, courts use the "best interest of the child" standard to determine which of the divorcing parents should have primary responsibility for the care of the children and which one should have only periodic visitation rights. Regardless of who has physical possession of the child, both parents remain responsible for the support necessary for the child. Some states are experimenting with joint custody by giving equal visitation and equal rights and responsibilities to both parents. This social experiment is too new to tell whether or not this procedure will resolve some of the conflicts surrounding parental rights after divorce.

The physician must remember that consent to treatment, other than to emergency treatment, is a right generally reserved for the custodial parent. In most cases the parent who only has visitation rights has limited rights to consent to the child's professional diagnosis and treatment. When dealing with children of a divorced family, physicians should know the law of their jurisdiction on these issues.

Some Guidelines

The following suggestions are designed to promote the treatment relationship in a family practice within the confines of the law and to assist the physician in this process:

1) Patients and family members who accompany patients should be informed of the family orientation of the physician. Clear guidelines should be established as to procedures in the event conflict occurs between professional standards, legal duties, and the need for treatment.
2) The patient and members of his or her family system must know exactly who is the client and the breadth of the physician's professional involvement. Family members need to understand the nature of a family-systems-oriented practice and the flexibility and adaptability which will be exercised by the physician.
3) Patients must be told of the limits of confidentiality.
4) Physicians should be familiar with the statutes that have implications for practice in the clients' state of residence. Many statutes are broadly written and may have to be interpreted in relation to their legislative history and judicial interpretation. A legal consultant may provide the interpretation.
5) Physicians should consider retaining an attorney to be on call for opinions and clarifications. The attorney should be familiar with family law and should have courtroom experience as well as theoretical grounding in the law.
6) Doctors need a close working relationship with members of their profession's local ethics committee. In marginal situations that do not involve a legal decision, advice from committee members who have a current working knowledge of professional ethics may be helpful.
7) It is advisable to keep abreast of new statutes that affect clinical practice, e.g., patients' rights laws, licensing laws, and limitations on research activities.
8) Physicians should be aware of all circumstances and all persons to be affected by treatment decisions and consider the impact upon them, both short- and long-term.

9) Straightforwardness and honesty remain excellent guides if the clinician is to avoid legal difficulties with clients.

Summary

A chapter such as this is no substitute for competent local legal advice. Knowledge of local practice must be gathered from individuals in the community who deal with these issues regularly. We therefore suggest that physicians consult a local resource, an attorney or law-school professor, who can give specific advice when a problem of legality is raised for which there is no other guidance. Just as they seek consultation from another expert physician for a patient with a difficult diagnosis, so should physicians seek outside advice when a legal issue arises. Our society has become increasingly litigation-conscious, as indicated by the dramatic rise of malpractice insurance premiums in the 1970s. Practicing within legal constraints, or going beyond them to the spirit rather than the letter of the law only after careful thought and weighing of responsibility, will do much to forestall legal problems.

Some issues covered by this chapter are well settled within the law; others are more volatile and subject to dispute among the states.

CASES

Caesar v. *Mountanos*, 542 F .2d 1064 (9th Cir. 1976).
Canterbury v. *Spence*, 464 F .2d 772 (D.C. Cir. 1972).
Cobbs v. *Grant*, 502 P .2d 1 (Calif. 1972).
In re Lifschutz, 467 P .2d 557 (Calif. 1970).
Natanson v. *Kline*, 350 P .2d 1093 (Kansas 1960).
State Department of Human Services v. *Northern*, 563 S.W.2d 209 (Tenn. Ct. App. 1978).
Tarasoff v. *Board of Regents of the University of California*, 529 P .2d 533 (Calif. 1974) 551 P .2d 334 (Calif. 1976).

REFERENCES

American Medical Association (1973). Principles of medical ethics. *American Journal of Psychiatry, 130,* 1057-1064.

American Psychological Association (1981). Ethical principles of psychologists. *American Psychologist, 36,* 633-638.

Bersoff, D., & Jain, M. (1980). A practical guide to privileged communication for psychologists. In G. Cooke (Ed.), *The role of the forensic psychologist*. Springfield, IL: Charles C Thomas.

Coleman, K., & Weinman, M. (1981). Conjugal violence: A comparative study in a psychiatric setting. In J.R. Hays, K. Roberts, & K. Solway (Eds.), *Violence and the violent individual.* New York: SP Medical & Scientific Books.

Everstine, L., Everstine, D., Heymann, G., True, R., Frey, D., Johnson, H., & Seiden, R.

(1980). Privacy and confidentiality in psychotherapy. *American Psychologist, 35*, 828-840.

Frankena, W.K. (1963). *Ethics*. Englewood Cliffs, NJ: Prentice-Hall.

Gelles, R. (1974). *The violent home: A study of physical aggression between husbands and wives*. Beverly Hills, CA: Sage Publications.

Hare, R.M. (1967). Ethics. In J. Macquarrie (Ed.), *Dictionary of Christian ethics*. London: SCM Press.

Hare-Mustin, R., Maracek, J., Kaplan, A., & Liss-Levinson, N. (1979). Rights of clients, responsibilities of therapists. *American Psychologist, 34*, 3-16.

Hays, J.R. (1975). The ethics of unobtrusive research. In J. C. Schoolar & C.M. Gaitz (Eds.), *Research and the psychiatric patient*. New York: Brunner/Mazel.

Hays, J.R. (1980). Sexual contact between therapist and client: Legal remedies. *Psychological Reports, 47*, 1247-1254.

Hays, J.R. (1981). Privacy and confidentiality. *American Psychologist, 36*, 914.

Hines, P., & Hare-Mustin, R. (1978). Ethical concerns in family therapy. *Professional Psychology, 9*, 165-171.

Hogan, D.B. (1979). *The regulation of psychotherapists* (Vol. 1). Cambridge, MA: Ballinger.

L'Abate, L. (Ed.). (1982). *Values, ethics, legalities and the family therapist*. Rockville, MD: Aspen Systems.

Margolin, G. (1982). Ethical and legal considerations in marital and family therapy. *American Psychologist, 37*, 788-801.

Shectman, F., Hays, J. R., Schuham, A., & Smith, R. (1982). Accountability and confidentiality in psychotherapy, with special reference to child treatment. *Clinical Psychology Review, 2*, 201-211.

Sinnett, E., & Thetford, P. (1975). Protecting clients and assessing malpractice. *Professional Psychology, 6*, 117-162.

NAME INDEX

SUBJECT INDEX